CHRONIC CARE, HEALTH CARE SYSTEMS AND SERVICES INTEGRATION

RESEARCH IN THE SOCIOLOGY OF HEALTH CARE

Series Editor: Jennie Jacobs Kronenfeld

Recently published volumes:

RESEARCH IN THE SOCIOLOGY OF HEALTH CARE
VOLUME 22

CHRONIC CARE, HEALTH CARE SYSTEMS AND SERVICES INTEGRATION

EDITED BY

JENNIE JACOBS KRONENFELD

Department of Sociology, Arizona State University, USA

2004

ELSEVIER
JAI

Amsterdam – Boston – Heidelberg – London – New York – Oxford
Paris – San Diego – San Francisco – Singapore – Sydney – Tokyo

ELSEVIER B.V.
Radarweg 29
P.O. Box 211
1000 AE Amsterdam
The Netherlands

ELSEVIER Inc.
525 B Street, Suite 1900
San Diego
CA 92101-4495
USA

ELSEVIER Ltd
The Boulevard, Langford
Lane, Kidlington
Oxford OX5 1GB
UK

ELSEVIER Ltd
84 Theobalds Road
London
WC1X 8RR
UK

First edition 2004

British Library Cataloguing in Publication Data
A catalogue record is available from the British Library.

ISBN: 0-7623-1147-9
ISSN: 0275-4959 (Series)

⊗ The paper used in this publication meets the requirements of ANSI/NISO Z39.48-1992 (Permanence of Paper). Printed in The Netherlands.

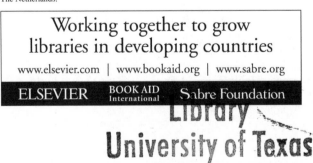

Working together to grow
libraries in developing countries

www.elsevier.com | www.bookaid.org | www.sabre.org

ELSEVIER   BOOK AID
International   Sabre Foundation

CONTENTS

SECTION III: LESSONS FROM BEYOND THE UNITED STATES

LIST OF CONTRIBUTORS

H. Armstrong	School of Social Work, Carleton University, Ottawa, Canada
P. Armstrong	Department of Sociology, York University, Toronto, Canada
Peri J. Ballantyne	Department of Public Health Science, University of Toronto, Ontario, Canada
Sandra L. Barnes	Department of Sociology & Anthropology and the African American Studies, Purdue University, Indianapolis, USA
Cornelia Beck	Departments of Geriatrics and Psychiatry and Behavioral Sciences & Alzheimer's Disease Center, University of Arkansas for Medical Sciences, USA
Cecilia Benoit	Department of Sociology, University of Victoria, British Columbia, Canada
Nancy Blythe	Department of Sociology, University of Victoria, British Columbia, Canada
Ivy Lynn Bourgeault	Health Studies Programme & Department of Sociology, McMaster University, Ontario, Canada
Melanie E. Campbell	Faculty of Medicine, University of Toronto, Ontario, Canada
J. Choiniere	Director of Policy, Practice and Research, Registered Nurses Association of Ontario, Canada

Neale R. Chumbler

Rehabilitation Outcomes Research Center, NF/SG Veterans Health System & Department of Health Services Administration, University of Florida, Gainesville, USA

Marisue Cody

VA HSR&D Center for Mental Healthcare and Outcomes Research, Central Arkansas Veterans Healthcare System & Department of Psychiatry, University of Arkansas for Medical Sciences, Little Rock, USA

Amy Dan

Ecological and Cultural Change Group, Michigan State University, East Lansing, USA

John Fortney

VA HSR&D Center for Mental Healthcare and Outcomes Research, Central Arkansas Veterans Healthcare System & Department of Psychiatry, University of Arkansas for Medical Sciences, Little Rock, USA

Boaz Kahana

Department of Psychology, Cleveland State University, Ohio, USA

Eva Kahana

Department of Sociology, Case Western Reserve University, Cleveland, USA

William Keck

Primrose Alzheimer's Living, Santa Rosa, USA

Kyle Kercher

Department of Sociology, Case Western Reserve University, Cleveland, USA

J. Lexchin

School of Health Policy and Management, York University, Toronto, Canada

Yen Ju Lin

Department of Health Administration, China Medical College, Taichung, Taiwan

S. Lindsay

Department of Sociology, University of Western Ontario, London, Canada

David Locker

Department of Community Dentistry, University of Toronto, Ontario, Canada

Man Wai A. Lun	Sociology Department, City University of New York, Old Bridge, USA
Rodney McAdams	Department of Health Sciences, Armstrong Atlantic State University, Georgia, USA
E. Mykhalovskiy	Department of Community Health and Epidemiology, Dalhousie University, Halifax, Canada
Ian Parker	Department of Physical Therapy, University of Toronto, Ontario, Canada
Maurice Penner	College of Professional Studies, University of San Francisco, California, USA
Susan J. Penner	Nursing Faculty, California State University, Hayward, USA
S. Peters	Department of Sociology, York University, Toronto, Canada
Eileen J. Porter	MU Sinclair School of Nursing, University of Missouri-Columbia, Columbia, USA
Teresa L. Scheid	Department of Sociology, University of North Carolina at Charlotte, USA
Gul Seçkin	Department of Sociology, Case Western Reserve University, Cleveland, USA
Kurt Stange	Department of Family Medicine, Case Western Reserve University, Cleveland, USA
Thomas T. H. Wan	Public Affairs Doctoral Program, University of Central Florida, Orlando, USA
Bill B. L. Wang	Director of Strategic Planning, National Defense Medical Center, Taipei, Taiwan
J. White	Department of Sociology, University of Western Ontario, London, Canada
Vic Willi	Center for Independent Living in Toronto, Canada

Karen Yoshida   Departments of Physical Therapy &
                         Rehabilitation Science, University of Toronto,
                         Ontario, Canada

Mary K. Zimmerman   Department of Sociology and Department of
                         Health Policy and Management, University of
                         Kansas, Lawrence, USA

HEALTH CARE SYSTEMS: ISSUES OF CHRONIC CARE AND SYSTEMS INTEGRATION

The theme of this volume is chronic care, health care systems and services integration. The volume is divided into three sections. The first section focuses on issues that relate to health care providers. The second section contains papers that deal with home and community based services for the elderly and those who need chronic care. The third section provides lessons from countries outside the United States related to the overall themes of chronic care, systems integration and services integration.

These are themes of growing importance in the U.S. health care system as well as in health care systems in most other developed nations. The aging of populations, already underway, and expected to increase in the coming decades will bring changes and challenges to the health care system. Many of these challenges relate to chronic care needs, since chronic care needs are more important in the elderly than in other population groups, although chronic care problems are not limited to the elderly. Once people reach their 40s and 50s, they begin to develop chronic problems. Chronic problems often require both more health care services and more complicated health care services, and thus place an emphasis on services integration.

AGING RELATED ISSUES

Aging is a growing concern in American society, whether one examines the issue in terms of growth of the elderly population, growth in expenses related to this population segment, or a concern about quality of life for people as they grow older. The population of the U.S. has aged throughout the twentieth century. While in 1900, only 4.1% of all Americans were over 65, the figure increased to 12.8% by 2000. The oldest old in the population, those 85 and over, increased even more, from only 590,000 people in 1900 to 3.7 million people in 2000. It is estimated that by 2030, when the baby boomers have become old, more than 20% of the U.S. population will be over 65. Some estimates are that those 85 and over will quadruple in size by 2030. Even given the reality that people are remaining physically healthy and may work longer than in the last generation, it is overwhelmingly clear that one of the major overall policy issues of the next several decades will be how to fund both the social and health services needs of the ever increasing elderly portions of the U.S. population. Nor is this issue of an aging population only a U.S. problem. Most developed countries are already experiencing this issue, and there are some European countries, such as Italy, that are already experiencing a declining population due to birth rates below replacement. When this happens in a country, then the elderly as a proportion of the population increase, and the issues of rising health care costs linked to changing population demographics become important policy issues in that country (Quadagno, 2005).

In the U.S., this is an important policy issue because an important portion of state and federal revenues are being used to help support the elderly. Leaving aside the issue of Social Security as the overall financial support system for many of the elderly, the costs for the federal and joint federal-state programs of Medicare and Medicaid for the elderly are large and continuing to grow. Medicaid is an important payer for some of these services, while at this point Medicare is less important. Use of private insurance is growing among some groups.

Most long term care services in the U.S. are now being provided outside nursing homes in conventional dwellings or group residential settings. One complicated issue in studying these issues today is there is not complete agreement on various definitions. Long term care refers to a range of services designed to help people with chronic conditions compensate for limitations in their ability to function independently. Typically, long term care does not involve high-tech medical care, but help with activities of daily living (ADLs) and instrumental activities of daily living (IADLs). The most advanced and medicalized long term care option is the nursing home. There are many regulations that govern such care. Generally, the most rapidly growing part of care for the elderly and for those with serious chronic health problems is not nursing home care.

A variety of home and group residential settings are more often the focus of care, along with the hospital for acute problems that arise from chronic health concerns. Home and community based services are one of the major locations for care for the elderly in the U.S. today, and are the topic of a number of the papers included in this volume. Clarity of specific definitions and terms begin to decrease as scholars and policy analysts discuss care outside of the hospital and nursing home. Turning first to group residential setting, terms used include assisted living facilities, continuing care retirement communities, supportive housing, shared housing, board and care homes, and independent living communities. Supportive housing is a more general term for a variety of group housing options that may assist the elderly with daily living. Home sharing has not fulfilled its expectations as a solution for many elderly. Board and care homes is a broad classification of facilities that provide meals, assistance with some daily activities and a supportive living environment. They can range from small home like facilities to larger hotel like operations. These facilities now serve many formerly hospitalized mental patients and there have been concerns about quality of care and maintenance of facilities. These facilities are generally less expensive than other alternatives to nursing home care, in contrast to assisted living and continuing care retirement communities (CCRCs), which often serve a more upscale clientele.

Assisted living has several different definitions. In its simplest definition, it refers to personal care services in a defined environment. An assisted living work group formed by the U.S. Senate Special Committee on Aging defined assisted living as a "Residential long-term care option that provides 24 hour personal care and supervision, but where residents have a right to make choices and receive services in a way that will promote the resident's dignity, autonomy, independence, and quality of life." Almost all sources agree that it is a type of residential long-term care designed primarily for older persons who require some ongoing assistance with daily activities. It has often been described as more consumer driven, in contrast with a more traditional model driven by health professionals. It does, in some ways, combine product (private apartment) with service (assistance with personal care). The assisted living facility is the fastest growing noninstitutional long term care alternative for frail older persons in the U.S. There is an assumption that these facilities tailor their services to an individual's needs and wants. A related type of option are CCRCs, multilevel facilities offering a range of living options generally including independent living apartments, units providing some assistance with tasks of daily living and an area of skilled nursing care. Many of these require a substantial upfront fee, in addition to a continuing monthly fee and are beyond the financial reach of many of the elderly. There are also independent living communities that have some of the same amenities but are generally geared toward a younger, healthier clientele. All of these facilities have been increasing in the U.S. over the past few decades, so that there is now a national organization, the Assisted Living Federation of America (ALFA), which is the largest association exclusively dedicated to the assisted living industry and the population it serves. ALFA represents over 5,000 for-profit and not-for-profit providers of assisted living as well as a diverse range of organizations involved in the assisted living industry. The organization has 41 state affiliates nationwide. ALFA promotes the philosophy of consumer choice and quality of life for seniors (Assisted Living Federation of American, 2004). Their current estimate is that one million Americans live in an estimated 20,000 Assisted Living residences. Other major organizations in the field include the American Association of Homes and Services for the Aging (AAHSA) which is committed to advancing the vision of healthy, affordable, ethical long-term care for America. The association represents 5,600 mission-driven, not-for-profit nursing homes, continuing care retirement communities, assisted living and senior housing facilities, and community service organizations. AAHSA estimates that its members serve one million older persons across the country.

For the elderly that wish to remain in their own homes and actually age in place, home and community based services (HCBS) are most important. These services include personal care, housekeeping, and case management in some cases. Since 1981, states in the United States, through their Medicaid programs can operate programs to provide such services as an alternative to more traditional nursing home options and use of these services has been expanding. Private long term care insurance is a growing option to cover costs of assisted living and of HCBS. Use of long term care insurance is expected to increase, partially because since 1997 there have been tax incentives in place to encourage such purchases. More employers are offering these options, as are private companies. Again, it is the more affluent elderly that are most likely to use such options, but understanding more about these options is important to developing a broader understanding of changing patterns and relationships of living choices, health care choices and system integration concerns.

CHRONIC CARE CONCERNS

Chronic conditions are health conditions that are expected to last a year or more. In general, to be considered a chronic health condition, the condition must also limit what one can do or require ongoing medical care. Some people have serious chronic conditions that both limit what they can do and require ongoing care. Severity is often related to the number of different conditions that a person has.

An estimated 128 million Americans live with one or more chronic conditions, disabilities, or functional limitations, 48% of the population. Over nine million of them have all three problems. For the 9.5 million persons with chronic conditions, functional limitations, and a disability, the costs and utilization of medical services in 1996 were nearly double, and the percent of persons going to school or work was half the rate compared to those with chronic conditions only (Anderson & Knickman, 2001).

All races and ethnicities are affected by disability, but minority groups have higher disability rates than White Americans. African Americans, American Indians and Alaska natives reported the highest disability rates, while White Americans, not of Hispanic or Latino descent, had a lower rate of disability despite having a higher median age.

When people have chronic conditions, it impacts how they view themselves, their health and the amount of health services that they use. In a series of recent polls of persons with chronic health care conditions conducted by Partnership for Solutions, people with any chronic conditions reported their health status to be fair or poor. People with serious chronic conditions had 65% reporting that their health status was only fair or poor (Chronic Conditions, 2004). People with chronic conditions often see many doctors, including a variety of specialists. In the same data set, 23% of people with chronic conditions saw four or more doctors compared to an even higher figure of 31% of those with serious chronic conditions. Of people with any chronic condition, 57% had seen a medical specialist in the previous year, while 80% of those with a serious chronic condition had seen a specialist. Nationally, as found in Medical Expenditure Panel Survey (MEPS), people with chronic conditions account for 38% of the non-elderly population and 69% of the expenditures spent on behalf of the non-elderly (Anderson & Knickman, 2001). Average per capita spending is $734 for those with no chronic conditions and $2,654 for those with chronic conditions.

Issues of care coordination are often of great concern for people with chronic care conditions. They need a variety of medical care and supportive services and need to have these services coordinated to produce high quality care. In the surveys of people with chronic health care conditions conducted by Partnership for Solutions, only 24% of people with serious chronic conditions reported that there was a doctor who coordinated their care versus 79% of all people with chronic conditions. Among family caregivers of people with chronic conditions, including those providing care to the chronically ill elderly, 45% expressed a preference to have someone other than themselves take the lead in the coordination of care to those for whom they provided assistance.

These basic definitions of chronic care and statistics about chronic care (and aging in the previous section) help to provide a general overview of some of the facts linked to aging, chronic care, and systems integration concern that are addressed in more detail and specificity in some of the specific chapters in this book. The next section of this chapter reviews the contents of each section and its chapters.

REVIEW OF THE OTHER SECTIONS OF THE BOOK AND THOSE CHAPTERS

This book includes three sections. The first section of the book focuses on health care systems and providers of care and includes five papers, most of which have a greater focus on an overall system issue or a provider of care concern. Section II includes four papers that focus more on home and community based services, and links to these types of special needs of the chronically ill or elderly. The last section of the book includes four papers that examine issues germane to the overall theme of the book, chronic care, health care systems and services integration, but does so from the framework of research about health care systems in other countries.

The first paper in Section I deals with the effects of care management, effectiveness, and practice autonomy on physicians' practice and career satisfaction. In this paper by Thomas Wan and his colleagues, the relationships of physician practice characteristics, case management effectiveness, autonomy and managed care involvement and physicians' practices and career satisfaction were examined. Studying a sample of 660 physicians from a 6,800 physician panel group, Wan and his colleagues find that there is not a statistically significant association between perceived effectiveness of care management and physician satisfaction, when practice characteristics and other perception factors are held constant. The study did find direct effects of practice characteristics and case management effectiveness on the practices of gate-keeping functions and earnings. While the study also examined contextual variables, career satisfaction was not related to any of the contextual variables studied and only two contextual variables (managed care penetration and median income in study communities) were related to physicians' practices.

Zimmerman and McAdams deal with a different aspect of health care systems, issues of publicly funded local health care in rural areas. The major thesis of the paper is that local public funding for health care is more extensive than previously recognized in rural areas of the U.S., and the presence of this public health funding plays an important role in the viability of rural health care systems. This paper particularly focuses on the impact of recent federal health policy on local community efforts to support the survival of rural hospitals. The Balanced Budget Act of 1997 (BBA) expanded Medicare's prospective payment system to non-acute care services, which promised reduced hospital reimbursement. One part of the legislation, the Critical Access Hospital Program, was specifically designed to counter the negative effect the broader legislation was expected to have. The study examines all 123 hospitals in Kansas in 1994, well before BBA legislation, and again in 2001. The study examines the hypothesis that counties receiving financial relief through participation in the Critical Access Hospital Program would show decreases in county subsidy levels compared to all other hospitals. Overall, despite participation in the federal program those hospitals received greater local public financial support and greater funding than the other community hospitals.

The next two papers relate to understanding the complexity of patient, neighborhood and service environments on health care experiences. The first paper does this with a focus on place, race and cost on the neighborhood experiences of residents in poor urban neighborhoods. This quantitative research study uses both bivariate and multivariate analyses to examine the impact of systemic factors such as the availability of health care providers and neighborhood poverty on individual health decisions made by African Americans, whites, Mexicans and Puerto Ricans living in poor Chicago neighborhoods. Residents in more impoverished areas are less likely to stay home ill. Having a regular physician increases the number of days home ill as well as days hospitalized. The paper also explores some complex differences in health profiles and providers as linked to race/ethnicity.

By contrast, older adults (ages 72 and up) are the focus of the paper by Kahana and her colleagues, with an emphasis on comparisons of HMO and fee-for-service enrollees. The paper compares the experiences of 100 elderly health maintenance organization enrollees and 315 older adults receiving fee-for-service care. They find that whichever care system elderly residents chose, they tend to focus upon the advantages of that system. Elders who choose fee-for-service care focus upon the desire to maintain control over physician choice, and believe that they are receiving superior care to HMO enrollees. Financial reasons were often an important factor in the choice of an HMO, but comprehensive coverage of services was also viewed as an advantage. The overall levels of satisfaction with physician care, confidence in physicians and availability of physicians was similar across the two groups. This was true even though HMO enrollees did have less continuity in health care more disruption in doctor-patient relationships.

The last paper in this section focuses, as did the first paper, on providers of care and their experiences. A topic of great recent interest in the U.S. has been the need for the inclusion of drug benefits for Medicare patients. This paper examines issues of outpatient drug benefits through the eyes of ten primary care providers and 12 pharmacists in the San Francisco area. Penner and Penner focus upon how each group of providers worked with pharmaceutical benefit management companies. Both groups of health care professionals reported problems in negotiating with the pharmaceutical benefit companies as a third party payer. They found the switches in formularies and multiple formularies to increase the work load for health professionals. The end of their paper links the experiences of these providers to the recent Medicare drug benefit law passed in 2003 and discusses some of the potential problems that might be expected, especially for those with chronic care needs.

The next section of the volume focuses on narrower, but important considerations, home and community based care and systems of care for the elderly and chronic care populations. The first two papers deal mostly with home care and home and community based services. The third paper looks at broader systems of service system integration, while the fourth paper examines the specific issue of mental health service utilization for family caregivers to community dwelling cognitively impaired seniors. Porter explores the topic of older persons' expectations of home care, an under explored topic among medical sociologists. The paper makes a theoretical and methodological contribution to further research in this area by reviewing theories of expectations and satisfactions and applying them to the construct of home care satisfaction. Lun's paper also deals with home based care, but it examines racial and gender differences in home and community based utilization of care. This paper uses data from the 1999 National Long Term Care Survey and applied the Andersen-Newman behavioral model to examine predictors of service use among four in-home and two community-based services. While race does not have a significant main effect on service use, gender does for certain services and there are also some interaction effects.

The Scheid paper looks at issues from a broader perspective. It describes efforts in one community to integrate services for individuals with chronic mental illness as well as a planning grant to integrate multiple chronic care systems for such problems as HIV, mental health, and substance abuse. The last paper in this section by Chumbler explores whether family caregivers with a strong sense of coherence who are caring for community dwelling older adults with cognitive impairments are less likely to use mental health services. This paper also uses an adaptation of the Andersen behavioral model, as did the Luna paper.

The last section of the book deals with lessons from beyond the United States. Three of the four papers deal with aspects of the Canadian health care system while one compares issues of advocating for patients in South Africa and the lessons for the U.S. In the first paper, Yoshida and her colleagues use a case study methodology to explore the key social and political factors that facilitated the emergences, development and achievement of the Ontario Self Managed Attendant Service Direct Funding Pilot. Using information from a different Canadian province, British Columbia, Blythe and Benoit explore the problem of late nephrology referral. Despite the fact that in the Canadian system all patients are entitled to receive necessary free health care for this problem, a substantial number of patients with chronic kidney disease experience late or no referral to nephrology care prior to needing renal replacement therapy. A number of social issues are important factors, such as race/ethnicity, English ability, marital status and proximity to care. Case study methodology is used in the third paper that examines access to essential medicines in the context of the HIV/AIDS pandemic in South Africa. For comparison, the paper also makes reference to diabetes care in the U.S. The paper emphasized the role of groups external to government in promoting access to essential medicines.

The last paper in Section III provides a very good end to the volume, since it focuses on very broad concerns in health care systems in modern countries. This paper focuses on the issue of negotiating care and compares the experiences of health care providers in Canada and the U.S. Bourgeault and her colleagues point out the linkages between the growth of managed care in the U.S. and the need for greater work in negotiation. Much of this work is delegated to nurses or administrative staff, and reflects some of the same gendered aspects of care that is found in other settings and among non-professional providers of care. The study reports on the experiences of physicians interviewed in the U.S. and Canada and on focus group interviews with groups of nurses in both countries. Interestingly, nurses often had to spend time on negotiating care in both systems, but in Canada the time was spent in securing care whereas in the U.S. the time was spent in securing payment for services. This insightful paper provides a good closing to the volume, and illustrates the complexity of care provision in modern societies, both in those with good national health care systems and even more so in a country such as the U.S. in which insurance and type of insurance is a major determinant of aspects of care.

Jennie Jacobs Kronenfeld
Series Editor

REFERENCES

Anderson, G., & Knickman, J. R. (2001). Changing the chronic care system to meet people's needs. *Health Affairs, 20*, 146–151.

Assisted Living Federation of America (2004). Website: http://www.alfa.org/.

Chronic Conditions: Public Perceptions About Health Care Access and Services (2004). http://www.partnershipforsolutions.org/DMS/files/polling_final.pdf.

Quadagno, J. (2005). *Aging and the life course: An introduction to social gerontology.* New York: McGraw-Hill.

SECTION I:
HEALTH CARE SYSTEMS AND
PROVIDERS OF CARE

THE EFFECTS OF CARE MANAGEMENT EFFECTIVENESS AND PRACTICE AUTONOMY ON PHYSICIANS' PRACTICE AND CAREER SATISFACTION

Thomas T. H. Wan, Yen Ju Lin and Bill B. L. Wang

ABSTRACT

The relationships of physician practice characteristics, care management effectiveness, autonomy, and managed care involvement, and physicians' practice and career satisfaction were investigated. A panel sample (N = 660) of 6800 physicians was made up of eleven physicians randomly selected from each of the sixty communities. Three latent constructs include care management effectiveness, practice autonomy, and openness in private practice. Multilevel modeling was performed. A statistically insignificant association was found between the perceived effectiveness of care management and physician satisfaction, holding the practice characteristics and other perception factors constant. The study demonstrated direct effects of practice characteristics and care management effectiveness on the practice of gate-keeping functions and on earnings. Only two contextual variables, managed care penetration and median income in the study communities, were related to physicians' practice.

Chronic Care, Health Care Systems and Services Integration
Research in the Sociology of Health Care, Volume 22, 3–24
Copyright © 2004 by Elsevier Ltd.
All rights of reproduction in any form reserved
ISSN: 0275-4959/doi:10.1016/S0275-4959(04)22001-4

INTRODUCTION

Successful physician practice depends on the physician's perceptions of care management's effectiveness and practice autonomy, and the physician's involvement in managed care. Numerous studies have documented the importance of physician satisfaction in effective clinical practice (Fennig et al., 2000; Konard et al., 1999; Schulz & Schulz, 1988). This empirical study is designed to identify the relative influences of physicians' personal characteristics, care management tools' effectiveness, managed care involvement, openness to accepting new patients, and contextual factors on their practice efforts and career satisfaction.

Lawler and Porter (1967) developed a systems view of work satisfaction as influenced by internal and external factors. In the same vein, Herzberg et al. (1959) conceptualized the determinants of job satisfaction as two broad types of factors – motivators (intrinsic) and hygienes (extrinsic). Intrinsic factors are personal perceptions of work values, incentives, and relationships with others, whereas extrinsic factors relate to the context and work environment (Akroyd et al., 1994; Koelbel et al., 1991). Similarly, physicians' career satisfaction is influenced by these factors. The following literature review is systematically organized under this framework to examine empirical evidence about the relationship of physician career satisfaction to both intrinsic and extrinsic factors.

RELATED RESEARCH

Physician satisfaction has been examined in both academic and practice fields for decades. At the end of the1980s, Reames and Dunstone (1989) interviewed nineteen physicians to identify the problems facing their profession: loss of autonomy (i.e. physicians' control over medical decisions), loss of control over the referral process, the threat of malpractice suits, ethical issues facing physicians in health maintenance organizations and reduced income. These concerns have been empirically investigated. For example, Burdi and Baker (1997) analyzed the level of physician satisfaction and autonomy, measured as physicians' perceived freedom to undertake eight identified activities of patient care, using a 1991 and 1996 survey of California physicians. It showed that in 1996 the young physicians were significantly less satisfied with their ability to spend enough time on patient care. Warren et al. (1998) surveyed 510 Arizona physicians and found that they were more likely to be satisfied when they wrote the orders that non-physicians must follow, when they were paid what they wanted, when patients more confidence in them, and when they did not need to subordinate their clinical judgment to that of non-physicians. Surveying 189 young physicians in the group and staff models of HMOs, Baker et al. (1994) found that the most important factors influencing physician satisfaction is the extent of perceived autonomy. However, working hours and yearly income were not found to be significantly related to physician satisfaction. In investigating the threat that bureaucratization of medical practice may lead to job dissatisfaction, Schulz et al. (1992) surveyed all 850 physicians in Dane County in 1986 to discover their perceptions of clinical freedom; their satisfaction with income, status in their profession, autonomy, resources, and professional relations; and their overall satisfaction. The authors found that perceptions of clinical autonomy and specific organizational settings were more predictive of satisfaction than other predictors. Age and gender also contributed to the differences in satisfaction.

Williams et al. (2003) describe an ideal job for a physician in ambulatory care as having good relationships with the staff and with colleagues, the ability to control time off, adequate material resources, and autonomy in decision-making. Studies also point out the importance of physicians' job satisfaction for their behavior. For example, using a sampling frame constructed from the American Medical Association's Physician Master File in the United States, and stratified into geographic regions of high and low penetration by managed care, non-Hispanic white vs. other physician ethnicity, and five specialty groupings, Williams et al. reported that physicians' perceived stress is negatively related to their job satisfaction, and that job satisfaction is positively associated with physicians' mental health. Job satisfaction is inversely related to intention to leave, to reduce work hours, to change specialty, or to leave direct patient care. Pathman et al. (2002) investigating five physician groups (2 specialty clusters and 3 age groups), found fourteen instances in which physicians in the lowest satisfaction quartile were more likely than those with average satisfaction to anticipate leaving. In only two cases were physicians in the highest satisfaction quartile less likely to anticipate leaving. In nearly all the physician groups, relative dissatisfactions with pay and with relationships with communities were associated with plans for leaving. For specific specialty and age groups, anticipated departure correlated with relative dissatisfaction with other selected areas of physicians' work.

Several studies have pointed out the effect of managed care involvement on physician practice and satisfaction. Surveying members of a physician-hospital organization at an urban teaching hospital in 1996 and 1997, Nadler et al. (1999) found that in terms of payment methods – fee-for-service vs. capitation, physicians were more satisfied with both methods of payment in 1997 than in 1996. In both years, fee-for-service was favored over capitation. After a year's experience, although satisfaction with capitation had improved, the perceived differences between capitation and fee-for-service had increased. Examining a large, academic, tertiary care hospital, Tyrance et al. (1999) found that physicians felt much less satisfaction with their ability to care for capitated patients than they felt with fee-for-service patients, especially in terms of their freedom to order necessary tests and make referrals. Multiple logistic regression found that a physician's overall satisfaction was predicted by patient load (OR = 2.7, 95% CI = 1.9–3.9), efficiency in resource utilization (OR = 1.5, 95% CI = 1.1–2.1), perceived employment stability (OR = 1.7, 95% CI = 1.3–2.2), and control over clinical time schedule (OR = 1.6, 95% CI = 1.2–2.0).

Schulz et al. (1997) surveyed all Dane County physicians in active HMO practice, in 1986 and 1993, and found that primary care physicians were more satisfied than subspecialists were with their HMO practices because of the income and the clinical freedom they had in an HMO practice. Declining in satisfaction with fee-for-service practice may result from the diminishing clinical freedom under insurance companies, increasing micromanagement of patient care.

Analyzing two cross-sectional surveys of physicians, Murray et al. (1997) examined the relationship of open-model versus closed-model practice settings to physician satisfaction in 1986 and 1997. In an open-model practice, physicians accept patients from multiple health plans and insurers; in a closed-model practice, physicians have an exclusive relationship with a single plan such as a staff or group model HMO. Overall, the physicians surveyed in 1997 were less satisfied with every aspect of their professional life than were the 1986 physicians, with statistical significance found in three areas: time spent with individual patients, autonomy, and leisure time. Open-model physicians were less satisfied than closed-model physicians with most aspects of practice.

Using a stratified random sample of 5704 primary care and specialty care physicians, Linzer et al. (2000) found that of the 2326 respondents, HMO physicians reported significantly higher satisfaction with autonomy and with administrative issues than did these other practice types: solo, small group, large group, or academic; the analysis controlled for specialty, gender, ethnicity, full-time versus part-time status, and time pressure during office visits. A study of market-level HMO activities with a national representative sample of physicians younger than 45 who had 2–9 years of practice experience in 1991 found no evidence that increased HMO activity adversely affected physician autonomy. Only limited evidence indicates that increased HMO activity reduces the satisfaction of specialist physicians, and there is no evidence that market-level HMO activities affected the satisfaction of generalists (Burdi & Baker, 1997). In examining the relationships of professional autonomy, compensation, and managed care with physician career satisfaction, Stoddard et al. (2001) analyzed the cross-sectional data generated from the 1996–1997 Community Tracking Study, a telephone survey of 12,385 physicians. Multivariate analyses demonstrated that, after controlling for all other factors, traditional core professional values and autonomy are the most important determinants of career satisfaction. Relative income is also an important independent predictor. Managed care, measured by the proportion of patient revenues generated from managed care, was shown to have an indirect effect on satisfaction through professional autonomy, but not through the resulting income reduction.

Physician satisfaction varies by gender. For example, female physicians were generally satisfied with their career (Frank et al., 1999). They were more likely than male physicians to be generalists or primary care physicians, and to be dissatisfied with the amount of time they had to spend with patients and colleagues, and with their ability to stay knowledgeable (Collins et al., 1997). Another study, however, found that female physicians were more likely than male physicians to report satisfaction with their specialties, and with patient and colleague relationships (McMurray et al., 1997).

Other factors that studies have identified as influencing physician satisfaction include physicians' age (Burdi & Baker, 1997; Leigh et al., 2003; Schulz et al., 1992), income (Schulz et al., 1992; Stoddard et al., 2001), group size (Hueston, 1998); medical abilities (Weinberg & Engasser, 1996); work stress (Frank et al., 1999); workload (Frank et al., 1999), specialty (Bates et al., 1998; Landon et al., 2003; Leigh et al., 2003), race/ethnicity (Frank et al., 1999), religion favor (Frank et al., 1999), professional control (Dunstone & Reames, 2001), specialty training certification (Fennig et al., 2000), practice settings (Breslau et al., 1978), regions (Leigh et al., 2003), managed care penetration (Hadley & Mitchell, 1997), and perceptions of the health care environment (Magee & Hojat, 2001).

Although previous studies have investigated many factors influencing the variation in physician satisfaction, the results have been inconclusive as far as the effects of managed care on physician practice are concerned (Baker & Cantor, 1993; Burdi & Baker, 1997; Murray et al., 1986, 1997). Also, inconsistent are the findings on gender, age, specialty, practice settings, medical liability insurance, and ownership of the practice as factors driving in physicians' practice. The determinants of physician career satisfaction may not be fully identified because the causal relationships are not well specified among physicians' perceptions of work settings, managed care environment, and career satisfaction. This conceptual dilemma is compounded by the diverse sample sizes and sampling frames used by researchers, and by inadequate analytic methods of handling the data. Moreover, most physician satisfaction studies rely on cross-sectional designs, which cannot investigate the dynamic nature of career satisfaction.

The present study employs a work satisfaction framework developed by Lawler and Porter (1967). The major thesis is that physicians' career satisfaction is directly influenced by practice autonomy, openness in private practice, managed care involvement, and their work efforts as gatekeepers and in generating patient

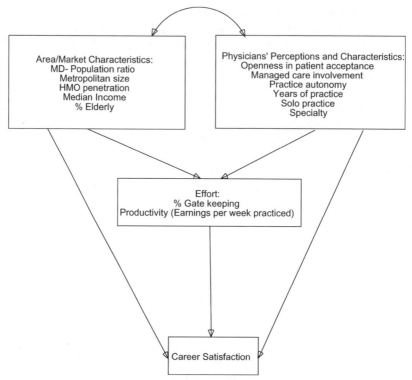

Fig. 1. A Model of Physicians' Career Satisfaction.

revenues, and is indirectly influenced by the perceived effectiveness of care management tools (Fig. 1). It is further postulated that managed care penetration and other contextual variables have no direct influence on career satisfaction.

METHODS

Data Sources

The data were drawn from the two-wave physician surveys conducted by the Community Tracking Study conducted for the Center for Studying Health System Change, in 1996 and 1998. The original study panel consists of approximately 6800 physicians with complete information in both surveys. Using the city/county codes, the survey data were merged with the Area Resource File to identify area characteristics such as managed care penetration, aging population, socioeconomic conditions, and physician-population ratio that may influence physician practice.

Study Design

Because physicians were nested in the study communities ($N = 61$), two-level multivariate modeling was performed. One community was excluded from the analysis because it did not have a county code, when the survey data were merged with the Area Resource File, which contains information on demographic, economic, health status, and health care resources at the county level (Health Resources and Services Administration, 1998). In order to accurately assess the effects of both individual physician attributes and contextual factors on physicians' career satisfaction, we randomly selected a subset of eleven physicians from each community, for a total of 660 physicians. This balance-design approach enables us to generate robust standard errors for testing the goodness of model fit and to avoid the Type I error in hypothesis testing (Arbuckle & Wothke, 1999; Heck & Thomas, 2000; Muthen & Muthen, 2001; Wan, 2002).

Measurement of the Study Variables

The three endogenous variables are: (1) the percentage of gate-keeping patients (PCTGATE) by a physician, serving as a gate keeper for medical care of patients; (2) productivity (PRODUCTI), calculated as annual earnings divided by total number of weeks worked; and (3) career satisfaction (CARSAT), ranging from the lowest level of satisfaction (scored 1) to the highest level of satisfaction (scored 5). Physician practice characteristics are: (1) years of medical practice after graduation (YRSPRAC); (2) percentage of earnings generated from practice in managed care (PMC); (3) openness in private practice (OPENNESS), measured by three indicators: willingness to accepting new patients covered by Medicare (NWMCARE), Medicaid (NWMCAID), and private insurance (NWPRIV); (4) perceived effectiveness of the following care management tools (care management effects): computerized clinical data (EFDATA), computer searches for treatment alternatives or practice guidelines (EFTREAT), use of formal practice guidelines (EFGUIDE), practice profiling (EFPROFI), and feedback from patient satisfaction surveys (EFSURV); and (5) practice autonomy, measured by five related indicators: having adequate time to care for patients (ADQTIME), having freedom in making clinical decisions (CLNFREE), the possibility of delivering high quality care (HIGHCAR), making decisions without worrying about financial incentives

(NEGINCN), and continuing patient relationships (PATREL). The contextual variables are the county/community characteristics: median income (INCOME97), HMO penetration (HMOPEN), elderly population (PCTAGED), and metropolitan size (METROSIZ). The detailed definitions of the study variables are presented in Appendix.

Analysis

Initially, we employed two-level structural equation modeling with latent variables, using the Mplus 2.12 computer program (Muthen & Muthen, 2001). The first-level analysis is based on individual physicians; the second-level analysis is based on the communities in which physicians were sampled. For a balanced design with equal numbers of subjects selected from each cluster, Mplus uses limited information, maximum likelihood estimator with robust standard errors to simultaneously decompose the variation in a set of endogenous variables into the variance components associated with each level of a data hierarchy, and explains the variation present at each level. For instance, some of the variance in career satisfaction may be explained by between-community differences (the community-level model for the $N = 60$ communities), while some of the variance may be explained by differences among individual physicians (the physician-level model for the $N = 660$ physicians). The structural equation model for the second (community) level frequently differs, in both specification and significance of parameter estimates, from the structural equation model for the first (physician) level.

The multilevel analysis adjusts for the design effect of the cluster sample (11 physicians randomly selected from each community), and indicates the strength of the design effect by providing intra-class correlations (ICCs) for all clustered variables. In our study, ICCs for physicians' career satisfaction, gate-keeping practice, and earnings/productivity were 0.035, 0.011, and 0.041, respectively. According to the rule of thumb suggested by Muthen and Muthen (2001), there is little cluster effect in the study variable if a design effect is less than 2, using a formula [1 + (average cluster size-1) × ICC] to compute the design effect for each variable. The computed values of design effect for the study variables were smaller than 2; therefore, we concluded no apparent design effect of the physicians nested in the study communities. Because the study physicians were independent, it is appropriate to perform a single-level rather than a two-level analysis of career satisfaction.

Prior to analysis, we examined patterns of missing data. We used mean imputation when there were less than 5% missing data. Structural equation modeling was conducted in two parts, using AMOS programs developed by Arbuckle and Wothke (1999): (1) using confirmatory factor analysis of several latent constructs such as care management effectiveness, practice autonomy, and openness in private practice to determine the construct validity of each latent variable as measured by multiple indicators; and (2) performing structural equation modeling of the relationships among exogenous variables (i.e. physician characteristics, perceived effectiveness of care management tools, openness to accepting new patients, managed care involvement, contextual factors, etc.) and endogenous variables (i.e. gate-keeping, earnings, and career satisfaction). The goodness-of-fit statistics of the study models are presented to show the adequacy of each model, with or without contextual variables as control variables, in explaining the variation in career satisfaction.

FINDINGS

A comparison was made for selected characteristics between the balance-designed sample ($N = 660$) and the original panel sample ($N = 6,800$) of physicians. Table 1 shows that no statistically significant differences were observed between the two sample groups. The sample appears to be very representative of the original panel sample. In this study sample, high overall career satisfaction (4.11 on average) was observed; the scores ranged from 1 (the lowest) to 5 (the highest). The average age of the physicians studied was 47.31. Most were white (82.12%), board certified (88.67%), and solo practitioners (90.91%). On average they practiced 47.40 hours

Table 1. Comparison Between the Balance-Designed Sample and the Original Panel Sample of Physicians, with Major Characteristics.

Characteristics	The Study Sample	The Original Panel Sample	*F*-Statistics Significance
Mean age	47.31	48.04	3.228 (ns)
% Male	77.79	79.54	1.130 (ns)
% Board certified	88.67	86.91	1.657 (ns)
% Solo practice	90.91	90.75	0.018 (ns)
Average weeks practiced	47.40	47.58	1.470 (ns)
% White	82.12	82.28	0.011 (ns)
% Practice revenues from managed care	47.77	46.16	2.129 (ns)
Mean overall career satisfaction score	4.11	4.11	0.014 (ns)

Note: A randomly selected sample (eleven physicians) from each of sixty communities constitutes the study sample of this analysis.

NS = Not statistically significant difference at the 0.05 level.

per week, and generated 47.77% of their earnings from practice under managed care.

Three latent variables – perceived effectiveness of care management tools, practice autonomy, and openness to accepting new patients from different insurance plans – were independently validated by confirmatory factor analysis. The results are presented in Figs 2–4. The factor loading (standardized coefficient) between the indicator (in the box) and the latent construct (in the circle) indicates the strength of the association or correlation. Only statistically significant loadings were included in each measurement model of the latent variable. In general, the models were reasonably well fitted to the data and demonstrated the construct validity of the measurements. It is interesting to note that the variable "openness" is not correlated with the variables of care management effectiveness and practice autonomy, whereas these two variables are positively correlated.

A structural equation model was developed, linking physicians' perceptions and characteristics to work effort and career satisfaction. This model assumed that the three latent predictor variables, years of medical practice (YRSPRAC), percentage of managed care revenues (PMC), and gender (MALE) directly affected work effort variables (PCTGATE and PRODUCTI), without any contextual variables included as control variables. Initially, we assumed that career satisfaction was directly influenced by work effort and by all of the predictor variables specified, with the exception of care management effectiveness: CARSAT = f

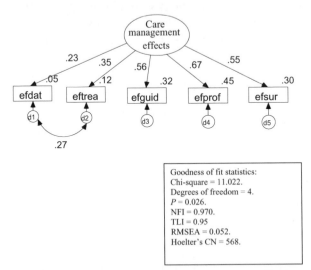

Goodness of fit statistics:
Chi-square = 11.022.
Degrees of freedom = 4.
$P = 0.026$.
NFI = 0.970.
TLI = 0.95
RMSEA = 0.052.
Hoelter's CN = 568.

Fig. 2.   The Measurement Model of Perceived Care Management Effectiveness: Physician Level Analysis.

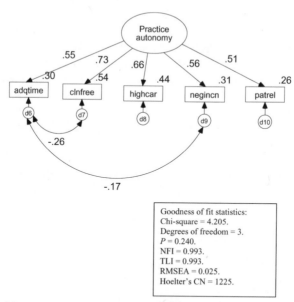

Fig. 3. The Measurement Model of Perceived Practice Autonomy: Physician Level Analysis.

(OPENNESS, YRSPRAC, MALE,SOLO, SPECIALTY, BOARDCT, PRACTICE AUTONOMY, PMC, PCTGATE, PRODUCTI). After performing several revisions of the generic model, we presented only a relatively well fitted model with statistically significant paths (standardized regression coefficients). The results

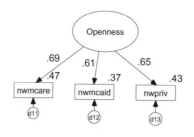

Fig. 4. The Measurement Model of Openness in Patient Acceptance: Physician Level Analysis.

with parameter estimates and goodness-of-fit statistics are presented in Table 2. Based on the analytical model presented in Fig. 5, the key findings are summarized as follows: (1) Career satisfaction was not directly associated with work effort variables or with perceived care management effectiveness; it was negatively influenced by percentage of managed care revenues (standardized regression coefficient $= -0.108$) and years of practice (-0.083), and was positively affected by openness to accepting new patients (0.108) and by practice autonomy (0.391). No gender effect on career satisfaction was observed. (2) Because physician characteristics such as solo practice, board certification, and specialty did not influence work effort or career satisfaction with statistical significance in the initial model, they were excluded from the final model. (3) The percentage of gate-keeping patients was positively influenced by perceived care management

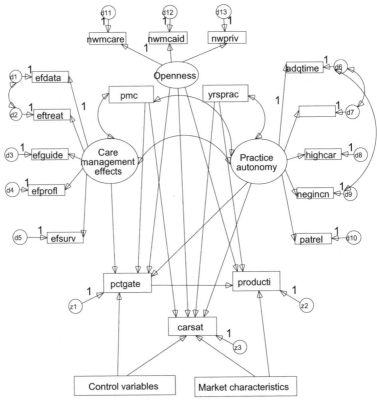

Fig. 5.   The Structural Equation Model of Physicians' Work Effort and Career Satisfaction.

The Effects of Care Management

Table 2. The Structural Equation Model of Predictors of Physician Work Effort and Career Satisfaction.

Variables	% Patients Gate-Kept (Y_1)		Productivity (Y_2)		Career Satisfaction (Y_3)	
	B	CV/P	B	CV/P	B	CV/P
Care management effectiveness	0.154	2.696*	–	–	–	–
% Revenues from managed care	0.358	9.711*	–	–	-0.108	-2.972*
Openness in patient acceptance	-0.152	-3.511*	0.082	1.856	0.098	2.256*
Years of practice			-0.181	-5.508*	-0.083	-2.291*
Practice autonomy	0.103	2.458*			0.391	7.480*
Male (=1; female = 0)	0.085	2.422*	-0.260	-7.229*	–	–
Y_1			-0.221	-5.823*	–	–
Y_2					–	–
R^2	0.202		0.158		0.185	

Note: B: Standardized regression coefficient; CV: Critical value; –: Variable is not included or is not statistically significant at the 0.05 or lower level; Goodness of fit statistics of the model: Chi-square = 293.023; Degrees of freedom = 138; P = 0.000; NFI = 0.850; TLI = 0.892; RMSEA = 0.042; Hoelter CN = 375.

*Significant at the $p \leq 0.05$ or lower level.

Table 3. The Structural Equation Model of Predictors of Physician Work Effort and Career Satisfaction: Market Characteristics as Control Variables.

Variables	% Patients Gate-kept (Y_1)		Productivity (Y_2)		Career Satisfaction (Y_3)	
	B	CV/P	B	CV/P	B	CV/P
Care management effectiveness	0.146	2.631[*]	–	–	–	–
% Revenues from managed care	0.370	10.170[*]	–	–	-0.110	-3.017[*]
Openness in patient acceptance	-0.167	-3.897[*]	0.079	1.797	0.098	2.254[*]
Years of practice	–	–	-0.178	-4.991[*]	-0.083	-2.296[*]
Male (=1; female = 0)	0.095	2.732[*]	-0.251	-7.007[*]	–	–
Practice autonomy	0.092	2.243[*]	–	–	0.390	7.487[*]
Area median income[a]	-0.106	-3.04[*]	–	–	–	–
HMO penetration (%)[a]	–	–	-0.113	-3.154[*]	–	–
Y_1			-0.182	-4.961[*]	–	–
Y_2			–		–	–
R^2	0.227		0.164		0.184	

Note: B: standardized regression coefficient; CV: critical value; –: Variable is not included or is not statistically significant at the 0.05 or lower level; Goodness of fit statistics of the model: Chi-square = 306.917; Degrees of freedom = 155; P = 0.000; NFI = 0.852; TLI = 0.901; RMSEA = 0.039; Hoelter CN = 398.

[*] Significant at the $p \leq 0.05$ or lower level.

[a] Market area characteristic at the county level.

effectiveness (0.154), percentage of managed care revenues (0.358) and practice autonomy (0.103). However, gate-keeping practice was negatively affected by openness to accepting new patients (−0.152). Male physicians (0.085) had a higher percentage of gate-keeping patients. (4) Physician practice income, measured by average earnings per week practiced, was negatively influenced by gate-keeping practice (−0.221) and by years of practice (−0.181), and was positively influenced by the openness of accepting new patients (0.082). Female physicians had higher average earnings per week than did male physicians. The total variances explained by the predictor variables for the three endogenous variables (PCTGATE, PRODUCTI, and CARSAT) are 20.2, 15.8, and 18.5%, respectively.

Several contextual variables were introduced in the analysis. They were area characteristics of the county where a physician practiced in 1997, namely physician-population ratio, metropolitan size, HMO penetration, median income, and percentage of elderly population residing in the county. However, the analysis showed that most of the contextual or ecological variables had no statistically significant influence on physicians' career satisfaction. Table 3 summarizes the results. Only two variables, serving as control variables, showed a negative influence on work effort variables: (1) HMO penetration negatively influenced practice income or earnings (−0.113); and (2) median income of the area negatively affected gate-keeping practice (−0.106).

In sum, relatively speaking, the most influential predictor variables for each of the three endogenous variables, respectively, are: (1) the predictor variable "practice revenues generated from managed care" for improving gate-keeping practice; (2) the variable "gate-keeping practice" for lowering physicians' earnings or productivity; and (3) the variable "perceived practice autonomy" for enhancing career satisfaction. Career satisfaction is not statistically related to work effort variables, gate-keeping or practice income.

DISCUSSION AND CONCLUSION

In 1999, the Institute of Medicine's report "To Err Is Human" drew great attention to improving professional practices, particularly related of physicians. It is increasingly debated whether physicians can still play a dominant role in medicine, retain public faiths in their professional authority and ability, and maintain control over their working conditions in terms of patients, labor, equipment, and facilities (Warren et al., 1998). Physicians' career satisfaction is an important subject to explore in order to optimize their functions and practice.

The present analysis has shed light on the relationship between variables related to physician practice and physicians' career satisfaction. The findings may help us understand how to improve physician satisfaction and work effort. Gate keeping is a major function of physician practice under managed care. Both the perceived effectiveness of care management and practice autonomy are positively associated with gate-keeping. Physicians who were open to accepting new patients or who practiced in an area with relatively higher median income were less likely to perform gate-keeping. However, it is surprising that HMO penetration did not explain the variation in gate-keeping practice. Perhaps, physicians' gate-keeping functions are ubiquitous in most areas, and so little variation in gate-keeping practice was observed in this study.

Physicians' earnings were negatively influenced by gate-keeping and by HMO penetration. The impact of managed care has been well demonstrated by such finding. An inverse relationship between years of practice and earnings, found in this study, is consistent to findings reported by previous studies (Goldberg, 1996). Many physicians have to accept new patients from all kinds of insurance plans in order to enhance their earnings. However, median income of the community where a physician practiced was not a statistically significant predictor of career satisfaction.

Practice autonomy was the strongest predictor of career satisfaction. This finding is consistent with other studies (Magee & Hojat, 2001; Schulz et al., 1992; Stoddard et al., 2001; Tyrance et al., 1999; Williams et al., 2003). Work efforts, the variables "gate-keeping" or "earnings," bear no significant relationship to career satisfaction. Higher revenues generated from managed care practice may not improve physicians' career satisfaction. This suggests a potential negative effect of managed care practice on career satisfaction. It is interesting to note that none of the contextual variables studied at the county level had any direct influence on physicians' career satisfaction. However, these variables may affect satisfaction indirectly through their joint influences on perceptions of autonomy, openness, and managed care practice.

Gender was not related to career satisfaction. Gender differences in both work effort variables were statistically significant. Male physicians had a higher proportion of gate-keeping patients and lower average earnings per week than did female physicians, when the effects of other predicator variables were controlled.

In conclusion, for the physician level analysis, reasonable objective measures of the effectiveness of care management are indispensable. It is essential to gather information from each practice on the actual use of care management tools and their relative effectiveness in enhancing productivity and the quality of care, to identifying the benefits and values added to clinical performance. At the market level, more carefully designed sampling strategies are needed to avoid the clustering effects of area characteristics. For instance, the physician sample can be drawn from the county-level roster of practitioners. A representative, small sample of physicians, perhaps 30–50 per county, can be randomly selected to generate a balance-designed national sample. Thus, a two-level analysis of determinants of physicians' work effort and career satisfaction may be properly conducted to tease out the variance components attributable to the individual physician and to market/area characteristics or predictor variables. In much of current thinking, the dissatisfactions of physicians' practice are attributed to managed care or to lack of control. That leaves problematic but essential areas unexplored, among them the roles of patient demand, market competition, and changing economic environments (Hoff, 2003). Learning more about the causal-specific links to multiple factors in career satisfaction and in physician productivity is urgent if we are ever to improve effectiveness and efficiency in private practice.

REFERENCES

Akroyd, D., Wilson, S., Painter, J., & Figures, C. (1994). Intrinsic and extrinsic predictors of work satisfaction in ambulatory care and hospital settings. *Journal of Allied Health, 23*(3), 155–164.

Arbuckle, J., & Wothke, W. (1999). *AMOS 4.0. User's guide*. Chicago: SmallWaters Corporation.

Baker, L., & Cantor, J. (1993). Physician satisfaction under managed care. *Health Affairs, 12*(Suppl.), 258–270.

Baker, L., Cantor, J., Miles, E., & Sandy, L. (1994). What makes young HMO physicians satisfied? *HMO Practice, 8*(2), 53–57.

Bates, A., Harris, L., Tierney, W., & Wolinsky, F. (1998). Dimensions and correlates of physician work satisfaction in a midwestern city. *Medical Care, 36*(4), 610–617.

Breslau, N., Novack, A., & Wolf, G. (1978). Work settings and job satisfaction: A study of primary care physicians and paramedical personnel. *Medical Care, 16*(10), 850–862.

Burdi, M., & Baker, L. (1997). Market-level health maintenance organization activity and physician autonomy and satisfaction. *American Journal of Managed Care, 3*(9), 1357–1366.

Collins, K., Schoen, C., & Khoransanizadeh, F. (1997). Practice satisfaction and experiences of women physicians in an era of managed care. *Journal of the American Medical Women Association, 52*(2), 52–56.

Dunstone, D., & Reames, H. (2001). Physician satisfaction revisited. *Social Science and Medicine, 52*(6), 825–837.

Fennig, S., Yuval, D., Greenstein, M., Rabin, S., & Weingarten, M. (2000). Job satisfaction among certified and non-certified general practitioners. *Israel Medical Association Journal, 2*(11), 823–827.

Frank, E., McMurray, J., Linzer, M., & Elon, L. (1999). Career satisfaction of U.S. women physicians: Results from the women physicians' health study. Society of general internal medicine career satisfaction study group. *Archives of Internal Medicine, 159*(13), 1417–1426.

Goldberg, J. (1996). Why some doctors make a lot, and some make little. *Medical Economics, 73*, 142–149.

Hadley, J., & Mitchell, J. (1997). Effects of HMO market penetration on physicians' work effort and satisfaction. *Health Affairs, 16*(6), 99–111.

Health Resources and Services Administration (1998). *Area resources file.* Rockville, MD: HRSA.

Heck, R., & Thomas, S. (2000). *An introduction to multilevel modeling techniques.* Mahwah, NJ: Lawrence Erlbaum.

Herzberg, F., Mausner, B., & Snyderman, B. (1959). *The motivation to work.* New York: Wiley.

Hoff, T. (2003). How physician-employees experience their work lives in a changing HMO. *Journal of Health and Social Behavior, 44,* 75–96.

Hueston, W. (1998). Family physicians' satisfaction with practice. *Archives of Family Medicine, 7*(3), 242–247.

Koelbel, P., Fuller, S., & Misener, T. (1991). Job satisfaction of nurse practitioners: An analysis using Herzberg's Theory. *Nurse Practitioners, 16*(4), 46–52.

Konard, T., Williams, E., Linzer, M., McMurray, J., Pathman, D., Gerrity, M., Schwartz, M., Scheckler, W., Van Kirk, J., Rhodes, E., & Douglas, J. (1999). Measuring physician job satisfaction in a changing workplace and a challenging environment. SGIM career satisfaction study group. Society of general internal medicine. *Medical Care, 37*(11), 1174–1182.

Landon, B., Reschovsky, J., & Blumenthal, D. (2003). Changes in career satisfaction among primary care and specialist physicians. *JAMA, 289,* 442–449.

Lawler, E., & Porter, L. (1967). The effects of performance on job satisfaction. *Industrial Relations, 7,* 20–28.

Leigh, J., Kravitz, R., Schembri, M., Samuels, S., & Mobley, S. (2003). Physician career satisfaction across specialties. *Archives of Internal Medicine, 162*(14), 1577–1584.

Linzer, M., Konrad, T., Douglas, J., McMurray, J., Pathman, D., Williams, E., Schwartz, M., Gerrity, M., Scheckler, W., Bigby, J., & Rhodes, E. (2000). Managed care, time pressure, and physician job satisfaction: Results from the physician worklife study. *Journal of General Internal Medicine, 15*(7), 517–518.

Magee, M., & Hojat, M. (2001). Impact of healthcare system on physicians' discontent. *Journal of Community Health, 26*(5), 357–365.

McMurray, J., Williams, E., Schwartz, M., Douglas, J., Van Kirk, J., Konrad, T., Gerrity, M., Bigby, J., & Linzer, M. (1997). Physician job satisfaction: Developing a model using qualitative data. *Journal of General Internal Medicine, 12*(11), 711–714.

Muthen, L., & Muthen, B. (2001). *Mplus User's guide.* LA: Muthen & Muthen.

Nadler, E., Sims, S., Tyrance, P., Fairchild, D., Brennan, T., & Bates, D. (1999). Does a year make a difference in changes in physician satisfaction and perception in an increasingly capitated environment. *American Journal of Emergency Medicine, 107,* 38–44.

Pathman, D., Konrad, T., Williams, E., Scheckler, W., Linzer, M., & Douglas, J. (2002). Physician job satisfaction, dissatisfaction, and turnover. *Journal of Family Practice, 51*(1), 593.

Reames, H. J., & Dunstone, D. (1989). Professional satisfaction of physicians. *Archives of Internal Medicine, 149*(9), 1951–1956.

Schulz, R., & Schulz, C. (1988). Management practices, physician autonomy, and satisfaction. Evidence from mental health institutions in the federal republic of Germany. *Medical Care, 26*(8), 750–763.

Schulz, R., Girard, C., & Scheckler, W. (1992). Physician satisfaction in a managed care environment. *Journal of Family Practice, 34*(3), 298–304.

Schulz, R., Scheckler, W., Moberg, D., & Johnson, P. (1997). Changing nature of physician satisfaction with health maintenance organization and fee-for-service practices. *Journal of Family Practice*, *45*(4), 321–330.

Stoddard, J., Hargraves, J., Reed, M., & Vratil, A. (2001). Managed care, professional autonomy, and income: Effects on physician career satisfaction. *Journal of General Internal Medicine*, *16*(10), 712–713.

Tyrance, P., Sims, S., Ma'luf, N., Fairchild, D., & Bates, D. (1999). Capitation and its effects on physician satisfaction. *Cost and Quality Quarterly Journal*, *5*(1), 12–18.

Wan, T. T. H. (2002). *Evidence-Based health care management: Multivariate modeling approaches*. Boston: Kluwer.

Warren, M., Weitz, R., & Kulis, S. (1998). Physician satisfaction in a changing health care environment: The impact of challenges to professional autonomy, authority, and dominance. *Journal of Health and Social Behaviour*, *39*(4), 356–367.

Weinberg, D., & Engasser, P. (1996). Dermatologists in Kaiser Permanente-northern California. Satisfaction, perceived constraints, and policy options. *Archives of Dermatology*, *132*(9), 1057–1063.

Williams, E., Linzer, M., Pathman, D., McMurray, J., & Konrad, T. (2003). What do physicians want in their ideal job? *Journal of Medical Practice Management*, *18*(4), 179–183.

APPENDIX
DEFINITIONS OF STUDY VARIABLES

Variable	Type	Definition
Predictor variables: Physician characteristics and perceptions		
Openness in accepting new patients (an exogenous latent variable)		
NWMCARE	O	Whether the practice accepts new patients who are insured through Medicare, including Medicare managed care patients (1: none; 2: some; 3: most; 4:all)
NWMCAID	O	Whether the practice accepts new patients who are insured through Medicaid, including Medicaid managed care patients (1: none; 2: some; 3: most; 4:all)
NWPRIV	O	Whether the practice accepts new patients who are insured through private or commercial insurance plans, including managed care plans and HMOs with whom the practice has contracts (1: none; 2: some; 3: most; 4:all)

Variable	Type	Definition

Perceived care management effectiveness (an exogenous latent variable)

EFDATA	O	Effect of use of computer to obtain or record clinical data such as medical records and lab results in the practice of medicine (5: very large; 4: large; 3: moderate; 2: small; 1: very small; 0: no effect)
EFTREAT	O	Effect of use of computer to obtain information about treatment alternatives or recommended guidelines in the practice of medicine (5: very large; 4: large; 3: moderate; 2: small; 1: very small; 0: no effect)
EFGUIDE	O	Effect of use of formal written practice guidelines such as generated by physician organizations, insurance companies or HMOs, or government agencies in the practice of medicine (5: very large; 4: large; 3: moderate; 2: small; 1: very small; 0: no effect)
EFFROFL	O	Effect of the results of practice profiles comparing your pattern of using medical resources to treat patients with that of other physicians in the practice of medicine (5: very large; 4: large; 3: moderate; 2: small; 1: very small; 0: no effect)
EFSURV	O	Effect of feedback from patient satisfaction surveys in the practice of medicine (5: very large; 4: large; 3: moderate; 2: small; 1: very small; 0: no effect)

Practice autonomy (an exogenous latent variable)

| ADQTIME | O | Agreement to the statement that respondent physician spends adequate time with patients during typical office/patient visits (5: agree strongly; 4: agree somewhat; 3: neither agree nor disagree; 2: disagree somewhat; 1: disagree strongly) |
| CLNFREE | O | Agreement to the statement that respondent physician has the freedom to make clinical decisions that meet his/her patient needs (5: agree strongly; 4: agree somewhat; 3: neither agree nor disagree; 2: disagree somewhat; 1: disagree strongly) |

Variable	Type	Definition
HIGHCAR	O	Agreement to the statement that respondent physician provides high quality of care to all his/her patients (5: agree strongly; 4: agree somewhat; 3: neither agree nor disagree; 2: disagree somewhat; 1: disagree strongly)
HIGHCAR	O	Agreement to the statement that respondent physician provides high quality of care to all his/her patients (5: agree strongly; 4: agree somewhat; 3: neither agree nor disagree; 2: disagree somewhat; 1: disagree strongly)
NEGINCN	O	Agreement to the statement that respondent physician makes clinical decisions in the best interests of patients without regard to the possibility of reducing income (5: agree strongly; 4: agree somewhat; 3: neither agree nor disagree; 2: disagree somewhat; 1: disagree strongly)
PATREL	O	Agreement to the statement that it is possible to maintain the kind of continuing relationships with patient over time that promote the delivery of high quality care (5: agree strongly; 4: agree somewhat; 3: neither agree nor disagree; 2: disagree somewhat; 1: disagree strongly)

Physician-practice-related variables

YRSPRAC	I	Practice experience in years
BOARDCT	O	Board certification status of physician (3: board certified; 2: board eligible only; 1: neither)

Physician performance

Productivity (PRODUCTI, an endogenous variable): EARN-INGS divided by WKSWEK

WKSWRK	I	Number of weeks physician spent practicing medicine in 1997
EAENINGS	I	Practice income in 1997

% of gate-keeping patients in practice (PCTGATE; an endogenous variable)

	I	Number of patients who are gate-kept by a physician per 100 patients in the practice in 1997

Variable	Type	Definition
Career satisfaction (CARSAT, an endogenous variable)		
	O	General satisfaction with overall medical career in 1998 (5: very satisfied; 4: satisfied; 3: neither satisfied nor dissatisfied; 2: dissatisfied; 1: very dissatisfied)
Control variables		
Physician characteristics		
GENDER	O	Gender of physicians (1: male; 0: female)
Community/area characteristics: Contextual variables		
MDPOPR	I	Physician-population ratio in a county
INCOME97	I	Median income in a county
PCTAGED	I	Percentage of elders (65+) in a county
HMOPEN	I	% Patients enrolled in HMOs in a county
METROSIZ	O	Metropolitan size (9 categories ranging from less than 2500 people to 1 million people)

Note: O = Ordinal scale; I = Interval scale.

PUBLIC SUPPORT FOR RURAL HEALTH CARE: FEDERAL PROGRAMS AND LOCAL HOSPITAL SUBSIDIES

Mary K. Zimmerman and Rodney McAdams

ABSTRACT

This paper focuses on the impact of recent federal health policy on local community efforts to support the survival of rural hospitals. Rural communities in the United States have an established tradition of providing public financial support to local hospitals. The Balanced Budget Act of 1997 (BBA) expanded Medicare's prospective payment system to non-acute care services, which promised reduced hospital reimbursement. Part of this legislation, the Critical Access Hospital (CAH) program, was specifically designed to counter the negative impact the broader legislation was expected to have. This study was designed to investigate the hypothesis that counties receiving financial relief for local hospitals through participation in the CAH program would show decreases in county subsidy levels compared to other hospitals. All 123 hospitals in Kansas were studied in 1994, well before BBA legislation, and again in 2001. Data on county-level health care spending for each of the two years were abstracted from all county budgets in Kansas. The amounts counties contributed to local hospitals were calculated and compared in terms of CAH versus non-CAH hospitals with attention to patterns of increase. Results showed that CAH hospitals, in spite of participation in the federal program, received greater local public financial

Chronic Care, Health Care Systems and Services Integration
Research in the Sociology of Health Care, Volume 22, 25–45
Copyright © 2004 by Elsevier Ltd.
All rights of reproduction in any form reserved
ISSN: 0275-4959/doi:10.1016/S0275-4959(04)22002-6

support and experienced greater funding increases than other community hospitals. The implications of these findings are discussed in terms of the circumstances of rural hospitals and recent changes in the CAH program.

The significant challenges of maintaining hospitals in rural areas are well known. In fact, their strength and survival have constituted an on-going central concern in national policy for much of the past century (Beaulieu & Berry, 1994; McAdams, 1996; Stevens, 1989; Zimmerman et al., 2004). From the consumer standpoint, having health care available in close proximity to home creates easier access and encourages continuity of care. On the other hand, low volumes and the proportionally high costs of keeping small hospitals open in rural areas are difficult to justify from a health care policy and management perspective. The tension between the health care needs of rural residents and the broader issues of health care markets and financing raise important questions about the role of government, both national and local, in providing solutions. In this paper, we consider how recent federal health care policies – in particular, the Critical Access Hospital program instituted in 1997 – have influenced patterns of local financial support. We examine the connections between federal programs and the local subsidies that have become a significant factor as well as a challenge to maintain in rural America.

RURAL HOSPITALS IN THE CONTEXT OF LOCAL COMMUNITIES

Rural hospitals are pivotal to local communities. Community hospitals in general and particularly those in rural areas have long been viewed, along with schools and religious organizations, as the foundation of community life. Moreover, rural communities and small towns carry on a well-established tradition of assuming responsibility for providing their hospitals some level of local financial support. Stevens (1989) observes that "the hospital which was built by local fund drives and community contributions was viewed as a community endeavor in spirit . . . affirmed as a local institution" (Stevens, 1989, pp. 122, 125). Going back to the early 1900s, community hospitals in rural areas of the United States have been built and maintained with local financial assistance.

Hospital financial viability remains a constant concern in rural America. Many rural hospitals continue to operate as local institutions, relying on a variety of revenue sources, including local tax funding, patient fees (whether from insurance or out-of-pocket) and charitable contributions to sustain operations. Nearly half (44%) of all hospitals in the United States are rural hospitals, although they account for only 21% of all hospital beds (Rural Health Research Center, 2003). This reflects the fact that many rural hospitals have fewer than 50 beds. These smaller rural hospitals also have lower occupancy rates. Hospitals in 2002 with fewer than 50 beds had an average occupancy rate of 38.5% while rates in larger hospitals ranged from 55 to 72% (U.S. Health Resources and Services Administration, 2002). Hospital occupancy measures the use of hospital beds and fixed assets and can therefore be viewed as a general indicator of financial viability (Gapenski, 2002).

The financial performance of rural hospitals declined in the late 1990s. Of those with fewer than 50 beds, 46% reported net losses in 1999 along with 32% of those with 50–99 beds (Rural Health Research Center, 2003). At the same time, rural hospital beds appeared to be decreasing. During the 1990s, over half (58%) of rural hospitals reduced bed size (Rural Health Research Center, 2003). The already vulnerable position of many of these rural hospitals was further threatened by the Medicare changes associated with the Balanced budget Act (BBA) of 1997 and the Balanced Budget Refinement Act (BBRA) of 1999. One part of this policy initiative, however, the Critical Access Hospital (CAH) program, was specifically designed to counter the negative impact that the broader legislation was expected to have on small, rural hospitals. In this paper, we focus on the CAH program in order to present evidence of its impact, and also to reveal the current relationship between the struggle in rural communities to sustain rural hospitals and the federal policies that provide the context. First, we place these recent events within their historical trajectory.

FEDERAL POLICIES AND RURAL HOSPITALS

Rural health financing issues became noticeable on the federal policy agenda beginning in the 1920s. Between 1930 and 1990, the U.S. government sponsored and/or lent strong support to five national initiatives with significant implications for rural health care financing: the 1932 report of the Committee on the Cost of Medical Care (CCMC), the Farm Security Administration of 1938, the Hill-Burton legislation of 1946, the "Great Society" legislation of the 1960s and the Rural Health Initiative of 1975 (see Zimmerman et al., 2004 for a more detailed account).

The first of these initiatives consisted of a study and report on health access issued in the early 1930s by the CCMC. The study, which cost nearly one million dollars, was funded by several private foundations, including Rockefeller and Carnegie. The report focused on four general areas: (1) incidence of disease and disability in the population; (2) the status of existing facilities; (3) family expenditures for services; and (4) incomes of service providers (Anderson, 1985). Although it didn't specifically address rural health care, the report expressly encouraged the expansion of health insurance, hospitals, and physician services to those Americans who lacked access (Starr, 1982). In the late 1930s, the Farm Security Administration (FSA) sponsored a program that was designed to provide medical care to low-income farmers. The FSA believed that many defaults on FSA loans were the result of paying health care expenses rather than making loan payments. To remedy the situation, the FSA encouraged the development of rural health cooperatives in underserved areas, which offered prepaid health care to as many as 600,000 people living in rural areas (Starr, 1982). Most of these cooperatives were short-lived, often attracting the criticism of the local medical community. This effort was terminated shortly after the end of World War II. Shortly thereafter, the Hospital Survey and Construction Act of 1946, commonly known as Hill-Burton, offered rural America a new approach to solving its health care problems. The new strategy involved the provision of federal financing for hospitals and medical facilities. Following World War II, many voluntary hospitals lacked the financial capital to expand, renovate, or modernize (Anderson, 1985). Furthermore, there were many people in rural areas that did not have access to hospitals. The Hill-Burton program authorized federal grants to survey, construct, and modernize hospitals and public health centers, awarding grants on a matching basis, with the federal government restricted to paying no more than two-thirds of the construction costs. Over the course of its duration, the Hill-Burton Program provided more than $4.5 billion in grant funds and $1.5 billion in loans to more than 6800 health care facilities, most of them located in rural areas (U.S. Health Resources and Services Administration, 2004). In exchange for federal funds, facilities were required to provide free care or reduce the cost of care to low-income patients (U.S. Health Resources and Services Administration, 2004).

Of the various federal initiatives, Titles 18 and 19 of the Social Security Act, better known as the Medicare and Medicaid programs, are commonly considered the most important public funding assistance that rural health care has received (Samuels, 1994). Providing comprehensive health care access for those over age 65 as well as for many low-income persons had a particularly significant impact on rural America because its population includes a disproportionate share of low income and elderly persons. Yet, Medicare and Medicaid were not developed specifically for rural areas and neither were other parts of the Kennedy-Johnson "Great Society" agenda, such as Community Health Centers, whose funds over time went primarily to central cities. Finally, in 1975, the Rural Health Initiative specifically addressed the previous imbalance in rural versus urban federal programming. It succeeded primarily because it focused on the unique health care needs of rural areas, a theme that was carried into the rural health financing policies of the next several decades.

In the 1980s and 1990s, health care cost containment strategies, beginning with Medicare prospective payment in 1983 and continuing with the rise of managed care and its various forms, placed increasing pressure on rural health care systems, especially hospitals (Davis et al., 1990). Arguably, no two pieces of legislation were more consequential than the BBA and BBRA. From a health care perspective, the chief purpose of the BBA was to slow Medicare spending and extend the solvency of the Medicare Trust Fund. It reduced Medicare reimbursement for inpatient hospital services and created prospective payment systems for other programs including skilled nursing, outpatient, home health and rehabilitation services and in 1999 long-term care and psychiatric services (National Advisory Committee on Rural Health, 2001). As a result of these changes, financial pressures intensified. Although other types of providers and health care organizations faced cuts under the BBA and BBRA, it is widely agreed that rural hospitals were particularly affected. Their responses included a range of altered organizational arrangements and strategies (Angelelli et al., 2003).

THE CRITICAL ACCESS HOSPITAL PROGRAM AND ITS IMPACT

One component of the BBA, the Medicare Rural Hospital Flexibility Program, was designed to benefit small, rural hospitals and improve access to care. This ongoing program established a new type of institution, known as a Critical Access Hospital (CAH). In exchange for more favorable reimbursement terms, hospitals under the CAH program were required to restructure as a limited-service inpatient facility. It was thought that converting to this type of facility would provide small, rural hospitals with a viable response to the possibility of reduced income resulting from BBA changes in reimbursement for hospital-based outpatient departments, home health agencies and skilled nursing facilities. To receive certification as a CAH, hospitals were required to meet a number of criteria (Dalton et al., 2000). The institution had to be a not-for-profit or public hospital located in a rural area, operate 15 or fewer acute care beds, provide 24-hour emergency care and limit length of stay to 96-hours for hospitalized patients. The BBA also allowed hospitals to have up to 10 additional swing beds to provide services to long-term care patients. In exchange for meeting these criteria, CAH's were reimbursed on a "reasonable cost" basis, rather than the usual prospective payment system used for inpatient and outpatient services under Medicare. Essentially, reasonable cost meant that the hospital was reimbursed for all allowable costs associated with the provision of services to Medicare patients. As another benefit, mid-level practitioners such as a physician's assistant, nurse practitioner, or clinical nurse specialist were allowed to provide inpatient care subject to supervision by a physician who was not required to be on site.

There are relatively few studies of the effectiveness of the CAH program, so it has been difficult to assess whether the program has improved the financial status of rural hospitals or promoted access. This is compounded by evidence suggesting that rural communities may have been slower than urban areas in developing their responses to the BBA changes (Mueller et al., 1999). Early reports, however, have indicated success (Hagopian, 1999; Reif & Ricketts, 1999; Stensland et al., 2000, 2004). One indicator of the success of CAH is the number of hospitals that have converted to critical access status. As of November 2003, 847 rural hospitals had become critical access facilities and 45 states had participated in the program (American Hospital Association, 2004). This exceeded preliminary estimates for potential conversions (Dalton et al., 2000). According to the American Hospital Association, CAHs represent 17% of all U.S. community hospitals and 39% of all rural U.S. community hospitals (American Hospital Association, 2004). This study focuses on the predominantly rural state of Kansas and offers a unique approach to assessing the impact of CAH policy. Kansas is an ideal setting for the study because it was one of the first states to certify critical access hospitals and currently is the state with the largest number of CAHs (American Hospital Association, 2004).

We have documented in earlier research that in the mid-1990s Kansas counties devoted between one-seventh and one-eighth of their annual budgets to support basic health services, such as ambulances, ambulatory care, mental health and nursing homes (Zimmerman & McAdams, 1999). The same study showed that Kansas counties contributed substantial amounts to their local hospitals in order to sustain operations (Zimmerman & McAdams, 1999). Ambulance, ambulatory care, and hospital services together accounted for 63% of total health care expenditures for the average Kansas county. This study suggested that local health care services in many rural areas depend on public tax support to remain viable. Contributions from local governments were quite substantial in some counties, reflecting both the financial pressure on local health providers and institutions as well as the continuing tradition of local funding support.

County budgets cannot expand indefinitely, especially in low income, rural areas. We found in the mid-1990s that the Kansas counties with the highest per capita health care expenditures were also those with the highest per capita incomes, suggesting that poorer counties regardless of need may not support local health services at the same level as wealthier counties. Since county subsidies to local hospitals appeared sensitive to the economic level of the county, we reasoned that they might also be sensitive to shifts in the local hospital's financial status. Recently, Stensland et al. (2004) studied the financial status of hospitals converting to CAH status in 1999 and 2000 and found that they benefited economically in the period directly following conversion. This provides evidence that CAH conversion does have the intended economic effect on rural hospitals. Accordingly, if financial pressures on rural hospitals are relieved, then they may require lower county subsidies (or at least less of an increase) in the subsequent period. Therefore, it makes sense to examine county subsidy levels for CAH compared to non-CAH hospitals during this period of conversion. Specifically, in this study, we hypothesized that counties receiving financial relief for local hospitals through participation in the CAH program should show decreases in county subsidy levels compared with other hospitals.

METHODOLOGY

A central purpose of the Critical Access Hospital program is to reduce the financial pressure on rural hospitals. In order to investigate whether participating as a CAH had a positive financial effect on rural hospitals over time, we looked at changes in local public subsidies for these hospitals. We reasoned that the amount of public tax funding provided by local communities to subsidize their hospital could serve as an indicator sensitive to the level of financial pressure on rural hospitals. Local subsidies exist in large part because rural hospitals need these funds in order to survive. If financial pressures decrease, then it is reasonable to assume that subsidy levels will not rise, or at least not show the same levels of increase of non-participating hospitals. On the other hand, without a way to reduce financial pressures, other (non CAH) community hospitals would be more likely to show greater increases in subsidy levels. For purposes of this study, local funding was defined as county-level public spending. Following this line of reasoning, we hypothesized that *county public spending levels to support rural hospitals participating in the CAH program would be lower over the study period than county public spending levels for other community (non CAH) hospitals.* In particular, we were interested in studying the years 1994 and 2001, which represent time periods a few years before and a few years after the BBA/BBRA program was implemented in 1997/1999. Accordingly, we looked at changes in levels of county spending for hospitals for those two years, comparing CAH to other rural community hospitals.

Site for the Study

Kansas was considered an appropriate site for the study based on the extent to which it is a rural state and due to the high level of participation of its hospitals in the Critical Access Hospital program. Standard measurement of rural versus urban based on the SMSA-non SMSA classification results in all but a handful of Kansas counties being considered rural. Thus, we chose to use the Urban Influence Codes (UIC) developed by the U.S. Department of Agriculture (Ghelfi & Parker, 1995) because they provide a more refined measure of rurality. Using this scale, which ranks counties from 1–9 according to how rural they are (with counties as designated as "9" the most rural), the median score for Kansas counties was "8." When the Kansas UIC median score was compared to the median scores for the neighboring states of Arkansas, Iowa, Missouri, Nebraska and Oklahoma, Kansas was found to one of the most rural. Kansas is also appropriate for the present study because it leads the nation in terms of the number of Critical Access Hospitals; 54 or 44% of the 123 community hospitals in the State participated in the CAH program at the time of this study (Kansas Department of Health and Environment, Office of Local and Rural Health, 2003).

Data Collection

Budget data for 1994 and 2001 were obtained for each of the 105 counties in Kansas as part of two larger studies of all county-level public expenditures for health care conducted in 1997–1998 and 2003–2004 (see Zimmerman & McAdams, 1999, 2003). Trained abstractors reviewed the final budget reports for each Kansas county for both study years and recorded all expenditures related to hospitals. To these amounts we also added the levied tax monies from several hospital special taxing districts, which were included in our definition of local public funding for hospitals. All but one of these districts were located within the boundaries of a single county so that the levied amount was added directly to the total amount of public spending for hospitals in that county. Where the district's jurisdiction extended over multiple counties, the amount collected was divided equally among them. Review of the entire budget for each county was necessary because some hospital expenses were listed as specific budget items or funds while others were categorized under the county's general fund.

Validity was enhanced by using an instrument for data collection that was pre-tested and validated, using the same set of trained abstractors for all data collection, and conducting telephone check backs with appropriate officials in each county for the purpose of clarifying and confirming any vague or questionable expenditure items. Reliability of measurement was tested using a process of repeat abstraction. Data were abstracted two separate times for a random sample of 10%

of the counties. Agreement was 98% between the two independent abstraction procedures, which shows that the method was highly reliable.

Variables

Using these budget data, hospital spending for each county was calculated in four ways: (1) *absolute amount of hospital spending in dollars*; (2) *absolute amount of hospital spending per capita*; (3) *absolute amount of hospital spending per admission*; (4) *absolute amount of hospital spending per hospital bed*. In addition, we collected data on several additional variables, which previous research has indicated are potentially important as factors related to the financial status of rural hospitals (Beaulieu & Berry, 1994; Lillie-Blanton et al., 1992; Moscovice & Rosenblatt, 1999). These variables include: (1) average hospital bed size; (2) average number of annual admissions; (3) average occupancy rate; (4) average age of county population (percent over 65); (5) average population change between 1960 and 2000; (6) average percentage of total admissions that are Medicare admissions; (7) average county population density (persons per square mile); and (8) the average distance between hospitals.

The first 3 variables – hospital bed size, annual admissions, and occupancy – relate to capacity and bed size. All three variables are general indicators of financial viability, i.e. smaller hospitals with lower occupancy rates tend to show poorer financial performance. These variables were used to look at differences in the amount of tax subsidy (county support) received by CAHs and other community hospitals. Medicare admissions were used to determine whether CAHs were more Medicare dependent and the amount of subsidy per Medicare admission. The average distance between hospitals was used as an indicator to determine whether CAHs are more isolated and have larger service areas than other community hospitals.

Two variables represent characteristics often associated with increased need or burden for rural health care – the *percentage of county residents 65 and older* and *population density*. Older individuals are thought to have greater health needs than younger individuals, with the potential of increasing use of health services. Low population density means relatively few users in the area proximate to the point of service. In order to maintain access for residents in low-density communities, rural hospitals are likely to have low utilization and inefficiencies, and require financial assistance. Thus, while an aged population may increase demand for rural hospitals, it is likely that such demand in low-density areas will serve simply to draw community attention to the need for local services without providing the volume necessary for their financial viability.

Data Analysis

The data for this study as described above were calculated for each county. The analysis was then conducted in two phases. First, county data were averaged across the state for each variable and the results compared for Critical Access Hospitals versus all other community hospitals. In the second phase, we examined changes over time in the amounts of county subsidies to both types of hospitals. Specifically, we analyzed the average percentage change in the amount of public tax expenditures going from the county to both CAH and non-CAH hospitals in Kansas, using the study years 1994 and 2001. These comparisons were conducted for percentage of change using three different hospital spending variables: *absolute amount of hospital spending, per capita tax subsidy*, and *subsidy per admission*. Finally, we looked in greater depth at hospitals of both types that received the largest amounts of county subsidies. We compared selected characteristics of the five CAH program hospitals that received the largest tax subsidy in 2001 with those of the five non-CAH program hospitals that received the largest tax subsidy in the same year.

FINDINGS

The results reported in Table 1 show a number of differences between the 54 Kansas hospitals that have Critical Access Hospital status and the 69 that do not. Consistent with program criteria, CAH hospitals have fewer beds, fewer admissions and

Table 1. Characteristics of Kansas Hospitals ($n = 123$) by Critical Access Hospital (CAH) Status, 2001.

Characteristic	Critical Access Hospitals ($n = 54$)	Other Community Hospitals ($n = 69$)
Average bed size	20	96
Average number of admissions (annual)	324	3,281
Average occupancy rate	15.1%	33.0%
% Of county population over 65 years of age	20.2%	16.2%
Average population change between 1960 & 2000	14.6%	30.7%
Average percentage of total admission that are medicare	68%	45%
Average county population density (persons per square mile)	9.7	55.8
Average distance between hospitals	23.2 miles	19.1 miles

an occupancy rate that is 50% lower compared to other community hospitals in Kansas. In addition, CAHs are located in markedly less densely populated counties; the average population density for CAH counties is 9.7 compared to 55.8 for other community hospitals (see Table 1). Counties with CAH hospitals have a slightly higher percentage of people over the age of 65 than do non-CAH counties. Consistent with the CAH criteria, participating hospitals had 50% more Medicare admissions.

Perhaps the most interesting variable shown in Table 1 is the average distance to the nearest hospital. This distance is 23.2 miles in the case of CAH program hospitals and 19.1 miles for other hospitals. According to CAH criteria, in order for a hospital to be designated a CAH it must be located more than a 35-mile drive from another hospital (U.S. Health Resources and Services Administration, 2004). This requirement can be waived by the State by finding the prospective Critical Access Hospital to be "a necessary provider of health care services to residents in the area." In Kansas, the 35-mile requirement has been waived for most of the Critical Access Hospitals.

The results of descriptive data, comparing hospital subsidies over all Kansas counties for both CAH and non-CAH hospitals for both study years, are reported in Table 2. These findings show that CAH facilities received considerably more local support than other hospitals during the study years. This finding is not surprising at the beginning of the period because these hospitals by definition are vulnerable and financially at high risk. In 1994, the 54 CAH hospitals in Kansas received a total of $12,265,017, which converts to an average subsidy of $227,130 per hospital, compared to a total of $5,932,998 for the 69 other community hospitals in the state, which converts to an average of $85,985 per hospital. By 2001, the total subsidy

Table 2. County Tax Subsidies for Kansas Hospitals ($n = 123$) by Critical Access (CAH) Status, 1994 and 2001.

	Critical Access Hospitals ($n = 54$)	Other Community Hospitals ($n = 69$)
Subsidy – 1994		
Total subsidy	$12,265,017	$5,932,998
Average subsidy per hospital bed	$9,174	$801
Average subsidy per admission	$605	$24
Average per capita subsidy	$32.60	$2.59
Subsidy – 2001		
Total subsidy	$16,970,194	$7,089,224
Average subsidy per hospital bed	$15,728	$689
Average subsidy per admission	$1,000	$27
Average per capita subsidy	$46.10	$2.99

amount had risen to $16,970,194 for the CAH hospitals ($314,263 per hospital) and $7,089,224 for the other community hospitals ($102,742 per hospital). When these increases are further analyzed in terms of the subsidy per hospital bed and the subsidy per hospital admission, the differences between subsidy amounts for CAH and non-CAH hospitals becomes even more pronounced. By definition, CAH hospitals have fewer beds and fewer admissions. As shown in Table 2, for example, the total amount of 2001 county dollars spent per CAH hospital bed in Kansas was nearly $16,000 compared to approximately $700 per bed in non-CAH hospitals. These data suggest that hospitals participating in CAH required greater financial support in 2001 than 1994, indicated by the fact that they continued to require significant public funding from their respective counties in order to operate. The data are also interesting in light of the Stensland et al. (2004) study, in which the authors acknowledged that only half the "dramatic changes" in the financial position of converting hospitals could be attributed to CAH status. The other half of the increase in revenue was due to non-Medicare sources, which could have included funding from county-level governments.

A central question in this study is what happened to county subsidies for both Critical Access and other community hospitals in Kansas between 1994 and 2001 in relation to BBA/BBRA and the federal CAH initiative. Although this latter policy was intended to give rural hospitals relief – and, according to earlier studies, did have an initial positive financial impact – our data show that subsidies increased for CAH as well as other hospitals during this period. The second phase of our analysis focused on the degree of this change. We calculated the percent change in county subsidies and compared CAH with non-CAH hospitals. Table 3 presents the findings for the two types of hospitals in terms of the percent change in *absolute amount of county subsidy, per capita subsidy*, and *subsidy per admission*. These results show that between 1994 and 2001 counties increased their public subsidy

Table 3.   Increases in Absolute Amount of Tax Subsidy, Per Capita Tax Subsidy and Subsidy Per Admission Provided to Critical Access Hospitals and Other Kansas Hospitals, 1994–2001.

	Critical Access Hospitals ($n = 54$) (%)	Other Community Hospitals ($n = 69$) (%)
Increase in absolute amount of tax subsidy (1994–2001)	39.4	19.5
Average increase in per capita tax subsidy (1994–2001)	41.4	15.4
Average increase in subsidy per hospital admission	65.3	14.0

for their local hospitals significantly more when the hospital was a participant in the Critical Access Hospital program than when they were not. For example, the absolute amount of county subsidy going to CAH program hospitals increased 38.4% over the seven-year period, while subsidies going to other community hospitals increased by only half that amount (19.5%). This finding is noteworthy because it contradicts what would be expected to occur, given the purpose of the CAH program. If the level of county subsidy is a valid indicator of financially stressed hospitals, then the CAH program has not been an entirely effective remedy for financially troubled hospitals. Moreover, without the increases in county tax support and the more generous cost-based reimbursement, perhaps many of these small, rural hospitals would have faced insolvency problems and possible closure.

Even more substantial discrepancies were found between the increases in CAH and non-CAH hospital subsidies when they were examined in terms of *per capita subsidy* as well as *subsidy per admission*. As Table 3 shows, over the seven year period of study, county subsidies to CAH hospitals per capita increased approximately three times more than those for other community hospitals. The differential increase was even more pronounced when viewed in terms of hospital admissions. Between the two study years, the county subsidy for CAH hospitals when analyzed *per admission* increased more than 65% compared to a much smaller 14% increase among non-CAH hospitals. Thus, the subsidy per admission increased five times more for hospitals participating in the Critical Access Hospital program than it did for non-participating hospitals.

While the average level of county subsidy across all CAH hospitals showed an increase, we wondered about CAH hospitals that may not have experienced an increase. Table 4 shows the 41 hospitals that received county subsidies in

Table 4. Changes in the Amount of Subsidy for Kansas Critical Access Hospitals That Received a County Subsidy ($N = 41$), 1994–2001.

Type of Change	Number of CAH Hospitals	% of All CAH Hospitals Receiving Subsidies ($n = 41$)
CAH Hospitals with an increase in subsidy of greater than 1% between 1994 and 2001	32	78
CAH Hospitals with a decrease in subsidy of greater than 1% between 1994 and 2001	9	22
CAH Hospitals with an increase of subsidy of greater than 25% between 1994 and 2001	20	49
CAH Hospitals with a decrease in subsidy of more than 25% between 1994 and 2001	4	10

terms of how many received increases versus decreases over the years of study. Thirty-two of these hospitals (78%) experienced increases and 20 of these (49%) experienced increases of greater than 25%. Nine hospitals (22%) experienced decreased county subsidies during this same period. These findings raise important questions about the true impact and consequences of this particular federal policy and also about the future of rural hospitals under the current organizational and financing arrangements operating within the American health care system. These issues will be considered in greater detail in the final sections of the paper.

The last phase of our analysis involved hospital-specific comparisons. Table 5 presents selected characteristics for the five most highly subsidized CAH hospitals and Table 6 presents similar data for the non-CAH hospitals for Kansas in 2001. Examining the most subsidized CAH hospitals reveals a startlingly high level of county public funding in a few cases. For example, Hospital A received $571 in local tax support on average from each of the county's 4,307 residents. Similarly, Hospital B received $300 per capita and Hospital C received $493 (Table 5). If extremely high levels of county subsidy indicate financial distress, then these 5 hospitals do not show the improvement (fiscal stress reduction) in 2001 that was intended by the objectives of the CAH program. Looking at the same variables among the other community hospitals (non-CAH) that received the most county public funding, the results show lower subsidy amounts – Hospital M had a per capita subsidy of $359 and Hospital N $238 whereas Hospital O received only $23 per capita (Table 6).

Comparing the two groups of hospitals produces another surprising result. It could be reasonably expected based on federal criteria that CAH hospitals would be located farther away from the nearest hospital than other community hospitals. This, however, did not turn out to be the case. Instead, they were actually situated slightly closer to the nearest hospital than non-CAH hospitals – an average of 25.6 miles apart for non-CAH hospitals compared to 21.8 miles apart for the CAH hospitals. Other comparisons, however, showed results that conformed to expectations. The most subsidized CAH hospitals were substantially smaller, with an average bed size of 14 compared to 39 for the most subsidized among the other hospitals. The most subsidized CAH hospitals also had fewer admissions and therefore much larger subsidies per admission compared to the other subsidized hospitals. Given their small size, they also received extraordinary subsidies per bed – with nearly $190,000 of public funding per bed per year in one CAH hospital and $109,000 per bed in another. County subsidies per bed in non-CAH hospitals were much lower, with the highest being $56,000.

There are several limitations associated with our methodology in this study. First, county-level subsidies to rural hospitals in any given year could include one-time amounts that result in the subsidy amount that year being larger than typical. For

Table 5. Kansas Critical Access Hospitals with the Largest Tax Subsidies, 2001.

CAH Hospital	Average Distance to Nearest Hospital (miles)	Total County Subsidy	County Population	Per Capita Subsidy	Total Admissions, 2001; Subsidy Per Admission	Total Acute Beds 2001; Subsidy Per Bed
Hospital A	29.4	$2,460,425	4,307	$571	101 Adm. $24,361	13-beds $189,263
Hospital B	31.8	$1,637,844	5,463	$300	475 Adm. $3,448	15-beds $109,190
Hospital C	24.2	$1,062,470	2,155	$493	220 Adm. $4,829	10-beds $106,247
Hospital D	10.6	$909,000	6,270	$145	193 Adm. $4,710	15-beds $60,600
Hospital E	13.1	$846,687	3,560	$238	283 Adm. $2,992	15-beds $56,446
Total and averages	21.8	$6,916,426	21,755	$318	1,272 Adm. $5,437	68-beds $101,712

Table 6. Kansas Other (Non-CAH) Community Hospitals with the Largest Tax Subsidies, 2001.

Non-CAH Hospital	Average Distance to Nearest Hospital (miles)	Total County Subsidy	County Population	Per Capita Subsidy	Total Admissions, 2001; Subsidy Per Admission	Total Acute Beds 2001; Subsidy Per Bed
Hospital K	18.2	$1,550,000	7,743	$200	668 Adm. $2,320	45-beds $34,444
Hospital L	42.0	$987,466	8,738	$113	701 Adm. $1,409	24-beds $41,144
Hospital M	25.1	$849,309	2,369	$359	456 Adm. $1,863	15-beds $56,620
Hospital N	34.5	$818,205	3,437	$238	1101 Adm. $743	40-beds $20,455
Hospital O	22.2	$644,213	27,947	$23	1874 Adm. $344	69-beds $20,455
Total and averages	28.4	$4,849,193	50,234	$97	4800 Adm. $1,010	193-beds $25,125

example, a hospital might purchase a piece of equipment or complete a renovation project that would not be repeated in subsequent years. For the two study years of 1994 and 2001, we took the expenditures for hospitals from budgets at face value and did not try to determine previous or subsequent trends. In addition, county subsidies are products of competing budgetary pressures, so the amounts provided to hospitals are determined in a context characterized by many types of expenditure demands. We only looked at health care expenses and did not look at changes in other budgetary categories.

Finally, the study is limited by studying the post BBA effects of the CAH program on county subsidies for hospitals only in 2001. Perhaps additional effects will be visible in subsequent years. Angelelli et al. (2003) suggest that strategies of rural hospitals in response to BBA/BBRA may have continued to evolve and that research extending at least to 2003 is required.

DISCUSSION

Kansas represents a major participant in the national Critical Access Hospital program. The results reported here show that many hospitals, both CAH and non-CAH, in the state receive county funding, sometimes considerable amounts. What our data show about CAH hospitals is that they are particularly small, low volume and financially vulnerable. This suggests that CAH hospitals in particular are likely to be actively struggling to remain open. On the one hand, the increases in county subsidies demonstrate strong community commitment and willingness to invest in maintaining rural hospitals. On the other, these efforts raise questions about the limits to which such efforts should be taken, especially given that CAH hospitals are no more isolated than other hospitals in the state. The relative proximity of highly subsidized CAH hospitals to neighbor hospitals raises the question of whether sustaining all these hospitals is necessary in order to meet the health care needs of the population. A case in point is Hospital A (Table 4), which received a 2001 county tax subsidy of $571 per capita although it has a neighboring hospital within 30 miles. In addition, Hospital A has only 13 beds and in 2001 reported less than 2 admissions per week. The other four highly subsidized CAH hospitals showed similar characteristics. These hospitals are among the most heavily subsidized, and raise questions about the appropriateness of some CAH designations.

Consolidation of hospitals in rural areas is a hotly contested issue and for that reason is often avoided. These data provide continuing evidence that this issue must continue to be engaged in discussions and policy formulation for health care services in rural America. Arguably, consolidating a number of small facilities into a single regional facility has both positive and negative aspects. On the positive side, a regional facility could take advantage of economies of scale, reduce service duplication, and provide a wider range of services and personnel. Another benefit of a larger regional facility is that it would be able to recruit and employ more physicians, nurses, and technical personnel at a single facility. A larger staff would reduce the burden that many rural health providers now face of being "on-call" for long periods of time.

The principle negative benefit of regionalization relates to economic development. Creating a regional hospital would eliminate the need for a number of smaller hospitals. Frequently, small hospitals are major employers and make significant contributions to the local economy (Doekson et al., 1998). Although it might reduce the tax burden on local communities and produce economies of scale in delivering health care services, a regional health system can also be detrimental for individual communities in the service area. The central question in this study is whether the Critical Access Hospital program of 1997 eased the financial situations of participating hospitals. As one way of looking at the program's positive impact, we have examined if public county subsidies to these hospitals decreased from 1997 to 2001 relative to other hospitals. Our study findings did not support this hypothesis. Not only did both types of hospitals receive increased county subsidies over the seven-year study period, but CAH hospitals received markedly larger increases. Participating hospitals were able to survive and remain open, but the program did not result in decreased local spending for their maintenance. Our data show increases in county subsidies to CAH hospitals between 1994 and 2001 that were twice what they were for non-CAH hospitals. Thus, for a number of these rural hospitals, a large amount of local support in combination with federal support is required to maintain them.

Such findings raise a number of important questions with respect to the CAH program and for current and future federal policies regarding rural hospitals. First, we have already mentioned the issue of whether all these marginal, rural hospitals should be saved. Perhaps consolidation might be possible, even though it is a politically contentious prospect. Second, is it possible that county subsidies are increasing because these are the hospitals with the greatest financial problems. Even with CAH reimbursement benefits, these hospitals may be profoundly weak. Thus, the impact of CAH cannot reduce the need for greater subsidies than for the other hospitals. Third, are communities willing to subsidize more because of participation in the CAH program? It could be possible that participation in CAH inspires confidence and a willingness to invest more local resources in rural hospitals. A fourth question deals with the issue of what will happen to these hospitals if counties can no longer provide subsidies. Counties with CAH hospitals are losing population and population loss has a debilitating effect on the local tax base. Will they falter despite the CAH program?

RECENT CHANGES IN THE CRITICAL ACCESS HOSPITAL PROGRAM AND IMPLICATIONS FOR THE FUTURE

The Medicare Prescription Drug, Improvement, and Modernization Act of 2003 has brought a number of changes to the Critical Access Hospital Program. Section 405 of the Act includes conditions that will enhance reimbursement, potentially expand bed size, and provide continued funding for the Medicare Rural Hospital Flexibility grant (FLEX grants) program (AHA, hospitalconnect, 2004). Flex grants are monies made available to states for rural health planning, rural network development and implementation, expansion of emergency medical services, and for designating Critical Access Hospitals (AHA, hospitalconnect, 2004). The Act provides for $35 million a year for FLEX grants through FY 2008.

Under the provisions of the Act, Critical Access Hospitals can have up to 25 beds designated as either acute care or swing beds. Under previous rules, hospitals could have no more than 15 acute care beds and 10 swing beds. Expanded bed capacity will allow greater flexibility in patient mix and provides the capacity to accommodate more admissions and patients.

In addition to increasing bed capacity, the Act also increases payment for both inpatient and outpatient services. Beginning in 2004, Critical Access Hospitals reimbursement will be increased from 100 to 101% of reasonable costs (Centers for Medicare & Medicaid Services, Medicare News, January 22, 2004). As a result of changes in reimbursement, payments to Critical Access Hospitals are expected to increase by $900 million over a ten-year period (Centers for Medicare & Medicaid, Medicare News, January 22, 2004).

As with most federal initiatives, the CAH program is a work in progress. One of the chief purposes of the program is to "improve access to hospital and other health services for rural residents of the state." In Kansas, it appears that program alone does not offer adequate leverage to keep many of the small, rural hospitals operational and solvent. Without the combination of tax subsidy and cost-based reimbursement, many rural hospitals would face a precarious operational climate. It also appears that both the CAH program and local tax subsidies offer a temporary remedy. Most of the CAH hospitals in Kansas operate in counties that are losing population. Of the 54 Kansas CAH hospitals, only 15 were located in counties that gained population between 1990 and 2000 (U.S. Census Bureau, 1990, 2000). Moreover, counties must increasingly balance health care expenditures with competing demands for monies for other types of services – demands that have been escalating as cost-cutting state governments shift programs to local communities.

In local communities without adequate patient populations and taxpayer rolls, some of the more vulnerable rural hospitals may be moving toward extinction. It seems clear that many of these hospitals will require more generous third party payments or tax subsidies if their service area populations continue to decline. Another looming financial problem facing CAH hospitals in Kansas is that their current physical plants were constructed during the 1960s and 1970s with Hill-Burton funding. As the physical plants age, funding will be needed for renovation, modernization, and new construction. Recently, while reflecting on the financial condition and the future of his critical access hospital, one administrator was heard to say: "it's not a pretty story, it's a story about rural health care."

ACKNOWLEDGMENTS

This research was supported in part by grant #47355 awarded to the authors by the Changes in Health Care Financing and Organization Initiative of the Robert Wood Johnson Foundation. The authors wish to thank the Policy Research Institute at the University of Kansas and Robert Lee, Pat Oslund, Alicia Reed, Brian Tongier and especially Lori Wiebold-Lippisch for their help at various stages of this research.

REFERENCES

Anderson, O. W. (1985). *Health services in the United States: A growth enterprise since 1875*. Ann Arbor, MI: Health Administration Press.

Angelelli, J., Fennell, M. L., Hyatt, R. R., & McKenney, J. (2003). Linkages in the rural continuum: The balanced budget act and beyond. *The Gerontologist, 43*(2), 151–157.

American Hospital Association (2004). www.hospitalconnect.com, April 13, Chicago, IL.

Beaulieu, J., & Berry, D. (1994). *Rural health services: A management perspective*. Ann Arbor: AUPHA/Health Administration Press.

Centers for Medicare and Medicaid (2004, January 22). CMS increases payments and expands flexibility for critical access hospitals in rural areas. *Medicare News*.

Dalton, K., Slifkin, R. T., & Howard, H. A. (2000). The role of critical access hospital status in mitigating the effects of new prospective payment systems under medicare. *The Journal of Rural Health, 16*(4), 357–370.

Davis, R. G., Zeddies, T. C., Zimmerman, M. K., & McLean, R. A. (1990). Rural hospitals under PPS: A five-year study. *The Journal of Rural Health, 6*(3), 286–301.

Doekson, G., Johnson, T., Baird-Holmes, D., & Schott, V. (1998). A healthy health sector is crucial for community economic development. *The Journal of Rural Health, 14*(1), 66–72.

Gapenski, L. G. (2001). *Healthcare finance*. Chicago: Health Administration Press.

Ghelfi, L., & Parker, T. S. (1995). *A new county-level measure of urban influence*. Staff Paper. Washington, DC: Rural Economy Division, U.S. Department of Agriculture.

Hagopian, A. (1999). Critical access hospitals and community development. In: *Rural Hospital Flexibility Program Tracking Project: Year Two Report*. Prepared by the Rural Policy Research Institute, University of Minnesota.

Kansas Department of Health and Environment (2003). Office of Local and Rural Health. www.kdhe.state.ks.us/olrh/KRHOPinKS.

Lillie-Blanton, M., Felt, S., Redmon, P., Renn, S., Machlin, S., & Wennar, S. (1992). Rural and urban hospital closures, 1985–1988: Operating and environmental characteristics that affect risk. *Inquiry*, *29*, 332–344.

McAdams, R. (1996). *Explaining health care innovation in Rural communities: A comparative, case study*. Unpublished Ph.D. Dissertation, University of Kansas.

Moscovice, I., & Rosenblatt, R. (1999). *Quality of care challenges for rural health*. University of Minnesota: Rural Health Research Center.

Mueller, K. J., Coburn, A., Cordes, S., Crittendon, R., Hart, J. P., McBride, T., & Myers, W. (1999). The changing landscape of health care financing and delivery: How are rural communities and providers responding? *Millbank Quarterly*, *77*, 485–510.

National Advisory Committee on Rural Health (May, 2001). Report: *Medicare reform: A rural perspective*. Washington, DC.

Reif, S., & Ricketts, T. (1999). The Medicare critical access hospital program: The first year. *The Journal of Rural Health*, *15*, 61–66.

Rural Health Research Center (2003). *Rural hospitals: New millennium and new challenges*. Minneapolis, MN: School of Public Health, University of Minnesota.

Samuels, M. E. (1994). Policy initiatives and issues in rural health services development. In: J. Beaulieu & D. Berry (Eds), *Rural Health Services: A Management Perspective*. Ann Arbor: AUPHA/Health Administration Press.

Starr, P. (1982). *The social transformation of American medicine*. Basic Books.

Stensland, J., Davidson, G., & Moscovice, J. (2004). The financial benefits of Critical Access Hospital Conversion for FY 1999 and FY 2000 Converters. Working Paper #51. Minneapolic, MN: Rural Health Research Center, School of Public Health, University of Minnesota.

Stensland, J., Moscovice, I., & Christianson, J. (2000). The financial viability of rural hospitals in the post BBA environment. Working Paper #33. Minneapolis, MN: Rural Health Research Center, School of Public Health, University of Minnesota.

Stevens, R. (1989). *In sickness and in wealth: American hospitals in the Twentieth Century*. New York: Basic Books.

U.S. Census Bureau (1990). Summary population and housing characteristics. U.S. Department of Commerce. Economics and Statistics Administration.

U.S. Census Bureau (2000). Summary population and housing characteristics. U.S. Department of Commerce. Economics and Statistics Administration.

U.S. Health Resources and Services Administration, Bureau of Health Professions (2002). Health professional shortage area primary medical care designation criteria. Washington, DC: U.S. Department of Health and Human Services.

U.S. Health Resources and Services Administration, Office of Rural Health Policy (2004). www.ruralhealth.hrsa.gov.

Zimmerman, M. K., & McAdams, R. (1999). What we say and what we do: County-level public spending for health care. *Journal of Rural Health*, *15*(4), 421–430.

Zimmerman, M. K., McAdams, R., & Halpert, B. P. (2004). Funding health services in the rural United States: Federal policies and local solutions. In: N. Glascow, L. W. Morton & N. Johnson (Eds), *Critical Issues in Rural Health* (pp. 211–224). Blackwell.

TOO POOR TO GET SICK?
THE IMPLICATIONS OF PLACE,
RACE, AND COSTS ON THE
HEALTH CARE EXPERIENCES OF
RESIDENTS IN POOR URBAN
NEIGHBORHOODS

Sandra L. Barnes

ABSTRACT

Literature suggests that the poor often face a myriad of health care constraints and health problems. This study uses bivariate and multivariate analyses to examine the effects of systemic factors such as the availability of health care providers and neighborhood poverty on individual health decisions for a sample of African Americans, Whites, Mexicans, and Puerto Ricans in poor Chicago neighborhoods. Results show that Medicaid usage and having a regular physician increase the number of days home ill and days hospitalized, while frequenting clinics decreases such activity. Additionally, residents in more impoverished urban areas are less likely to stay home ill. Differences in health profiles and providers are also evident based on race/ethnicity. These findings illustrate the important relationship

Chronic Care, Health Care Systems and Services Integration
Research in the Sociology of Health Care, Volume 22, 47–64
Copyright © 2004 by Elsevier Ltd.
All rights of reproduction in any form reserved
ISSN: 0275-4959/doi:10.1016/S0275-4959(04)22003-8

between macro-level factors and specific health choices many residents in
poor urban areas make at the micro-level.

Literature suggests that obtaining adequate, affordable, accessible health care continues to undermine the health of many poor persons due largely to systemic problems associated with under-serviced communities with limited health care facilities (Auerbach & Krimgold, 2001; Cebrun, 1997; Duncan et al., 1995; Karger et al., 2003; Lykens & Jargowsky, 2002; Schram et al., 2003). The problem is particularly acute for poor urban residents who are typically women and racial/ethnic minorities (Hersch & White-Means, 1993; Seccombe et al., 1994; Smith, 1993). And although residents in poor urban areas are more likely to experience chronic health problems than their counterparts in other areas, they are less likely to seek treatment or take part in preventive health care (Billingsley, 1992; Lewin-Epstein, 1991; Sabol, 1991; Stobino et al., 1992). Health-related social problems are often exacerbated by other macro-level challenges associated with chronic poverty such as crime, neighborhood segregation, and social isolation (Anderson, 1999; Billingsley, 1992; Massey & Denton, 1993; Wilson, 1996).

Much of the research on this subject focuses on the implications of the lack of health insurance and general health care services for residents in poor urban areas; fewer studies empirically examine the relationship between place and specific health care experiences and decisions made by residents in poor urban areas when they become ill or injured. This research focuses on the relationship between accessibility and the number of days persons stayed home ill or were hospitalized in 1986 for 2490 African American, Mexican, Puerto Rican, and White residents in poor urban Chicago neighborhoods. I also explore their health profiles and health insurance options. I am particularly interested in *who* residents frequent for primary care, *where* they frequent, and *how* these factors influence staying home ill and hospitalization. The overall research goal is to examine ways in which macro-level system issues associated with limited health care options and poverty affect the individual decisions of urban residents (i.e. micro-level issues). This project adds to the literature by empirically examining whether such health care experiences are affected by neighborhood poverty or differ by race/ethnicity. In addition, findings can be used to inform health policy analysts of ways in which residents in poor urban areas negotiate medical choices given economic constraints. Results will also inform us about possible implications of welfare reform and the 1996 Personal Responsibility and Work Opportunity Reconciliation Act (PRWORA) on the health care experiences of persons in impoverished urban areas.

HEALTH CONDITIONS, HEALTH CARE, POVERTY, AND RACE/ETHNICITY

Macro-Level Issues and Individual Choices

Rather than performing a traditional theory test, this project is grounded in the body of literature that informs our understanding of the relationship between poverty, race/ethnicity, and health care issues. When considering these three broad areas of inquiry, it is important to examine where impoverished persons go for medical attention when they become sick, who they rely on, and how they pay for services. These three issues are also important because they inform the larger discourse on the relationship between structure and agency for residents in poor urban areas (Wilson, 1987, 1996). Studies show that, compared to their middle and upper class counterparts, the poor tend to: have higher rates of untreated illnesses, feel sicker, and become disabled more frequently and for longer periods of time (Billingsley, 1992; Erwin, 1996; Lykens & Jargowsky, 2002). In addition, a variety of health problems have been attributed to the nexus of place and poverty. Poor nutrition, neighborhood pollution, poor sanitation, inadequate housing and clothing, and stress have been associated with potentially devastating physical and socio-psychological consequences (Auerbach & Krimgold, 2001; Billingsley, 1992; Cockerham, 1995; Fox, 1989; Navarro, 2002; Wilson, 1987). Given these problems, it is not surprising that, among the poor, mortality rates are higher for almost every disease. Additionally, the ability to get quality, affordable health care is exacerbated by the effects of neighborhood concentrated poverty (Berk et al., 1991; Billingsley, 1992; Wilson, 1987, 1996).

Other findings show that patients who are considered less profitable are often directly or indirectly denied treatment. For example, Marmor (1994) and others contend that medical facilities can avoid the poor by simply establishing locations away from low-income neighborhoods, electing not to provide services frequently requested by the poor (i.e. drug counseling, AIDS services, certain types of emergency care) or refusing admission to persons who are unable to pay (Cockerham, 1995). Furthermore, doctors are often scarce in poor neighborhoods and many residents do not have transportation to visit physicians outside their immediate locale (Bullough, 1972; May, 1975; Weiss & Greenlick, 1970). Such conditions result in deleterious consequences for the poor who are ill or potentially ill. The poor are also more likely to delay medical treatment and be without a primary caregiver – which often results in costlier subsequent treatment if conditions become chronic (Billingsley, 1992).

When we consider how persons pay for health care, according to U.S. Census data, during the period 1999–2000, on average, 14.5% of all persons in the U.S. were without health insurance coverage for a given year. Figures by race/ethnicity for this period were; 13.3% for Whites, 18.5% for Asians, 19.2% for African Americans, and 33.0% for Hispanics (U.S. Bureau of Census, 2000, 2001, 2002). The number of uninsured had fallen in 1999 and 2000, but rose by approximately 1.4 million in 2001 (U.S. Bureau of Census, 2002). In 2001, figures were 14.6% for the entire U.S. population and 13.6, 18.2, 19.0, and 33.2% for Whites, Asians, African Americans, and Hispanics, respectively. These figures, attributed to increased unemployment, fewer employer-sponsored health care programs, and increased expenses for existing employer programs, would be higher save Medicaid and the State Children's Health Insurance Program (SCHIP) (Park et al., 2002; U.S. Bureau of Census, 2002). Research has also uncovered the rapidly increasing number of employed poor without health coverage. The "working poor" are often the most negatively affected because most do not qualify for Medicaid, many cannot afford employer-sponsored or subsidized health plans, and most cannot pay for their own coverage should they become under-employed or unemployed (Berk & Wilensky, 1987; Duncan et al., 1995; Seccombe, 1996; Smith, 1993). National data also show that about 84% of persons without insurance are employed or are the dependents of employed persons (House Energy and Commerce Subcommittee on Health and Environment, 1993).

Scholarship suggests that health care inequities exist based on race/ethnicity and persons who need health care service the most are often the least likely to receive them (Erwin, 1996; Lykens & Jargowsky, 2002). The poor, in general, and African Americans, in particular, are at greatest risk of receiving inadequate medical attention or emergency treatment. According to research on U.S. hospitals, less than 50% of African Americans and poor patients deemed very sick were admitted to intensive-care units, while about 70% of White and poor Medicare recipients were admitted. Similar patterns of inequitable medical care have also been observed in federal Veterans Administration hospitals (Blakeslee, 1994). Fewer studies examine these issues for poor Hispanics, but similar findings are emerging (Lykens & Jargowsky, 2002).

Like earlier studies, this project examines the affects of health care coverage on health decisions. Unlike other studies, I also consider the implications of the types of neighborhood health care facilities that are available, health care practitioners and locations that are frequented, neighborhood poverty, as well as race/ethnicity on the number of days respondents: (1) stay home when ill or injured; and are (2) hospitalized in a year. Thus this project reflects a test for possible macro-micro linkages by considering two individual-level outcome variables within the larger social context of impoverished urban neighborhoods. I hypothesize that both the number of days home and in the hospital will be: (1) undermined by neighborhood and household poverty; (2) less for non-Whites than for Whites; (3) directly related to access to no-cost/low cost health care; (4) inversely related to Medicaid receipt; (5) directly related to having a regular physician; and (6) inversely related to primary use of emergency room facilities (Lewin-Epstein, 1991; Lykens & Jargowsky, 2002; Wilson, 1996). The next section describes the sample, study variables, and methodology.

RESEARCH METHODS

Data

The 1986 Urban Poverty and Family Life Survey of Chicago (UPFLS) is an in-depth study of residents in poor urban neighborhoods that includes attitudinal and behavioral variables at the neighborhood and household level. The sample of 2490 respondents contains 364 non-Hispanic Whites, 1183 African Americans, 489 Mexicans, and 454 Puerto Ricans, aged 18–44 who, in 1986, lived in Chicago census tracts in which at least 20% of the residents were below the poverty line in 1980. The sample was selected in two phases. Initially, all poverty census tract blocks in Chicago were grouped based on the modal representation of the four racial/ethnic groups. After blocks were sorted based on ethnicity and tract, 100 blocks were randomly selected to coincide with the number of 1980 census households in each block. Block units with the most households had a greater probability of selection. Once the census tract blocks had been selected, every housing unit in each of the chosen blocks was identified and included in a list from which an equal probability sample of households was selected. While the first phase was based on a random sample of dwelling units, the second screening phase disproportionately selected from poverty tracts with high concentrations of non-Hispanic Whites, Mexicans, and Puerto Ricans. Given their lower relative representation in the population, all eligible non-Hispanic Whites were selected for final interview. Response rates ranged from 73.8% for non-Hispanic Whites to 82.5% for African American parents. Although these data are somewhat dated, findings will be important given my emphasis on factors such as place (example, types of facilities available, limited facilities) and race/ethnicity – two factors intricately tied to health care issues for urban residents. Although these data would be dated for a study on certain urban issues that have changed significantly since 1986 (i.e. certain effects of welfare usage given welfare reform), given my focus on somewhat more static factors such as place (i.e. types of available facilities, neighborhood poverty) and race/ethnicity that remain central to poor urban living, emergent findings will be germane to the continued discourse on health care issues for residents in poor urban locales.

Dependent Variables

Two continuous dependent variables examine respondents' health experiences based on the questions; "During the past 12 months about how many days did illness or injury keep you in bed more than half of the day?" and "In total, how many days were you in the hospital in the past 12 months?" Values range from 0 to 365 days. Mean values (standard deviations) for the two variables, *Stay Home Ill* and *Hospitalization*, are 6.18 (0.46) and 0.93 (0.15), respectively. The reader should note the strengths and limitations of using single-item questions. The former variable is broad in its reference to illness or injury. Due to the limitations of this secondary data source, I am unable to ascertain the specific health issues faced by the respondents (i.e. broken leg, flu). And although hospitalization is a more salient event, a one-year recall period for illness and injury resulting in days sick may be affected by recall bias for some persons. Thus it is important to consider the implications of recall on the *Stay Home Ill* variable. However, both variables are beneficial in their ability to specifically and directly identify illness and hospitalization experiences during a given period as reported by respondents.

Independent Variables

Control and Health-Related Variables

Four health-related variables are considered. A dummy variable identifies whether respondents have a regular physician. To test the possible effects of where respondents seek health care, I consider whether persons visit a private physician's office (reference variable), hospital, clinic, emergency room, or some other/no facility. [As examples of the difference between the aforementioned variables, a respondent may have a regular physician that she visits at the physician's office. A respondent might visit a doctor in a clinic rather than at a physician's office or a respondent may tend to frequent a local clinic, emergency room, or hospital for care. Other combinations are possible.] Dummy variables also assess whether residents have access to a no-cost/low-cost health care facility and whether they receive Medicaid or not (the reference category for the latter variable consists of persons with medical insurance and the uninsured). The reader should note that, in 1986, prior to welfare reform, Medicaid recipients included persons with disabilities as well as those in poverty. Lastly, respondent's self-described health

Table 1. Selected Study Variables and Health Profiles by Race/Ethnicity ($N = 2,490$).

Variables	Race/Ethnicity			
	Afr. Am.	White	Mexican	P. Rican
Demographics				
1. Percent female	57.7^P	65.5^M	53.2^{WP}	68.0^{AM}
2. Percent married	38.1^{WMP}	65.6^{AMP}	84.1P^{AW}	57.1^{MAW}
3. Number of children	2.1^{MP}	2.3^{MP}	3.1^{AWP}	2.7^{AWM}
4. Percent H. school grad.	57.1^{MP}	62.2^{MP}	17.0^{AWP}	30.9^{AWM}
5. Neighborhood poverty	35.8^{WMP}	27.7^{AP}	28.3^{AP}	31.1^{AWM}
6. Household income range	$10–15K^W	$15–20K^{AMP}	$10–15K^{WP}	$10–15K^{WM}
7. Average age	30.99 ^{WMP}	34.01^{AMP}	32.39^{AW}	32.35^{AW}
8. Percent employed	83.03^{WM}	94.20^{AMP}	90.42^{AWP}	78.70^{WM}
Health profile (in past 12 months)				
9. Self-assessed health status[*] (% excellent or good)	83.97	84.85	70.29	8.50
10. Mean days home ill	7.96 (46.67)	12.76 (62.21)	2.57 (10.02)	8.93 (51.50)
11. Means days in hospital	0.89 (6.78)	1.83 (12.43)	0.11 (3.66)	1.20 (7.33)
12. Mean visits to doctor	5.54 (11.62)	7.10 (14.36)	3.38 (7.67)	7.10 (13.92)
13. Regular doctor[*] (% "Yes")	74.02	75.97	71.05	75.55
Health insurance				
14. % Medicaid[*]	41.21	20.17	6.17	34.73
15. % W/O health insurance[*]	54.80	67.87	47.94	52.76
16. % Employed adults w/o health insurance	29.06	15.00	39.19	18.75
Health care providers				
17. % No-cost/low-cost in area	45.50	20.05	18.42	16.02
18. Type of Providers[*]				
% Private doctor	28.45	55.96	56.76	63.00
% Hospital	33.99	16.34	16.19	15.42
% Neighborhood/govt. clinic	18.40	8.03	13.32	8.81
% Emergency room	13.29	5.54	2.05	2.20
% Other/no regular care	5.88	14.13	10.45	10.36

Note: Standard deviations provided in parentheses. A = Mean or percentage is significantly different from that of African Americans: $p < 0.05$; W = Mean or percentage is significantly different from that of Whites: $p < 0.05$; M = Mean or percentage is significantly different from that of Mexicans: $p < 0.05$; P = Mean or percentage is significantly different from that of Puerto-Ricans: $p < 0.05$.

[*]χ^2 differences by race/ethnicity at $p < = 0.05$.

status is examined based on the categories: (1) poor; (2) fair; (3) good; (4) very good; or (5) excellent.

To study possible effects of neighborhood poverty on days ill or hospitalized, I incorporate a continuous poverty indicator based on the official "poverty line" used by the U.S. Census. This measure is considered due to its wide use and appeal as a

Table 2. Linear Regression Coefficients for Days Stayed Home Ill and Days Hospitalized.

	Days Home Ill	Days Hospitalized	
	Model 1	Model 2	Model 3
Race/Ethnicity			
African American	−3.80 (2.17)	−1.14 (0.78)	−0.67 (0.73)
Mexican	−8.11 (2.13)***	−2.30 (0.81)**	−1.29 (0.74)
Puerto rican	−5.60 (2.32)*	−1.75 (0.84)*	−1.02 (0.76)
Other controls			
Neighborhood poverty	−0.14 (0.04)***	−0.02 (0.01)	−0.00 (0.01)
Household income	0.09 (0.15)	−0.04 (0.06)	−0.06 (0.05)
Sex (1 = Female)	0.94 (0.86)	0.03 (0.36)	−0.13 (0.35)
HS graduate (1 = Yes)	0.36 (1.22)	−0.27 (0.35)	−0.26 (0.31)
Married (1 = Yes)	−1.99 (1.10)	0.03 (0.35)	0.33 (0.31)
# Kids in HH	1.14 (0.79)	0.11 (0.23)	−0.07 (0.22)
HH Total	−0.53 (0.26)*	−0.02 (0.10)	0.05 (0.09)
Age	0.10 (0.08)	0.00 (0.03)	−0.01 (0.02)
Employed (1 = Yes)	1.01 (1.22)	0.46 (0.50)	0.25 (0.46)
Health controls			
Health (5 = excellent)	−5.04 (0.81)***	−1.21 (0.23)***	−0.54 (0.15)***
Regular doctor (1 = Yes)	2.81 (1.02)**	1.05 (0.35)**	0.67 (0.30)*
No-cost/low-cost provider in area (1 = Yes)	1.17 (1.00)	0.39 (0.31)	0.29 (0.30)
Medicaid (1 = Yes)	3.09 (1.31)*	1.23 (0.41)**	0.80 (0.35)*
Health care providers			
Hospital (1 = Yes)	−0.00 (1.29)	−0.43 (0.38)	−0.50 (0.37)
Neighborhood clinic (1 = Yes)	−5.28 (1.25)***	−1.87 (0.36)***	−1.18 (0.32)***
Emergency room (1 = Yes)	1.72 (2.29)	0.59 (0.71)	0.36 (0.63)
Other/no regular care (1 = Yes)	−2.52 (1.02)*	−0.51 (0.50)	−0.22 (0.44)
Days home Ill			0.13 (0.03)***
R^2	0.10	0.07	0.21
N	2,268	2,273	2,261

*$p < 0.05$.
**$p < 0.01$.
***$p < 0.001$.

statistical baseline estimate (Wilson, 1987, 1996). Based on sociological literature on the urban experience and bivariate correlations, demographic control variables include: four race/ethnicity dummy variables (African American, White, Mexican, and Puerto Rican, where White is the reference category); dummy variables to identify high school graduates, sex, age, whether respondents are employed at least 30 hours weekly, and married persons; a continuous household income variable ranging from $0 to $45,000; and, continuous variables to determine number of children and total persons in the household. It should be noted that controlling for age (life course issues), sex (child-bearing for females), and employment status (such persons are somewhat more likely to have health insurance) enable me to indirectly adjust for important factors that have been shown to affect health care decisions (Auerbach & Krimgold, 2001; Navarro, 2002; Sawhill et al., 2002). A total of twenty independent variables are examined. Minimal multicollinearity is evident among the independent variables (survey questions and bivariate correlations provided upon request).

Table 3. Summary of Model Results for Days Home Ill and Days Hospitalized by Place, Race, and Cost Variables.

	Days Home Ill	Days Hospitalized	Days Hospitalized
Place			
Consistent doctor	Significant (+)	Significant (+)	Significant (+)
Low-cost provider			
Hospital			
Clinic ER	Significant (−)	Significant (−)	Significant (−)
Other/None	Significant (−)		
Neigh. Poverty	Significant (−)		
Race			
African American			
Mexican	Significant (−)	Significant (−)	
Puerto Rican	Significant (−)	Significant (−)	
Cost			
Medicaid	Significant (+)	Significant (+)	Significant (+)
Other health controls			
Health status	Significant (−)	Significant (−)	Significant (−)
Days home Ill	−	−	Significant (+)

Note: Each column is a model summary. "−" means variable is not used in the model; "+" = increases and "−" = decreases days home ill or days hospitalized for significant variables, other variables are insignificant.

Methodology

Sample means and proportions and *t*- and χ^2-tests are presented to determine whether health profiles vary by race/ethnicity (Table 1). During the modeling phase, I regress the two dependent variables on the twenty control and health-related variables. I use multiple linear regression analysis because the two dependent variables, number of days home ill and hospitalized, are continuous (Table 2, Models 1 and 2). In the final model, I include the dependent variable that identifies the number of days respondents spent home ill to determine whether it helps to explain days hospitalized (Model 3). Overall findings are summarized in Table 3. After an overview of the sample demographics and health profiles, regression findings, conclusions, and policy implications are provided.

FINDINGS

Demographics and Health Care Profiles

Because research suggests residents in urban areas may respond differently to exposure to poverty (Billingsley, 1992; Wilson, 1987, 1996), it is important to consider whether varied health profiles emerge as well. The demographic profiles presented in Table 1 show that, regardless of race/ethnicity, over 50% of respondents are female. In addition, a greater percentage of African Americans are unmarried as compared to their counterparts. Relative to the other groups, the number of children for Hispanics is slightly greater although most respondents are of similar ages (30–34 years old). A disproportionately lower percentage of Mexicans and Puerto Ricans have high school diplomas as compared to the other two groups. Review of neighborhood and household economic indicators show that most respondents live in moderately poor neighborhoods (20–39.99%), have average annual household incomes of less than $15,000, and over three-fourths of respondents are employed.

Variables 9–13 summarize health profiles. The vast majority of persons consider themselves to be in excellent or good health. However, health status does not coincide with the number of days ill. Although a greater percentage of people from minority groups have fair or poor health, a greater percentage of Whites, followed by Puerto Ricans were bedridden in the 12 months prior to the interview (12.76 and 8.93 days, respectively). Mexicans, followed by African Americans are the least likely to remain home in bed or to spend time in the hospital due to illness. Mexicans and African Americans are least likely to visit a doctor or medical personnel and over one-fourth of respondents do not have a regular physician. Next, Variables 14–16 show whether health coverage varies by race/ethnicity.

African Americans are more likely to receive Medicaid (41.21%). Results show that a greater percentage of employed African Americans (29.06%) and Mexicans (39.19%) are without coverage. Furthermore, Variable 17 illustrates that over 45% of African Americans and a substantially lower percentage of non-African Americans have access to no-cost/low-cost health care providers. Lastly, Variable 18 presents the most common places respondents visit to get regular health care. The majority of Puerto Ricans, Whites and Mexicans visit a private doctor for treatment, while less than one-third of African Americans do. In contrast, African Americans rely on hospital outpatient care at twice the rate of the three other groups. In addition, almost 20% of African Americans use neighborhood clinics and 13% of Mexicans do so. A significantly higher percentage of African Americans also frequent hospital emergency rooms. Based on these profiles, there is need to consider the specific number of days respondents are home ill or hospitalized and whether they differ when characteristics such as race/ethnicity, poverty, Medicaid, and health care locations are considered together.

Regression Model Results for Health Care Experiences

Days Stay Home Ill

The modeling objective is to determine those variables that explain the number of days at home due to illness or injury and days hospitalized. Information on this subject will help to better understand some of the macro-level factors that influence the behavior of residents in poor urban neighborhoods when they actually become ill. According to results presented in Table 2 (Model 1), differences exist in the number of days respondents stay home due to illness or injury based on race/ethnicity. Although Puerto Ricans ($b = -5.33$, $p = 0.05$) and Mexicans ($b = -8.14$, $p = 0.001$) spend fewer days home ill than Whites, there is no significant difference between outcomes for Whites and African Americans, even after considering other controls. When I consider neighborhood and household economic indicators, neighborhood poverty, rather than household economics, significantly influences the number of days one is home ill and suggests that, regardless of household economic status, respondents from more impoverished neighborhoods stay home ill *fewer days* than their counterparts in less impoverished areas. Similarly, persons from larger households tend to spend fewer days home ill.

When I consider the influence of health-related indicators, as expected, healthier respondents spend fewer days home ill. However, persons who frequent the same physician tend to spend more days home ill than those without a regular physician suggesting the influence of having a regular physician on both health maintenance and preventive care. The relationship between subsidized health care and how persons respond to illness or injury is supported here because the number of days home ill is directly related to whether respondents receive Medicaid. Next, the number of days home ill is significantly influenced by *where* persons seek medical care. Respondents who primarily frequent a neighborhood clinic, other care facility, or who don't seek care regularly stay home ill *fewer* days than persons who frequent a personal doctor. This result points to both the possible effects of the quality of health care locations at the disposal of residents and the choices some persons make to ignore their health needs (Billingsley, 1992; Wilson, 1996). The significant variables account for 10% of the linear variability in the dependent variable ($R^2 = 0.10$). Given that days home ill could reflect a variety of illnesses, it is also important to consider situations that warrant hospitalization.

Hospitalization
Several similar patterns are evident when I consider number of days hospitalized (Table 2, Model 2, $R^2 = 0.07$). Mexicans and Puerto Ricans spend fewer days in the hospital than Whites; so do healthier respondents. Similar to the results from Model 1, a significant difference is not apparent between hospitalization experiences for Whites and African Americans. However, unlike the model the focuses on days home ill, the type of neighborhood in which one resides does not affect hospitalization. Furthermore, household economic status remains insignificant, and unlike the first model, household size is no longer an important predictor.

A review of the health-related indicators show that, similar to the first model, having a regular physician is directly related to the number of days hospitalized; respondents who go to a private doctor for medical care tend to spend *more* days in the hospital than persons without such a primary caregiver. Because lengthier hospital stays are generally correlated with greater chances of recuperation and wellness, this result illustrates the important benefits of having a regular physician to monitor the caregiving process. Type of health care coverage continues to be important. Medicaid receipt is directly related to number of days hospitalized such that respondents who receive Medicaid ($b = 1.23$, $p = 0.01$) tend to spend more days in the hospital than non-Medicaid recipients – suggesting the importance of subsidized health care for some residents in poor urban areas as a means to help make medical attention possible. Lastly, the type of facility frequented is important and the data show that persons who seek medical attention primarily at a clinic tend to spend fewer days in the hospital as compared to their counterparts who tended to frequent a private doctor ($b = -1.87$, $p = 0.001$). Although this result is not an indictment of urban clinics in general, it does suggest differences in hospitalization outcomes based on where residents frequent for their health care needs.

In Model 3, I include the dependent variable, *Stay Home Ill*, as a control to examine its influence on days hospitalized. As expected, its inclusion improves the model's explanatory ability three-fold ($R^2 = 0.21$) and shows that, regardless of race/ethnicity, neighborhood poverty, and household economics, the number of days respondents are home due to illness or injury directly influences the number of days hospitalized. This finding suggests the "leveling effects" of illness as well as the possible implications of unattended health issues because, increased illness at home increases the tendency for hospitalization and overshadows other important demographic (i.e. race/ethnicity), household (i.e. income), and neighborhood (i.e. area poverty) conditions. However, place remains important and clinic use continues to decrease days hospitalized. In addition, having a regular physician and receiving Medicaid continue to be associated with more days hospitalized.

DISCUSSION

These findings inform the literature regarding linkages between systemic health care issues and choices made by residents in poor urban areas in Chicago. When health profiles are considered broadly, these findings show that White residents in poor urban areas tend to take more days off due to illness, have slightly longer hospital stays, and seek medical consultation more than non-Whites. Given that a greater percentage of minorities, particularly Mexicans and Puerto Ricans, consider themselves to be in only "fair" or "poor" health, this suggests that, even in poor neighborhoods among the poor and near poor, health status and health concerns tend to be addressed more readily by Whites. Race/ethnicity is also related to the type of medical care selected. African Americans tend to use health care options often considered less comprehensive such as outpatient hospitals and clinics and emergency rooms more frequently than their counterparts. Studies suggest that these options are often the most expensive service providers and also offer limited or little "hospitable" amenities due to their often crowded, noisy, chaotic environments. If the quality of services tends to be better at private facilities, then Whites and other non-African Americans in the sample are at an advantage because the majority of these groups receive treatment at a private physician's office (National Center for Health Statistics, 1992).

When I consider the specific hypotheses based on multivariate tests, results show that the number of days home ill is inversely related to neighborhood poverty, but neither dependent variable is directly influenced by household economics as studied here (but the reader should note the relationship between the two variables in that as the percentage of poor households increases in a neighborhood, so does neighborhood poverty). This result illustrates the possible effects of neighborhood concentrated poverty that can overshadow household finances (Wilson, 1987, 1996) and that factors other than personal finances influence health decisions and alternatives (Marmor, 1994).

Model results also show that the number of days home ill and days hospitalized vary by race/ethnicity. Although Mexicans and Puerto Ricans consistently spend fewer days home ill or hospitalized than Whites, no significant difference is apparent between the experiences of Whites and African Americans. These findings about race/ethnicity are important in light of the fact that most of the other demographic variables (i.e. sex, marital status, age, household size) are not predictive. However, readers should recognize the relationship between certain demographic variables and race/ethnicity. As one example, although sex is not predictive here, a disproportionate percentage of African Americans in poor urban neighborhood are female. And although the variable that identifies access to no-cost/low-cost care does not appear important here, it is clear that the type of medical personnel respondents regularly visit and location are predictive. Persons who frequent a private doctor have more days home ill or hospitalized (regardless of the doctor's locale). This result illustrates the importance of personalized care that is often more consistent via a private physician rather than at other sites. However, where residents frequent such a caregiver, specifically in a clinic, appears to consistently undermine the health experiences studied here. Lastly, contrary to the hypothesis, Medicaid recipients actually spend more days home ill or hospitalized than their counterparts suggesting that government-subsidized health care assistance for the poor and disabled indirectly serves to free up resources to address personal illnesses and seek medical attention.

One additional modeling observation should be noted. Regardless of the demographic, economic, and health-related controls, the variable that identifies whether persons are generally in good/excellent health is consistently important here and reduces number of days ill or hospitalized. This result illustrates the importance of preventive care to minimize potential health challenges and possible undue economic hardship should poor urban residents become ill (Auerbach & Krimgold, 2001; Karger et al., 2003; Lykens & Jargowsky, 2002; Schram et al., 2003). And just as preventive care is influenced by proactive decisions made by urban residents at the micro-level, my findings show the necessity to candidly consider structural constraints beyond the control of persons that also undermine preventive care and foster the types of chronic health conditions that may further economically entrench the poor (Billingsley, 1992). Model findings also suggest the importance of considering other variables that influence health care decisions of residents in impoverished areas (as indicated by the R^2 values) in addition to those examined here. Table 3 visually summarizes the modeling results in light of my focus on place, race, and costs.[1]

CONCLUSION

Given the varied problems faced by many residents in poor urban neighborhoods, what factors influence their health experiences and choices? Are problems related to macro-level system issues such as health care locations, access to low-cost care, or neighborhood poverty? These are the research issues studied here. First, these findings illumine important issues regarding ways to address chronic health problems among residents in poor urban spaces, how these problems are linked to systemic issues such as poverty and limited health care options, and some of the implications for residents' daily lives. These findings also support the importance of preventive care, even in impoverished neighborhoods. Because the number of days home ill improves the ability to explain days hospitalized, it appears that chronic illness (implied here by increased days home ill) serves as an "equalizer" across broad demographic differences (i.e. regardless of race/ethnicity or household or neighborhood economic context) and increases the likelihood of hospitalization. However, preventive care involves both residents being proactive relative to their health as well as addressing structural forces that undermine adequate, affordable, accessible health care options. Another important finding here are the implications of having a regular doctor and Medicaid receipt (Bradsher, 1995; Lykens & Jargowsky, 2002). This suggests that even among the impoverished and regardless of race/ethnicity and neighborhood poverty level, more consistent monitoring by a healthcare provider and the financial resources to get treatment (for one's self or children) may reduce delays in addressing health issues (Wilson, 1996). Furthermore, the negative relationship between frequenting clinics supports the need for additional and/or improved health care facilities in impoverished areas (Billingsley, 1992; Stobino et al., 1992).

These findings illustrate the importance of considering, not only "who pays" for the health care of the poor, but also who residents frequent and where they seek treatment. Much of the discourse on this subject has focused on the former question; additional studies are needed of the two latter ones. For example, despite the eighteen states that are planning or have already adopted plans for Medicaid cut-backs, it has been suggested that Congress should fortify existing Medicaid and SCHIP programs and funnel unused SCHIP funds back into the program (Park et al., 2002). Some suggest increased usage of HMO models (although HMOs do not address the health care needs of millions of underemployed) (Nowacheck et al., 1994; Pear, 1995). And still others suggest new managed-care models and non-traditional alliances between the public and private sectors and urbanites based on existing community assets (Cebrun, 1997; Grogan & Proscio, 2000; Kretzmann & McKnight, 1993). Varied solutions are needed. In some instances, the most pressing challenge appears to be how to move beyond the discourse and empirical evidence that often conceals the everyday costs and quality of life problems associated with illness, delayed treatment, and available quality medical care. Welfare reform initiatives and innovations in child support enforcement such as the 1996 PRWORA tends to focus on the "who pays" issue. However, my findings suggest that, such changes should also be informed by social policy to address macro-level health disparities and ultimately establish more health care facilities in impoverished areas, improve existing ones, and provide incentives for physicians to establish practices in such locales.

NOTE

1. In models not provided here (upon request), I also consider how various interaction variables might help explain the number of days home ill and days hospitalized. First, I consider possible interaction effects to explain the number of days home ill based on the following: (1) sex X race/ethnicity to examine, for example, whether the number of days home ill differs for African American females as compared to White males; (2) race/ethnicity X health care location to consider whether, for example, whether African Americans who frequent a doctor at a private office are more likely to stay home ill than Whites who frequent clinics; and (3) sex X health care location to consider, for example, whether females who frequent a doctor at a private office are more likely to stay home ill than males who frequent emergency rooms. However, due largely to multicollinearity, the predictive power for each of the models does not improve and none of the interaction terms are significant. Next, because the number of days home ill increased the number of days hospitalized, I am interested in whether the number of days hospitalized would be affected by interactions for the following: (1) days home ill for females as compared to males to assess whether sick females are more or less likely to be hospitalized than sick males; (2) days home ill by race/ethnicity to assess, say, whether sick African Americans are more or less likely to hospitalized that sick Whites; and (3) days home ill by health care location to consider whether sick respondents who frequent a doctor at a private office are more likely to be hospitalized than sick persons who frequent clinics or emergency rooms. In each of the interaction models, although the overall model's predictive power improves [R^2 (home ill X sex) = 0.23, R^2 (home ill X race/ethnicity, for the four groups) = 0.21, and R^2 (home ill X health location, for the five locations) = 0.25], none of the interaction terms are significant. It should be noted that, despite of the inherent multicollinearity issues associated with considering interaction terms, the variable that identified number of days home due to illness remains significant and positively influences days hospitalized in each model. The continued salience of days home ill as a precursor to hospitalization, even after considering interaction controls, further supports the implications of unchecked health problems and the importance of preventive care.

ACKNOWLEDGMENTS

This study was based on data from the University of Chicago's Urban Poverty and Family Life Survey of Chicago, William Julius Wilson, principal investigator, conducted by the national Opinion Research Center and supported by grants from the Carnegie Foundation, the Ford Foundation, the Rockefeller Foundation, the William T. Grant Foundation, the U.S. Department of Health and Human Services, the Chicago Community Trust, the Lloyd A. Fry Foundation, the Joyce Foundation, the MacArthur Foundation, the Spencer Foundation, and Woods Charitable Trust. My use of these data was an independent secondary analysis.

REFERENCES

Anderson, E. (1999). *Code of the street: Decency, violence, and the moral life of the inner city.* New York: W. W. Norton.

Auerbach, J., & Krimgold, B. (Eds) (2001). *Income, socioeconomic status, and health: Exploring the relationships.* Washington, DC. National Policy Association: Academy for Health Services Research and Health Policy.

Berk, M., Cunningham, P., & Beauregard, K. (1991). The health care of poor persons living in wealthy areas. *Social Science & Medicine, 32*(10), 1097–1103.

Berk, M., & Wilensky, G. (1987). Health insurance coverage of the working poor. *Social Science and Medicine, 25,* 1183–1187.

Billingsley, A. (1992). *Climbing Jacob's ladder: THE enduring legacy of African-American families.* New York: A Touchstone Book.

Blakeslee, S. (1994). Poor and black patients slighted, study says. *New York Times,* April 20, p. B9.

Bradsher, K. (1995). Rise in uninsured becomes an issue in Medicaid fight. *New York Times,* August 27, pp. A1, A20.

Bullough, B. (1972). Poverty, ethnic identity and preventive health care. *Journal of Health and Social Behavior, 13,* 347–359.

Cockerham, W. C. (1995). *Medical sociology* (6th ed.). Upper Saddle River, NJ: Prentice-Hall.

Cebrun, A. (1997). The role of managed care: The national and Tennessee experiences. *Journal of Health Care for the Poor & Underserved, 8*(3), 384–387.

Duncan, P., Seccombe, K., & Amey, C. (1995). Changes in health insurance coverage within rural and urban environments – 1977 to 1987. *Journal of Rural Health, 11*(3), 169–176.

Erwin, P. (1996). Health planning and health care for the poor: The internal ethic of public health. *Journal of Health & Social Policy, 7*(3), 47–63.

Fox, R. (1989). *The sociology of medicine.* Englewood Cliffs, NJ: Prentice-Hall.

Grogan, P., & Proscio, T. (2000). *Comeback cities: A blueprint for urban neighborhood revival.* Boulder, CO: Westview Press.

Hersch, J., & White-Means, S. (1993). Employer-sponsored health and pension benefits and the gender/race wage gap. *Social Science Quarterly, 74*(4), 850–866.

House Energy and Commerce Subcommittee on Health and Environment (1993). *Medicaid sourcebook: Background data and analysis.* Washington, DC: U.S. Government Printing Office.

Karger, H. J., Midgley, J., & Brown, C. (Eds) (2003). *Controversial issues in social policy.* Boston: Allyn and Bacon.

Kretzmann, J. P., & McKnight, J. L. (1993). *Building communities from the inside out: A path toward finding and mobilizing a community's assets.* Chicago: ACTA Publications.

Lewin-Epstein, N. (1991). Determinants of regular source of health care in Black, Mexican, Puerto Rican, and Nonhispanic White populations. American Sociological Association conference paper.

Lykens, K., & Jargowsky, P. (2002). Medicaid matters: Children's health and medicaid eligibility expansions. *Journal of Policy Analysis and Management, 21*(2), 219–238.

Marmor, T. R. (1994). *Understanding health care reform.* New Haven, CT: Yale University Press.

Massey, D. S., & Denton, N. A. (1993). *American apartheid: Segregation and the making of the underclass.* Massachusetts: Harvard University Press.

May, J. J. (1975). Utilization of health services and the availability of resources. In: P. Anderson, J. Kravits & O. W. Andersen (Eds), *Equity in Health Services* (pp. 131–149). Cambridge: Ballinger.

National Center for Health Statistics, U.S. Department of Health, Education, and Welfare (1992).

Navarro, V. (Ed.) (2002). *The political economy of social inequalities: Consequences for health and quality of life.* Amityville, NY: Baywood Publishing.

Nowacheck, P. W., Hughes, D. C., Stoddard, J. J., & Halfon, N. (1994). Children with chronic illness and Medicaid managed care. *Pediatrics, 93*, 497–500.

Park, E., Ku, L., & Broaddus, M. (2002). Children losing health coverage. *Families USA*, Sept. 19.

Pear, R. (1995). H. M. O.'s refusing emergency claims, hospitals assert. *New York Times*, July 9 (pp. 1–22).

Sabol, B. (1991). The urban child. *Journal of Health Care for the Poor & Underserved, 2*(1), 59–73.

Sawhill, I., Weaver, K., & Kane, A. (Eds) (2002). *Welfare reform and beyond: The future of the safety net.* Washington, DC: Brookings Institution.

Schram, S., Soss, J., & Fording, R. (Eds) (2003). *Race and the politics of welfare reform.* Ann Arbor: University of Michigan Press.

Seccombe, K. (1996). Health insurance coverage among the working poor: Changes from 1977 to 1987. *Research in the Sociology of Health Care, 13*, 199–227.

Seccombe, K., Clarke, L., & Coward, R. (1994). Discrepancies in employer-sponsored health insurance coverage among Hispanics, Blacks, and Whites: The effects of sociodemographic and employment factors. *Inquiry, 31*, 221–229.

Smith, R. B. (1993). Health care reform now. *Society, 30*(3), 56–65.

Stobino, D., Wulff, L., & Cornely, D. (1992). Follow-up of the use of local health department clinics for preventive care among young children. *American Journal of Preventive Medicine, 8*(3), 178–181.

U.S. Bureau of Census. Current Population Survey (2000, 2001, 2002). *Annual Demographic Supplement.* Washington, DC: U.S. Government Printing Office.

U.S. Bureau of Census. Current Population Survey (2002, Sept. 30). Health Insurance in America: Number of Americans with and without health insurance rise (press release).

U.S. Bureau of Census. Statistical Abstract of the United States (2000). Washington, DC: U.S. Government Printing Office.

Weiss, J. E., & Greenlick, M. (1970). Determinants of medical care utilization: The effect of social class and distance on contacts with the medical care system. *Medical Care, 8*, 456–462.

Wilson, W. J. (1987). *The truly disadvantaged: The inner city, the underclass, and public policy.* Chicago: University of Chicago Press.

Wilson, W. J. (1996). *When work disappears: The world of the new urban poor.* New York: Alfred A. Knopf.

CHANGING HEALTH CARE EXPERIENCES AND PERSPECTIVES OF OLDER ADULTS: COMPARISON OF HMO AND FEE-FOR-SERVICE ENROLLEES

Eva Kahana, Amy Dan, Boaz Kahana, Kyle Kercher, Gul Seçkin and Kurt Stange

ABSTRACT

This paper examines the health care experiences of older adults over a · five-year period, including continuity in care, changes in health insurance coverage, and satisfaction with care.

Face-to-face interviews were conducted annually with 415 older adults (mean age = 84, range = 72–105), 100 of whom were originally health maintenance organization (HMO) subscribers and 315 of whom were receiving fee-for-service care. Several predictors of health care experiences were examined, including personal characteristics, health status and health care variables. Coverage type (HMO or fee-for-service) was the most consistent predictor. HMO subscribers were more likely than fee-for-service recipients to experience changes in insurance (both negative and positive changes) and discontinuity in physician care, although satisfaction with care did not vary among HMO and non-HMO members. Two-thirds of HMO subscribers and

Chronic Care, Health Care Systems and Services Integration
Research in the Sociology of Health Care, Volume 22, 65–80
© 2004 Published by Elsevier Ltd.
ISSN: 0275-4959/doi:10.1016/S0275-4959(04)22004-X

nearly one-third of fee-for-service recipients reported changes in insurance coverage over the five-year study period. In terms of perspectives on HMO care, the most frequently mentioned advantage of HMO care among those in HMOs was diminished costs, while fee-for-service subscribers did not believe there were any advantages to being in an HMO. Those not in HMOs viewed loss of physician choice and poor quality care as major disadvantages of HMOs. Results of this study demonstrate that older adults commonly experience changes in their health care coverage and physician care. They adapt to these changes through positive appraisals of the type of case they receive.

INTRODUCTION

This paper reports on the experiences of community dwelling older adults (ages 72+) in obtaining health care. The perspectives of 100 elderly health maintenance organization (HMO) subscribers are compared to those of 315 older adults receiving fee-for-service care. We are particularly interested in how receiving care from different types of health care organizations (HMOs and traditional fee-for-service care) shapes health care experiences and perceptions of health care delivery. The impact of discontinuity in care and changes in health insurance coverage on satisfaction with care is also considered. It is particularly important to understand the health care experiences and perspectives of older adults in and out of managed care because this age group uses a disproportionate amount of health care services (Lee & Kasper, 1998). In addition, access to care, continuity of care, and quality of care are critical to older adults, many of whom are managing multiple chronic illnesses and are facing life-threatening and disabling conditions. Our study takes advantage of longitudinal data over a five-year period to consider changes in insurance coverage and in organization type from which health care is obtained.

BACKGROUND

Major changes in the U.S. health care system, reflected in the advent of managed care in the past twenty years, represent one of the major forms of social change in recent years (Wilkerson et al., 1997). Managed care was seen as a potential solution to the health care system's problem of escalating costs because it aims to reduce expenses by controlling costs and efficiently providing only necessary services (Callahan, 1998). A Health Maintenance Organization (HMO) is a prevalent type of managed care plan that provides health services to enrollees for a set fee (Pickard, 1997). Health care professionals, researchers, and the public have expressed concern, however, that managed care may compromise health care quality in order to cut costs (Miller & Luft, 1994), by reducing patient choices, continuity of care, access to specialists, and the amount of time patients can spend with physicians (Mechanic, 1998; Reschovsky & Kemper, 1999/2000; Tudor et al., 1998). Evidence, to date, comparing quality of fee-for-service and HMO care is inconsistent (see Miller & Luft, 1994, 1997 for reviews of this literature). HMOs have been found to use costly tests and procedures less frequently (Miller & Luft, 1997) and to reduce access to specialists by having primary care physicians serve as gatekeepers (Lin et al., 2000; Waitzkin & Cook, 2000). On the other hand, there is some evidence that HMO enrollees are more satisfied with financial aspects of care than fee-for-service recipients (Kasper & Riley, 1992; Miller & Luft, 1997). Since Medicare introduced managed care as an option in the early 1980s, over five million older adults have enrolled in managed care programs (Encinosa & Sappington, 1999). This equates to about 13% of Medicare recipients' ages 75–84 and 10% of those 85 and older (Centers for Medicare and Medicaid, 1997).

Many studies have found that older adults are generally satisfied with their medical care (Adler, 1995; Freeman et al., 1987; Meng et al., 1997; Tudor et al., 1998), and that they report higher levels of satisfaction compared to other age groups (Blendon et al., 1998; Owens & Bachelor, 1996). While largely satisfied with their care, Medicare recipients in HMOs are more likely than fee-for-service subscribers to report access problems (Meng et al., 1997; Nelson et al., 1997). Obtaining more extensive information about health care experiences of elders who utilized different types of health care services is thus critical to understanding the influence of organizational context on care delivery (Owens & Bachelor, 1996). To accomplish this aim, we examined data obtained from both close-ended and open-ended questions.

Continuity of physician care is also an important determinant of quality of care and satisfaction with care, especially when patients are managing multiple illnesses. A patient who does not have a regular primary care physician or is shuffled from one physician to another is less likely to receive high quality of care compared to patients who have a long-term relationship with their physician. A longer patient-physician relationship can foster better interpersonal relationships (Love et al., 2000) and increase the knowledge patients and physicians have of one another, which in turn can result in better quality of care and patient quality of life outcomes (Hanninen et al., 2001). Our own past research also pointed to difficulties experienced by patients who were forced to change physicians, based on changing insurance coverage (Kahana et al., 1997). The predictors and health care outcomes of continuity are examined in this study.

Specifically, we focus on older adults' perspectives on their health care experiences in the context of the type of health care coverage they receive (HMO or fee-for-service). Our research questions explore the ways in which older adults in HMOs and older adults in fee-for-service care view managed care, what they see as advantages and disadvantages of belonging to HMOs. We also consider changes experienced by respondents in health care delivery over a five-year period, and their satisfaction with the health care they have received.

SAMPLE

Data from 415 older adults were obtained as part of an ongoing longitudinal study of late life adaptation to frailty and aging. Study participants were originally randomly selected from three retirement communities in Clearwater, Florida (see Borawski et al., 1996; Kahana et al., 2002 for a more detailed description of sample selection procedures). To be eligible for participation in the study, respondents had to be at least 72 years old and had to be able to complete a 90-minute interview. We have conducted face-to-face interviews with respondents annually since 1989. For this paper, data collected from 1997 to 2001 are analyzed. During this five-year period, more extensive information about health care experiences was ascertained than in prior years.

Two-thirds of the sample is female ($N = 278$), and the vast majority are white, reflecting the composition of the retirement communities. The mean education level of respondents is 13.7 years (standard deviation = 2.6; range = 6–23), and the mean age of respondents at time 1 is 84 years (S.D. = 4.5), with an age range of 72–105. Forty-four percent of the sample is married, one half is widowed, 3% has never been married, and 1% is divorced. At time 1, 66% reported being in good or excellent health, and only 8% said they were in poor to very poor health. The remaining 26% reported being in fair health. Respondents averaged 3.9 health conditions in the initial wave of data collection (S.D. = 2.0; range = 0–11). The vast majority of respondents were not seriously impaired instrumental activities of daily living [IADLs] (as measured by the OARS scale).

DATA COLLECTION AND DATA ANALYTIC STRATEGY

Face-to-face interviews were conducted annually in respondents' homes. A series of questions about medical care experiences in the prior year were asked in each interview over the five-year period examined. All respondents were queried about changes in their primary care physician, changes in their health care coverage during the prior year, and satisfaction with aspects of physician care. In 1997, older adults were also asked to describe their understanding of managed care and to evaluate HMO care compared to fee-for-service health care.

Data from both close-ended and open-ended questions were used in this paper to obtain maximum information on older adults' perceptions and experiences with the health care system. The open-ended data were analyzed by identifying common themes. These themes were then coded, with multiple themes per respondent permitted for each of the questions to analyze closed-ended survey data. We conducted a series of multivariate regression analyses to examine predictors of various health care experience outcomes. In each regression, we included personal characteristics of age, marital status (married or unmarried), education level and gender as control variables. Health status was another predictor variable. Health status was measured as the total number of health conditions (e.g. diabetes, heart disease) based on the Older Americans Resource Study (OARS) Illness Index and IADL functional limitations (George & Fillenbaum, 1985). The IADL functional limitations were measured on a 1–4 scale (1 = "no difficulty" to 4 = "great difficulty"). Items included difficulty getting from room to room, going out of doors, walking up and down stairs, doing own housework, preparing meals, and shopping for groceries.[1] The third set of predictors were various indicators of health care (e.g. number of primary care physician visits, satisfaction with physician care, and HMO/fee-for-service enrollment). Ordinary least squares (OLS) regression was used for continuous outcomes, and logistic regression was used for dichotomous outcomes. To understand patterns of movement between different types of health care organizations, we created a three-category outcome (i.e. in HMO care for all five years, fee-for-service for all five years, and change between HMO and fee-for-service care over the five years) consequently multinomial logistic regression was used.

RESULTS

Health Care Organization Membership

Seventy-six percent of respondents ($N = 315$) received fee-for-service care at time 1. The remaining 24% ($N = 100$) received care from an HMO. All respondents were eligible for Medicare. In a multivariate analysis in which the predictors of age, gender, marital status (married versus unmarried), education level, and health status were regressed on HMO/fee-for-service membership, only education was a significant predictor. HMO subscribers tended to be less educated than non-subscribers. One-fifth of all respondents received care only from an HMO over the five years examined ($N = 80$), and 69% only had fee-for-service care for the period considered ($N = 286$). Five percent switched from fee-for-service to HMO care over the five years, and 4% left their HMO for fee-for-service coverage. The remaining 3% changed delivery type at least twice.

Respondents who left an HMO over the five-year period were asked to indicate why they left ($N = 29$). About half of these older adults left their HMO because of dissatisfaction with the care provided or a desire for more physician choice. The other half left their HMO because of insurance changes or personal financial reasons. Not surprisingly, the respondents who left because of dissatisfaction held very negative views about HMOs. As one respondent stated, "[while receiving care under an HMO] I needed to go to a different hospital. HMO wouldn't approve a transfer until the doctor at [other hospital] insisted and threatened a lawsuit. Wouldn't let my cardiologist operate. They [the HMO] brought in their own doctor." A second respondent also explained her personal experiences under HMO care; "HMOs are poorly run – run for money. They didn't take my health problems into consideration." Those who left for insurance or financial reasons did not have such pessimistic perspectives.

Elderly Patients' Perspectives on the Health Care System

In this section, we explore older adults' views on HMO care. These viewpoints and understandings may shape the decision to join, not join, or leave HMOs. Respondents were asked to directly compare HMO and fee-for service care. As presented in Table 1, HMO subscribers judged care by their organization to compare favorably (49%) or to be equivalent to traditional fee-for-service care (43%). Fee-for-service patients, in contrast, overwhelmingly evaluated HMOs

Table 1. How Does Care in an HMO Compare to Care from Fee-For-Service?

	HMO Respondents ($N = 72$)[a] % (N)	Non-HMO Respondents ($N = 216$)[a] % (N)
HMO care is . . .		
Worse	6 (4)	70 (152)
The same	43 (31)	7 (16)
Better	49 (36)	2 (4)
Don't know	3 (2)	20 (44)
Chi-square	181.68	$p < 0.001$

[a] The number of cases used in this analysis is less than the total sample size because some respondents were not asked this question (it was not in the earliest version of the questionnaire).

as providing inferior care (70%) ($p < 0.005$). In addition, one-fifth (20%) of non-HMO subscribers said they could not compare HMO and fee-for-service care, while only 3% of non-enrollees said that. The only other statistically significant predictor in the multivariate analysis is satisfaction with physician care; respondents who were satisfied with their own physician were more likely to give favorable views of HMOs (regardless of whether they belonged to HMOs).

Older adults were asked to describe their understanding of "managed care" and to state the advantages and disadvantages of HMOs. This information provides a better understanding of older adults' attitudes toward HMOs. Respondents' definitions of managed care varied according to whether or not they were HMO members. The majority of both groups associated managed care with HMOs (83% of HMO subscribers and 57% of those outside HMOs said this). Generally, those receiving fee-for-service care defined managed care in more negative terms than those receiving their health care from HMOs. For the majority of elderly respondents, definitions of managed care tended to be constructed around issues of control. To some, participation in managed care/HMOs signified loss of personal control for the patient in choosing doctors (2% of HMO and 10% of non-HMO participants). Conversely, for others control was reframed more positively as reflecting being cared for by the health care organization (15% of HMO and 19% of non-HMO members).

Negative perceptions of managed care by those who did not join HMOs included prevalent views of loss of control by patients. These views are reflected in such respondent comments as, "HMOs tell you what to do"; "they [i.e. managed care] control your affairs"; "managed care puts rules on you and regulates your visits"; and "you have to use their doctors and nurses." A minority of respondents receiving fee-for-service care reflected a more cynical view of managed care based on their profit motive (2%). Examples of this perspective include, "business is running the medical side"; "an HMO will manage you for a profit"; and "HMOs are trying to make more money."

Positive perceptions of managed care reflected an alternative, more benign construction of loss of control redefined as being cared for. Examples include, "we are taken care of"; "someone manages my health care"; "it is like a retirement home that takes care of my needs"; "someone handles my affairs"; and "they send me where I need to go." This redefinition of loss of control as being cared for was exhibited both by HMO (15%) and non-HMO (19%) patients. Some frail older adults in HMOs expressed views that reflected their sense of dependency and attributions of beneficent control, which go beyond realistic levels of care HMOs could provide. Examples of such definitions of managed care include, "if I am bedridden someone will take care of me"; and "[HMOs are] good when you can't take care of yourself."

Table 2. Perceived Advantages and Disadvantages of HMO-Based Care.

	HMO (N = 92) % (N)	Non-HMO (N = 286) % (N)
Advantages		
No known advantage	4 (4)	75 (215)
Diminished costs	87 (80)	22 (63)
Enhanced benefits/coverage	22 (20)	2 (7)
Good medical care	20 (18)	1 (2)
Better access to care	4 (4)	0 (0)
Greater convenience of services	1 (1)	1 (2)
Better choice/control	1 (1)	0 (0)
Disadvantages		
No known disadvantage	63 (58)	25 (71)
Diminished benefits/coverage	3 (3)	1 (3)
Poor medical care	8 (7)	21 (61)
Decreased access to care	14 (13)	9 (27)
Confusion/inconvenience	3 (3)	1 (3)
Lack of choice/control	8 (7)	47 (135)
Not trustworthy/self-serving	0 (0)	8 (23)

Note: Percentages do not sum to 100 because respondents were permitted to provide multiple advantages and disadvantages.

Table 2 depicts the perceived benefits and disadvantages of HMO-based care that respondents reported. Major differences in perceptions of HMO care were identified by those who joined and those who did not join these organizations. Diminished costs comprised the major perceived advantage of HMO membership as endorsed by 87% of HMO members and 22% of fee-for-service enrollees. The two other primary advantages of HMO care mentioned by HMO enrollees were better coverage (22%) and quality medical care (20%). These reported advantages are consistent with other research findings that many older adults enroll in HMOs to obtain prescription drug coverage, which significantly reduces their health care costs (Rector, 2000). In contrast, only 3% of those in the fee-for-service sector cited quality of care and better coverage as advantages of HMO care.

While the majority of those in HMOs said there were no disadvantages to this type of coverage (63%), decreased access to care was the most prevalently reported problem (14%). Examples of access problems described by HMO subscribers include, "I can't see a doctor right away"; "you have to go to a primary care doctor before you can go to a specialist"; "your problems are not addressed as quickly" and "I have trouble getting appointments." A small number of HMO enrollees (8%) identified diminished control over physician choice as a disadvantage. One patient said, "I don't like my doctor, but I can't change since he's the HMO doctor." Others complained of having to "use their [i.e. HMOs] list of doctors."

Reflecting unfavorable views of HMOs, three-fourths of fee-for-service recipients did not believe there were any advantages to HMO care. Fear of loss of control represented an overriding disadvantage seen by 47% of this group. Fee-for-service subscribers repeatedly made comments like, "I don't want to be told what doctor to see"; "they send you from one doctor to another"; and "you can't choose doctors. I have so many things wrong with me, it would be difficult not to have my doctors."

Poor quality medical care (reported by 21% of non-enrollees), decreased access to care (9%), and a general lack of trust in HMOs (8%) were also cited as disadvantages of HMOs relative to fee-for-service care by those who were not enrolled in HMOs. Some fee-for-service consumers based their perspectives of HMOs on other people's experiences or media reports. Examples include, "my doctor told me the care isn't as good"; "all I hear are complaints from members"; "I don't like what I read"; and "the publicity is bad." Examples of negative beliefs about the type of health care provided to HMO subscribers given by our fee-for-service respondents include, "they refuse to give you important procedures like bypass surgery"; "they won't let you see a doctor when you need to"; "they are for profit, not for the patient's welfare"; and "it's a money making scheme! Why it is run by a business instead of doctors!" One-quarter of fee-for-service patients, however, said there were no disadvantages to HMO care.

Changing Health Care System Experiences of Elderly Respondents

Costs and Access to Care

We now move from a discussion of respondents' general perceptions of health care to their personal experiences. Thirty-nine percent ($N = 163$) of the sample reported changes in their health care coverage during the five-year period. Analyses examined predictors of the total number of coverage changes experienced, the total number of negative changes, the total number of positive changes, and of specific types of changes noted.

Type of health care organization and functional limitations were the only two statistically significant predictors of the number of total, negative, and positive coverage changes. Older adults experiencing greater functional limitations tended to report fewer changes in insurance coverage (positive or negative) compared to those who had fewer functional limitations. HMO subscribers were significantly more likely than fee-for-service subscribers to report changes in coverage (66 and 30% respectively). Interestingly, HMO enrollees were more likely to report both

Table 3.   Reported Changes in Health Care Coverage Over a 5-Year Period.

	HMO ($N=100$) % (N)	Non-HMO ($N=315$) % (N)
Reported a change in health care coverage	67% (67)	30% (96)
Chi square	69.9	$p < 0.001$
Type of change		
Positive changes		
Diminished costs	32% (32)	12% (88)
Enhanced benefits/coverage	29% (29)	4% (14)
Better access to care	4% (4)	0% (0)
Negative changes		
Increased costs	14% (14)	12% (39)
Diminished benefits/coverage	26% (26)	7% (21)
Diminished access to care	21% (21)	6% (19)

Note: Percentages do not sum to 100 because respondents identified multiple changes in coverage.

positive changes in insurance coverage (50%) and negative changes in coverage (46%) compared to fee-for-service enrollees (22 and 15% respectively).

Table 3 summarizes the changes in health care coverage. Changes centered on costs of care and benefits. Twelve percent of fee-for-service and 14% of HMO patients indicated that their health care costs increased. The most frequently mentioned categories of increased costs were higher premiums for health insurance, higher deductibles, and increased co-pay. One-third of HMO subscribers said that their costs actually diminished (compared to 12% of fee-for-service respondents).

One of the clearest differences between HMO and fee-for-service subscribers was in reported changes in health care benefits (see Table 3). While 29% of HMO enrollees received enhanced benefits and coverage over the study period examined, only 4% of fee-for-service recipients reported enhanced benefits and coverage. Enhanced benefits generally included coverage for prescription drugs and other ancillary services, such as optical and dental coverage. In contrast, 7% of fee-for-service and 26% of HMO enrollees reporting changes mentioned diminished benefits and coverage. Types of diminished benefits reported mirrored examples of enhanced benefits with reduced dental and prescription coverage most frequently stated.

One-fifth of HMO and 6% of fee-for-service respondents reported diminished access to care in the prior year. In contrast, no fee-for-service and only 4% of HMO patients reported greater access to care over the five-year period. Specific examples of access problems include, "it is harder to see the doctor, and it takes more time to see a specialist"; "it takes a longer time to get appointments and see the doctor"; "my doctor is busier so he hired a nurse practitioner"; and "I need referrals for everything, including emergencies now."

(Dis)Continuity in Physician Care

Over the five-year period, 31% of the sample changed primary care physicians once, 11% changed twice, and 2% changed physicians three times. Multivariate analysis revealed that HMO membership and dissatisfaction with physician care predicted greater discontinuity in physician care. Personal characteristics, health status, and number of physician visits were not significant predictors of discontinuity. Over the five-year period 44% of HMO members and 38% of those receiving fee-for-service care throughout the five years reported changing their primary care physician at least once. Sixty-three percent of those who moved between HMO and fee-for-service care changed physicians one or more times.

While some older adults changed their primary care physicians because their physicians retired, died, or moved, many changed physicians due to organizational factors (e.g. insurance changed its policies or coverage). There were differences between HMO and fee-for-service patients in experiencing forced physician changes; about 30% of those who had been receiving HMO care over the five years and who moved between fee-for-service and HMO care experienced forced change. In contrast, only 4% of those receiving fee-for-service care over the entire period changed doctors for organizational reasons ($\chi^2 = 61.2, p < 0.001$). Similar percentages of fee-for-service, HMO and those moving between the two types of health care delivery systems changed physicians because of dissatisfaction (overall = 14%).

Dissatisfaction with care and HMO membership were the only statistically significant predictors of length of the physician-patient relationship before changing physicians. HMO subscribers and less satisfied individuals had a shorter relationship with their physicians compared to fee-for-service and more highly satisfied older patients. Average number of years with physicians was 7.2 years for the former group and 11.1 years for the latter group.

Satisfaction with Physician Care

Three aspects of the doctor-patient relationship were considered: how older adults rate their overall relationship with their primary physicians (range: 1 = "very poor" to 5 = "excellent"), how much confidence they have in their physicians (range: 1 = "not at all" to 5 = "very much"), and the extent their physicians are available to answer their questions (range: 1 = "not at all" to 5 = "very much"). As other studies have found (Kasper & Riley, 1992; Meng et al., 1997; Ward, 1987), most older adults in our sample reported having a good relationship with their physician (mean = 4.1, S.D. = 0.9), great confidence in their physician (mean = 4.0, S.D. = 0.9), and generally thought their physicians were available to answer questions (mean = 3.9, S.D. = 1.1). These three items form a highly reliable scale of satisfaction with physician care (α = 0.93). No differences existed in satisfaction with physician care by personal characteristics, health status, number of visits to the physician, and HMO/fee-for-service membership.

We also considered how older adults' satisfaction with care was affected by changes in primary care physicians. It is important to keep in mind when reading these results that older patients largely rated their satisfaction with care quite high, so changes described are typically small and changing satisfaction levels still quite high. Half of those who experienced a change in their primary care physician rated their satisfaction with care lower than they did the prior year before the change. About one-third were more satisfied with physician care after the change, and one-fifth had similar levels of satisfaction with the care received both before and after the change. The reason for the change in physicians affected satisfaction somewhat, with those experiencing forced discontinuity tending to report more dissatisfaction after the change, although this was not always the case.

DISCUSSION

We recognize that social changes in health care in the U.S. during the past ten years have been "massive and complex, involving and affecting the situation for clients, their families, and other caretakers (including health care providers), and health care organizations" (Pescosolido et al., 1997, p. 70). The present paper explored the impact of these changes, which Pescosolido and colleagues term "aftershocks," by providing information about the ways elderly patients perceive and respond to the changes in the health care delivery system. We found that elderly persons have diverse ways of confronting the complex and changing health care system. Elderly patients' major instrumental coping strategy relates to joining HMOs or remaining in the fee-for-service system. They also appear to focus on the advantages of the system they opted for, and they generally perceive a sense of control and maintain optimism about their care. Those maintaining fee-for-service care note they did not join HMOs because they wished to maintain control over their health care through physician choice and believed they were receiving superior care to HMO members. In contrast, many who joined HMOs did so because of financial reasons or because they either did not mind having less control over their health care or positively reframed their perspectives on HMOs if they lost control.

We found it useful to consider both advantages and disadvantages of HMOs from patients' perspectives. Accordingly, we recognize that even if negative aspects of HMO care reported in the literature (e.g. gatekeeping and restricted provision of expensive procedures) (Miller & Luft, 1997) pose a threat to quality of health care received, older adults receive benefits from HMO care in terms of reduced health care costs and more comprehensive coverage of services. Based on the totality of their health care experiences, many elderly patients value such attractions of HMOs.

Our findings support observations of prior research (Kasper & Riley, 1992; Tudor et al., 1998) that HMO enrollees tend to be satisfied with structural aspects of their care, primarily those involving costs-savings and greater coverage for certain services. These benefits serve as strong incentives for joining HMOs for community dwelling elderly. Additionally, both HMO and fee-for-service subscribers reported similar levels of overall satisfaction with physician care, confidence in their physicians, and availability of physicians.

High satisfaction by HMO beneficiaries may reflect a selection effect, whereby individuals with more positive attitudes toward HMOs are more likely to join. Alternatively, HMO subscribers may reflect a reality that the cost advantages of obtaining health care from HMOs surpass concerns about lack of health care continuity or access limitations. Furthermore, we cannot overlook health benefits accruing from greater coverage of medication and ancillary services by HMOs, which may be viewed as counteracting negative aspects of care posed by high costs of non-covered services.

Of course we must also consider counterpoints to such benefits posed by risks to the health of older persons belonging to HMOs. HMO enrollees had less continuity in health care and experienced forced changes. Disruption in physician-patient relationships and shorter duration of physician-patient partnership threatens the physician-patient relationship and represent cause for concern. Discontinuity of health care in HMOs may pose hidden problems for older adults (Franks et al., 1992). High quality medical care rests in large part on whether patients receive services as disjointed commodities within a fractionated system, or as integrated care within the context of an ongoing, trusting and responsive relationship with a physician (Kahana et al., 1999). The older adult's personal physician can minimize prospects of poor quality care as s/he can provide a broad spectrum of services and guides access to more specialized services when needed, within the context of a relationship that is developed over time (Stange et al., 1998). Greater continuity has been found to enhance patient compliance (Safran et al., 1998) and quality of life (Hanninen et al., 2001). Interestingly though, HMO and fee-for-service enrollees did not differ in their level of satisfaction with care. Forced physician changes, however, tended to result in lower levels of satisfaction with physician care, although satisfaction was still generally high.

Regarding the generalizability of this research, our study is based on a representative sample of old-old adults living in independent households in Sunbelt retirement communities. Nevertheless, this is a generally healthy population. Experiences of health care problems may be far more apparent in sicker populations where patients are most likely to encounter challenges posed by the changing health care system. Additionally, sicker populations of elders are known to be less extensively pursued by HMOs to become members (Morgan et al., 1997). Accordingly, negative health care experiences in our sample should be viewed as conservative.

This study considered elderly patients' reported health care experiences and did not include independent data on the actual care they received. Since patient satisfaction is an important component of quality of health care (Adler, 1995; Lee & Kasper, 1998), results regarding differences and similarities in reported experiences by elderly HMO and fee-for-service patients provide useful information. Furthermore, self-reports of discontinuity in care or of increases in co-pay are likely to reflect actual occurrences. Nevertheless, self-report data should ultimately be compared to independent observations or chart reviews to establish concordance between alternative indicators of care.

In sum, managed care was introduced to the American health care system to help control escalating costs. Findings of this study show that many older adults join HMOs for financial reasons and because they believe they are receiving quality care. Those who had not joined HMOs tended to believe the care was inferior to traditional coverage and did not like the reduced control over physician choice that may accompany HMO membership. While increasing physician choice may be a more difficult obstacle to overcome, if HMOs could better demonstrate to the public that the care provided under their sponsorship is of good quality, they could potentially increase their enrollments. Furthermore, increasing continuity of care should be a goal of the health care system, especially for older patients. Improving continuity of care can result in higher quality of care.

NOTE

1. Self-assessed health was also included as a predictor but was not a statistically significant predictor in any of the models, so we did not include it as a predictor in the results we present to streamline the number of predictors.

REFERENCES

Adler, G. S. (1995). Medicare beneficiaries rate their medical care: New data from the MCBS. *Health Care Financing Review, 16*(4), 175–187.

Blendon, R. J., Brodie, M., Benson, J. M., Altman, D. E., Levitt, L., Hoff, T., & Hugick, L. (1998). Understanding the managed care backlash. *Health Affairs, 17*(4), 80–94.

Borawski, E., Kinney, J., & Kahana, E. (1996). The meaning of older adults' health appraisals: Congruence with health status and determinants of mortality. *Journals of Gerontology, 51B,* S157–170.

Callahan, D. (1998). Managed care and the goals of medicine. *Journal of the American Geriatrics Society, 46*(3), 385–388.

Centers for Medicare and Medicaid Services (1997). Data tables: The characteristics and perceptions of the Medicare Population, 1997. www.cms.hhs.gov/.

Encinosa, W. E., & Sappington, D. E. M. (1999). Adjusted community rate reforms to promote HMO participation in Medicare + Choice. *Health Care Financing Review, 21*(1), 19–29.

Franks, P., Clancy, C. M., & Nutting, P. A. (1992). Gatekeeping revisited – protecting patients from overtreatment. *New England Journal of Medicine, 327,* 424–427.

Freeman, H. E., Blendon, R. J., Aiken, L. H., Sudman, S., Mullinix, C. F., & Corey, C. R. (1987). Americans report on their access to health care. *Health Affairs, 6*(1), 6–18.

George, L. K., & Fillenbaum, G. G. (1985). OARS methodology. A decade of experience. *Journal of the American Geriatrics Society, 33,* 607–615.

Hanninen, J., Takala, J., & Keinanen-Kiukaanniemi, S. (2001). Good continuity of care may improve quality of care in Type 2 diabetes. *Diabetes Research and Clinical Practice, 51*(1), 21–27.

Kahana, E., Kahana, B., Kercher, K., & Chirayath, H. (1999). A patient-responsive model of hospital care. In: J. J. Kronenfeld (Ed.), *Research in the Sociology of Health Care, 16,* 31–54.

Kahana, E., Lawrence, R. H., Kahana, B., Kercher, K., Wisniewski, A., Stoller, E., Tobin, J., & Stange, K. (2002). Long-term impact of preventive proactivity on quality of life of the old-old. *Psychosomatic Medicine, 64*(3), 382–394.

Kahana, E., Stange, K., Meehan, R., & Raff, L. (1997). Forced disruption in continuity of primary care: The patients' perspective. *Sociological Focus, 30*(2), 177–187.

Kasper, J., & Riley, G. (1992). Satisfaction with medical care among elderly people in fee-for-service care and an HMO. *Journal of Aging and Health, 4*(2), 282–302.

Lee, Y., & Kasper, J. D. (1998). Assessment of medical care by elderly people: General satisfaction and physician quality. *Health Services Research, 32*(6), 741–758.

Lin, C. T., Albertson, G., Price, D., Swaney, R., Anderson, S., & Anderson, R. J. (2000). Patient desire and reasons for specialist referral in a gatekeeper-model managed care plan. *American Journal of Managed Care, 6*(6), 669–678.

Love, M. M., Mainous, A. G., Talbert, J. C., & Hager, G. L. (2000). Continuity of care and the physician-patient relationship: The importance of continuity for adult patients with asthma. *The Journal of Family Practice, 49*(11), 998–1004.

Mechanic, D. (1998). Managed care, rationing, and trust in medical care. *Journal of Urban Health, 75*(1), 118–122.

Meng, Y. Y., Jatulis, D. E., McDonald, J. P., & LeGorreta, A. P. (1997). Satisfaction with access to and quality of health care among Medicare enrollees in a Health Maintenance Organization. *Western Journal of Medicine, 166*(4), 242–247.

Miller, R. H., & Luft, H. S. (1997). Does managed care lead to better or worse quality of care? *Health Affairs, 16*(5), 7–25.

Miller, R. H., & Luft, H. S. (1994). Managed care plan performance since 1980. A literature analysis. *Journal of the American Medical Association, 271*(19), 1512–1519.

Morgan, R. O., Virnig, B. A., DeVito, C. A., & Persily, N. A. (1997). The Medicare-HMO revolving door – the healthy go in and the sick go out. *New England Journal of Medicine, 337*(3), 169–175.

Nelson, L., Brown, R., Gold, M., Ciemnecki, A., & Docteur, E. (1997). Access to care in Medicare HMOs, 1996. *Health Affairs, 16*(2), 147–156.

Owens, D. J., & Bachelor, C. (1996). Patient satisfaction and the elderly. *Social Science and Medicine, 11*, 1483–1491.

Pescosolido, B. A., Wright, E. R., McGrew, J., Mesch, D. J., Hohmann, A., Sullivan, W. P., Haugh, D., DeLiberty, R., & McDonel, E. C. (1997). The human and organizational markers of health system change: Framing studies of hospital downsizing and closure. In: J. J. Kronenfeld (Ed.), *Research in the Sociology of Health Care* (pp. 69–95). Greenwich: JAI Press.

Pickard, R. B. (1997). Leaving care, needing care? Vulnerable elderly and HMOs. In: J. J. Kronenfeld (Ed.), *Research in the Sociology of Health Care* (pp. 207–232). Greenwich: JAI Press.

Rector, T. S. (2000). Exhaustion of drug benefits and disenrollment of Medicare beneficiaries from managed care organizations. *Journal of the American Medical Association, 283*(16), 2163–2167.

Reschovsky, J. D., & Kemper, P. (1999). Do HMOs make a difference? Introduction. *Inquiry, 36*(4), 374–377.

Stange, K. C., Jaen, C. R., Flocke, S. A., Miller, W. L., Crabtree, B. F., & Zyzanski, S. J. (1998). The value of a family physician. *Journal of Family Practice, 46*, 363–368.

Tudor, C. G., Riley, G., & Ingber, M. (1998). Satisfaction with care: Do Medicare HMOs make a difference? *Health Affairs, 17*(2), 165–176.

Waitzkin, H., & Cook, M. A. (2000). Managed care and the geriatric patient-physician relationship. *Clinics in Geriatric Medicine, 16*(1), 133–151.

Ward, R. A. (1987). HMO satisfaction and understanding among recent Medicare enrollees. *Journal of Health and Social Behavior, 28*(12), 401–412.

Wilkerson, J. D., Devers, K. J., & Given, R. S. (Eds) (1997). *Competitive managed care. The emerging health care system.* San Francisco: Jossey-Bass Publishers.

THE FORMULARY, PHYSICIAN, AND PHARMACIST: MANAGING AND DELIVERING OUTPATIENT DRUG BENEFITS

Maurice Penner, Susan J. Penner and William Keck

ABSTRACT

Pharmaceuticals are essential for the management of many chronic conditions. As a result, it is important to examine how the administration of pharmaceutical benefits affects physicians and pharmacists providing chronic care services. In the 1990s, HMOs and PPOs began to more aggressively manage outpatient pharmaceutical benefits, leading to the growth of pharmaceutical benefit management companies (PBMs).

In this exploratory study, 10 primary care physicians and 12 pharmacists in the San Francisco area were interviewed in 1999, and 11 more pharmacists in 2004, on how they worked with PBMs and their controls on prescribing and dispensing. Responses indicated major problems for both health professionals in negotiating with the PBM as a third party payor, in coping with switches and multiple formularies, and in added work for the health care professional. Increased risk to chronically ill patients for poorer outcomes is an important related problem with PBMs.

The Medicare drug benefit law passed in 2003 will likely result in similar problems for many beneficiaries, including those with chronic care needs. The

Chronic Care, Health Care Systems and Services Integration
Research in the Sociology of Health Care, Volume 22, 81–97
Copyright © 2004 by Elsevier Ltd.
All rights of reproduction in any form reserved
ISSN: 0275-4959/doi:10.1016/S0275-4959(04)22005-1

paper proposes some policy solutions to reduce PBM problems for physicians, pharmacists and the Medicare population.

Beginning in the early 1990s, HMOs and PPO health plans asserted greater control over insured outpatient drug prescribing. Health plans began setting limits on payment for prescribed medications, along with several other cost controls. Many contracted with pharmaceutical benefit management companies (PBMs), or performed their own drug management functions. For retail pharmacies and prescribing physicians, these changes include the PBM as a third party payor influencing the physician prescribing and the pharmacist dispensing a drug. PBMs control costs by using a formulary, or list of approved drugs based on effectiveness and cost criteria.

Typically, when a physician prescribes a new drug, the patient takes the prescription to a pharmacy approved by the health plan. Before the pharmacist fills the prescription, the patient is asked to provide an insurance card to receive the drug benefit. For the insured, the health plan or designated PBM website is contacted for insurance coverage information and approval procedures. The patient's insurance and drug information are entered by the pharmacy staff, and the website's software adjudicates the claim. Decisions are made regarding approval of the drug, the contracted price for reimbursement, and the amount of patient co-payment to be collected.

However, many approval requests are denied. The PBM responds, sometimes with an approved substitute prescription ("switch"). The pharmacist explains to the patient that another drug is covered if this switch is made, otherwise the patient can self pay and try to get the original drug covered with a future appeal. If the drug switch is from a brand name to a cheaper generic version of the same drug, the pharmacist is authorized to make the switch as long as the prescription does not prohibit a substitute. For switches to a different drug (usually in the same drug class), a physician authorization is required. Almost all insured patients refuse the self pay option for these initial refusals, resulting in additional work for both pharmacy and physician office staff, and frequently, dispensing delays for the patient.

In this paper, we discuss the additional work and other problems associated with these procedures. Observations are based on interviews with 10 primary care physicians and 12 pharmacists practicing in the San Francisco Bay Area in 1999, and 11 additional pharmacists in 2004. There was very little benefit apparent to them or their patients from this change in drug management.

Those administering the newly enacted Medicare prescription drug benefit will likely use a similar structure, set of controls, and incentives. Insurance plans (HMOs, PPOs, and Medigap plans) and their owned or contracted PBMs will administer the benefits. There will be different formularies for each major plan, resulting in drug switching delays and other problems for chronically ill patients, as well as additional work for pharmacies and physician offices.

BACKGROUND

HMOs and self-insured employers use a variety of strategies for controlling pharmaceutical costs. Initially they focused on lowering administrative expenses by moving from patient submitted paper claims to electronic pharmacy claims that are submitted online. They also negotiate discounts with retail pharmacies and offer lower-cost mail-order services for drugs used to control chronic conditions. Retail pharmacies want the business from HMOs and will usually agree to accept the "maximum allowable cost" schedule for brand name drugs. Together, these three steps, though important, create only modest savings.

In a second phase, health plans lower unit costs by encouraging the use of generic substitutes, frequently paying the pharmacies more for the pharmacist's time (called the "dispensing fee") for generics vs. brand name drugs. At the same time, HMOs limit the number of brand name drugs on the formulary, creating closed formularies. HMOs also negotiate rebates with drug companies based on sales of their drugs to the HMO's members. A large HMO such as United Healthcare or Aetna, each with nearly 10 million members, has substantial market power. If a drug company's major drugs are not on that HMO's formulary, it can mean the loss of a significant amount of business. As a result, drug companies frequently rebate between 5 and 25% of the average wholesale price of their drugs to large HMOs, or to large PBMs that negotiate similar agreements with drug companies. Health plans may operate their own PBMs or contract with a PBM. According to a drug company representative, rebates can reach 50% for drugs that are no better than others in its drug class and have no generic equivalent. Data are not available on PBM rebate amounts; however, using data from industry reports on Medicaid rebates and anonymous sources, Smith (2004) estimates these at 9.3% of third party drug expenditures.

Several HMOs have opened up their formularies, but require higher co-payments for non-formulary medications. For example, in 1998 Cigna went from $5 for generic or preferred brand name drugs (full price for non-preferred drugs) to $5 for generic, $15 to $20 for preferred (formulary) brand name drugs and $35 to $40 for non-formulary brand name drugs.

By 2000 all HMOs and 74% of employer-sponsored plans used PBMs (Smith, 2004). The majority of large employers are self-insured, paying the cost of their employees' health care who are not in HMOs. Costs for outpatient drugs have soared from 6–9% of a health plan's total costs in the mid-1990s to 10–14% by 1998. It exceeded 20% in 1999 and continues to grow. From 1999 to 2002 outpatient drug spending had increased from $104 billion to $162 billion (Smith, 2004).

The major reason for this increase is the plethora of new and very expensive drugs. Many of these new drugs are far more effective than older and less expensive medications. On average they cost three to four times more than older drugs. A study by the Centers for Medicare and Medicaid Services found over two thirds of the 1994–2002 increase was due to prices, with less than a third due to increased use and intensity (Smith, 2004).

PBMs use their market power to reduce costs via manufacturers' rebates, and they set low prices for retail pharmacy reimbursement. According to a report appearing in Managed Healthcare Executive (Anonymous, 2003), in the U.S. there are 12 firms or subsidiaries of insurance plans that each have over 2 million covered lives for management of outpatient drug benefits. The top two firms cover 62 million and 36 million lives (Medco and WellPoint Pharmacy Management), respectively. To get reimbursement for insured drug purchases, pharmacies are required to use computers to contact the HMO's PBM. The pharmacy does not get paid by the HMO unless the prescription is pre-approved by the PBM. This gives the PBM the opportunity to suggest, and often require substitution of a cheaper drug before filling the prescription.

Sometimes the PBM does not allow the original prescription to be filled. In these cases, the pharmacist may call the physician's office to request approval for a substitute that the PBM has suggested. Frequently, the patient needs to follow through with the physician's office. As a clinical pharmacist with a large HMO notes: "a retail pharmacist who used to fill 100 scripts a day ten years ago now fills 200 to 300. Rite-Aid and Walgreens have significantly lower reimbursement from health plans so they have to make it up with higher volume. The pharmacists do not have the time to help out patients."

METHODS AND SAMPLE

In 1999, we interviewed 10 primary care physicians and 12 pharmacists using a convenience sample, frequently relying on graduate health administration students and their referrals. All of the subjects practice in the San Francisco Bay Area. The physicians included 7 in private practice and 3 who were practicing in community health centers. The pharmacists included a managed behavioral health company psychopharmacologist, 10 retail store pharmacists, and the former manager of a Kaiser HMO retail pharmacy serving enrolled Kaiser members. Physician interviews covered all areas of managed care utilization management, such as preadmission and concurrent inpatient reviews and preauthorization requests, including non-formulary drug approvals. The pharmacists interviews focused on their experiences with PBMs and health plans administering outpatient drug benefits. In 2004, we interviewed 11 San Francisco Bay Area pharmacists.

The purpose of this paper is exploratory, to better understand the procedures that must be followed and the problems both physicians and pharmacists face, as well as the benefits. Implications for patients and for recent changes to Medicare are derived from this study.

PHYSICIAN ISSUES

All 10 physicians interviewed in 1999 complained about the loss of authority in making medical decisions, a finding supported by other studies (Avorn, 2002). They had little to complain about regarding preadmission and concurrent inpatient utilization reviews for hospital stays, with higher levels of dissatisfaction regarding preauthorization for outpatient medical tests (especially MRIs). All of the physicians found PBM controls and denials to be highly problematic both in staff and physician work to review and make requested changes, and further lessening of their authority to make medical decisions.

Primary care physicians indicated denials and requested switching to less costly drugs for around 20–30% of new prescriptions, as well as additional denials and requested switches when formularies change. Physicians often get approval for a denied drug if they appeal and provide strong medical justification. The community health center physicians reported somewhat fewer problems as their insured prescribing was largely limited to Medicaid, as few of their patients have commercial insurance. However, there are several competing Medicaid plans in each of the 8 most populous California counties, resulting in some of the problems encountered by prescribers when confronted by differing formulary restrictions.

Most of the physicians we interviewed had not appealed a PBM denial in the past week; none had appealed more than one per week. Several discussed their discomfort with some of the marginal cases where an appeal might help the patient. One of them is a primary care physician who started practicing in Los Angeles in the mid-1980s in a large medical group that had primarily HMO patients. He stated that he believes in managed care, but is disappointed with its management of drug benefits.

He pulls out a chart. "These are the most frequently prescribed drug classes for primary care physicians and this lists which drugs are on the formulary – that is what they will pay for. There is quite a variation between the HMOs I have to work with. This is my biggest headache." The chart is published by his medical group that contracts with eight HMOs. The chart lists 11 frequently prescribed drug classes, including antidepressants, hormone replacements and calcium channel blockers. In the 11 drug classes, only hormone replacements and antihistamines had at least one single drug in common for all eight HMOs. This means primary care physicians need to know about several drugs for the drug classes they prescribe the most.

The problem is that it takes time for physicians to learn about unfamiliar medications. Knowledge about drugs comes from experience in managing patients' diseases and learning how the drug works in practice.

"Sometimes I know a drug will be denied, and I do a prior authorization request to get the patient the drug. It takes me and my medical assistant 15–20 minutes, sometimes more – from reviewing the patient's chart, filling out the paperwork, and calling the PBM. I do around one a week. But the major action is from the prescriptions the PBM denies. They used to tell me what they would approve, but that changed over the past six months. Now they do not tell me. This can be quite a problem if I cannot figure it out from the formulary chart, if it is not listed there."

Drug switching can save large amounts of money on pharmaceuticals but, according to another respondent: "it can be very dangerous and it is rampant. This is contrary to everything we teach in medicine, which is know a few drugs, know them well, pick the best medicine for your patient, and do not change unless it is medically indicated. But now with so many new drugs, doctors need to learn about them plus those on the numerous HMO and PPO formularies."

The idea that physicians should know a few drugs and know them well was the original concept behind formularies. "It is an old concept, and in a hospital setting it allowed physicians and other prescribers to get used to a limited number of drugs. Managed care has taken the concept from the hospital to the community environment and we are not quite sure that the transition has worked as well as it could."

Restrictive formularies and PBM denials have significantly added to the workload of physician offices. We interviewed office staff and physicians on this matter. When the PBM denies a drug without a generic equivalent, the pharmacist must call the physician office or tell the patient to do it. Another primary care physician estimated that for "about 30% of all of my new prescriptions, I have to change the original prescription because the PBM denied it. This takes up my time as well as my office staff. When the pharmacist or patient phones my medical office assistant with a denied prescription that needs a substitute, the assistant needs to pull the patient's chart for me, contact the PBM and find what is acceptable, but I cannot agree until I review the patient's chart. If I find the substitute unacceptable, I pick up the phone and explain why I need this drug." He estimates around 50–75% of a medical office assistant's time is spent on PBM denials and requested switches for a 5 physician group. After the PBM call, the assistant must call the pharmacy with the substitute and notify the patient that the prescription can be filled.

We asked pharmacists and physicians if there were any benefits for them or for their patients from PBMs. For example, since patients can use different pharmacies the PBM has the most complete data on what the patients are taking. Are PBMs using computer software to determine possible problems from two different physicians prescribing duplicate medications in the same drug class, then notifying the physicians of this possible problem? Sometimes this occurs, but more often PBMs send reports on the average cost for drugs by that primacy care physician, suggesting the use of a less expensive drug for selected conditions.

Another respondent stated that primary care physicians can reduce denials by listing their preferred drugs in each drug class they prescribe the most, then comparing it with the formulary for each HMO or PPO. Constructing a chart that lists these by health plan is the initial step. But if there is little overlap between the health plan formularies, the best the physician can do is to spend time learning more about the drugs that can be prescribed and determine under what conditions these are acceptable. Before prescribing a drug, the physician can refer to the list and determine if prior authorization is needed.

A large medical group of over 100 employed physicians uses computer technology to avoid formulary problems and speed approval of prescribed drugs. None of this group's physicians were interviewed for this study; however, an administrator there commented on an earlier draft of this paper. He explained that beginning in the late 1990s the group trained their physicians for a new requirement to use computers to order prescribed drugs. The patient's insurance number and health plan triggers software to compare the drug ordered to those approved by that patient's insurance plan. If approved, the computer transmits the order to the patient's pharmacy. This system significantly reduced physician and office staff work for formulary problems, and has support from other experts (Avorn, 2002). Information on the prescribed drug can be accessed prior to prescribing; however, physicians will still need to learn more about infrequently prescribed medications to maximize patient welfare.

PHARMACIST ISSUES

Twelve pharmacists were interviewed in 1999, including 10 retail store pharmacists, a psychopharmacologist for a large managed behavioral healthcare company, and the manager of a Kaiser health plan retail pharmacy.

Some PBMs do a better job than others, according to a pharmacist for large retail drugstore chain with several years of experience before the implementation of intensive formulary management. She cares enough about her patients to spend an hour on the telephone with physicians' offices trying to get denied prescriptions changed so her patients can start taking their medications. "When the PBM denies the prescription because it is not on the formulary, some will work with you to figure out an alternative. If the drug is not covered, sometimes I have to call and ask what is covered. Some will not, and tell you to call the HMO to find out what is covered. That is another telephone call for me."

Other pharmacists respond: "The major problem is a delay in getting the medication. Between 15% and 20% of all new (insured) prescriptions at my store cannot be filled at the time the patient presents the prescription to me – unless the patient wants to self pay for it. The denials are usually for the most expensive drugs, so this often is not an option for the patient."

Some PBMs are very slow. "The biggest one for my patients just went through a period where they did not review anything for a week. That is a long delay in getting needed treatment, but the usual delay is a day or two."

PBMs can also be inconsistent. "The one I work with the most is a real problem. It depends on who reviews it. Sometimes things that get approved are a real surprise. Some will not talk with me at all and say the doctor has to call them. But there is one I work with that will actually call the doctor. This really helps when the doctor is slow to call them."

Several pharmacists shared "horror stories" such as this one. "A large HMO's PBM really has had problems. At one point they were paying for things that they did not have to cover. When they realized they were making mistakes, the next month they corrected these mistakes and did not pay for the medicines that their members were already taking. I confronted them on this. They admitted that paying for it was a mistake, and now they were correcting this. But what about the patient who has to change medicines? When you are stabilized on a medication, I do not recommend you arbitrarily switch medications."

"I have one patient who is frail and has had repeat angioplasties. She goes in the hospital every couple of months. She took her retirement for disability and told me she was going on Medicare and needed to pick an HMO for cost reasons. I advised her to call each HMO and find out which of her medications they would cover. She did this and decided to go with a large national HMO. Come January first, they had a new formulary and her medications were switched because she could not afford to pay for her current medicines out-of-pocket. I think people are getting used to switching because it happens so often and for financial reasons they have no choice."

PBMs make arbitrary decisions for cost reasons that may not be best for the patient. "When I started working in Indiana, Seldane, a non-sedating antihistamine, had just come on the market. I had a patient who was on 20 medicines but not all of them every day. The PBM reasoned that the patient did not need a non-sedating antihistamine at night and could take an over-the-counter medication. The thirty day supply was set at 30 instead of the 60 normally dispensed. While this saves money it adds confusion to an already complicated regimen. Now they are doing the same thing with similar drugs, such as Claritin and Allegra. I take Claritin myself for my allergies. I have tried all of the over-the-counter antihistamines, and they all knock me out."

Another problem is the thirty day requirement on refills. "For maintenance drugs we can only fill a thirty day supply which cannot be refilled until the patient's supply is practically exhausted. Often patients have one day to get their refills before their supply runs out. What happens if it is on a Sunday when my store is closed? And then there is the rules affecting vacations that last over thirty days. One HMO lets you dispense a vacation supply once a year. You can only go on one long vacation a year unless you self pay."

For some drugs, PBMs limit the number of doses dispensed each month. One HMO limits the number of doses of an injectable drug for migraines to 6 per month. "I had a patient who demanded at least 10 doses yesterday. He became livid when I explained that 6 was all I could dispense. Migraines can be very scary and painful. I would not want to be out of my medications if I had migraines."

"Some will not pay for drugs prescribed by dentists, such as antibiotics for patients with artificial heart valves when they see the dentist. If the patient needing the antibiotics gets endocarditis, the patient goes in the hospital, which is costly, and endocarditis is frequently fatal. They also do not cover a special plastic tube for asthmatics that they attach to their inhalers to get the medication up in their mouth. It is very effective and easier to use than using the inhaler itself. It gets the medicine deeper in the lungs."

Pharmacists said the only benefit to them of PBMs is online billing and knowing what is not covered by the HMO before they fill the prescription. For patients a benefit is that the PBM requires documentation from the physician that the patient is able to safely use an injectable drug before allowing it to be dispensed. "They verify with the doctor that the patient can use it before they will authorize an injectable. Overall, while PBMs save money for the HMO, they are the biggest headache in my life. Filling prescriptions does not take that long. When it takes you a 15 minutes, you are not waiting for us to count the pills. What we are doing is calling the PBM or the doctor to try to get a prescription filled that the PBM denied online."

While PBMs can sometimes be slow, inconsistent, and difficult, physicians sometimes add to the problem. "There are times patients have to wait for days until the physician calls me with a substitute. I have one prescription that has been pending for over two weeks. I have left multiple messages for the doctor." The pharmacist suggested that physicians "give us a diagnosis and medical justification for the prescription and we can fill out the prior authorization for the original prescription and often get it approved. But not all physicians are willing to do this."

Sometimes patients need to keep calling the physician's office to get a denied prescription approved or changed. Otherwise they may never get drug treatment started. "In my pharmacy about 5% of all the prescriptions initially denied by the PBM do not get filled because the doctor or patient did not follow up."

In 2004, we began a follow-up study that so far includes a re-interview of a pharmacist from the original sample and interviews with 11 additional pharmacists from a San Francisco area city (Santa Rosa). The re-interviewed pharmacist reports, "both the patients and physicians have changed somewhat but PBMs are about the same" in problems such as requiring drug switching for reimbursement, inconsistency in some PBMs for administering benefits, and difficulty in getting a live voice on the telephone who is empowered to change a PBM decision.

"The physicians have gotten more cooperative in being responsive to reviewing patient charts and approving PBM-required substitutes. Also fewer of the patients are surprised when they have to wait for PBM approval or for their physician to approve suggested substitutes. Some of my patients understand it is easier but more expensive to pay out of pocket and try to get it approved later for at least future reimbursement. But the problems remain, including requiring substitutes for current drugs when health plans change, even when they are stabilized on another medication."

The 2004 group differed little in their reports on PBM operational problems (difficulty in getting a live voice, especially a pharmacist for problem resolution, and administrative inconsistency). However, several report that these problems have decreased somewhat as their work experience with PBMs increases. Physician responsiveness to denials remains a major problem causing dispensing delays and slightly reduced rates of drug treatment.

The 2004 group was asked to estimate PBM-caused work for them and their staff and patient issues. They report a PBM-caused workload ranging from 8 to 60 hours a week per pharmacy with a median of 20–30 weekly hours. The average delays resulting from PBM denials range from a half to 3 days. Of denied prescriptions, around 5% never get filled at that pharmacy, according to 9 of the 11. They stated that around half of delays are due to waits for physician approvals or appeals. One respondent finds "it is 48–72 hours to hear back from the physician on a refill." Generally the pharmacist initiates the switch request and communicates via faxes but "misplacements are common which causes further delay; also some claim they don't have the time to deal with non-paying situations – this physician work is not on billable time."

Sometimes delays are caused by PBM limits on dosages. "All too often, I type in the information for say a 50 mg dose, and insurance only pays for 25 mg, so the patient waits 3–5 days, often the time to get the physician to appeal, if willing." The 2004 and 1999 interview responses are very similar concerning PBM-caused problems for pharmacies and patients.

MENTAL HEALTH ISSUES

A large managed mental health company developed a strategy to overcome formulary restrictions for one line of its business. When an employer contracts with this company to manage mental health services for its employees, the employer carves out mental health services from its HMO and PPO contracts. As a result, the HMOs and health insurance plans do not provide and are not at risk for mental health services. The managed mental health care company assumes risk or is responsible for managing mental health benefits.

A clinical pharmacist working for the managed mental health company who we interviewed in 1999 explains, "the large employers that we serve are definitely aware of formulary issues. When we contract with these employers, we require the HMOs and PPOs to cover any drug prescribed by our network of psychiatrists. This contractual requirement works surprisingly well. In my year at the company I am not aware of a single formulary complaint. But we have another line of business serving the members of our large, national HMO. The HMO's formulary rules – not our psychiatrists. We went through a lot of arguments last year on changing the formulary. Initially they were not going to grandfather in those already stabilized on mental health medications so they would have to switch. It is a very large HMO and this would affect hundreds of thousands of members taking these medications. When the psychiatrists and primary care physicians learned about this proposal, they screamed. So they ended up keeping the same drug on the formulary."

"I do not believe in formularies. They end up causing a lot of extra time for prescribers and a period of delay for the patient to get the medication. It is frustrating for me to be on the formulary committee for the HMO's psychotropic medications. They say that they are looking at the clinical ramifications of not having this medication on the formulary, but ultimately it always comes down to what is this going to mean on a per member cost?"

"The PBM for our HMO has gone to a prior authorization system for many drugs in the SSRI drug class. That may not be a very good idea for a person with a diagnosis of depression to have treatment delayed. Approximately 15% of patients with a clinical diagnosis of depression will attempt suicide."

For mental health drugs, restrictive formularies pose a special problem. The managed mental health care company pharmacist explains, "Primary care physicians prescribe 75% of these drugs, but study after study finds they do not prescribe as effectively as psychiatrists. This is understandable given the wide range of drugs primary care physicians prescribe and their ever-increasing number."

"In a drug class with 20 different drugs a primary care physician is usually familiar with only a few. When one of these is denied by the PBM, these physicians may be unfamiliar with the side effects of the suggested substitute, agree to it, but the patient may not get better as a result. This may be part of the reason for the low refill rate on antidepressants in the HMO that owns us. Typically treatment of depression with antidepressants is a nine month course of treatment. In our HMO less than 65% have their antidepressant medication refilled after the first thirty days. Then at 60 days it drops off to 50%." Part of the reason may be due to prescribing low-cost antidepressants with unpleasant side effects.

Kaiser's Single Formulary

Most of these problems disappear for a large group staff model HMO that operates its own pharmacies. Physicians need only to learn one formulary, they also can bypass its restrictions automatically, simply by using the non-formulary prescription form. In one of its busiest pharmacies where 2000 prescriptions are filled each day, as many as 30% of all prescriptions are not on the formulary.

According to the pharmacy's manager, interviewed in 1999, "it usually is not this high, but this year there are so many new drugs, especially in 1998 and 1999. But first the pharmacy and therapeutics committee must review these before they are added to the formulary. They only add new drugs every six months and may require more research before adding it. But the doctors know that some of the new drugs are so superior that it is best not to wait. For example, many of our doctors have found Cozaar, a new anti-hypertensive combination drug more effective in controlling high blood pressure for many patients that were not benefiting from other drugs. For Asians and African Americans who have a higher incidence of hypertension, they are also more likely to have it suddenly go out of control. For them, Cozaar has been especially beneficial. Also there are brand-new drug treatments for arthritis. Many of our physicians think this is superior, so the patient gets it."

This liberal policy of not requiring prior authorization for non-formulary drugs is balanced by routine profiling of physician prescribing to detect patterns of inappropriate care. For example, physicians are identified who frequently prescribe a non-generic drug when the generic ones are just as effective. "But that is generally not a problem with our doctors. And it helps that patients need to pay much of the cost difference between the generic and non-generic drug. They know this before they come to my pharmacy. I know that some patients want a particular drug, think it is better, and convince the physician to prescribe it for them. That is the major reason most of the time when generics are not used and one is available. As for the physicians, their performance is evaluated annually to determine next year's salary and this includes where they stand on adhering to the formulary. The overall responsibility falls on the chief of that department. Here is the graph for your department, if you are outside of the guidelines, then there has to be a justification."

"Our physicians find staying within formulary much easier than at other health plans. First, they know the formulary well. They only have to know one, not the ten or more drug lists that many private practice doctors must deal with. In addition, the buying power for this large HMO means steep discounts on many drugs. While most of the competition has a few drugs in each drug class on their formularies, we have ten. It is really a better system for the patients and physicians. I worked in retail pharmacies and still do a little work for my friends in their pharmacies. These [non-Kaiser] patients can experience delays in getting their medicines."

DISCUSSION

This is an exploratory study based on data collected in 1999 and 2004, from small San Francisco Bay Area convenience samples. Some PBMs serve limited geographic areas and may significantly differ in service quality. However, this geographic area has long had very high rates of HMO enrollment, with HMOs first using PBMs before PPO use became widespread. Thus these pharmacists and physicians should have more experience working with PBMs vs. many other U.S. areas.

Table 1 summarizes the problems with PBMs identified by the physicians and pharmacists, with implications for patients. The problems are organized across the three dimensions of the effects of the PBM as a third party, effects of switching formularies, and added work and risk for all parties involved. Solutions are included for each of these dimensions, based on the comments by physicians and pharmacists in the study.

These interviews indicate several problems for physicians, pharmacists, and patients from current drug benefit management practices. All three parties now must spend more time to get a prescription approved by the PBM, then filled and ready for the patient to pick up. Physicians, pharmacists and their staff must be willing to spend time as patient advocates or increase the risk of poorer patient outcomes when prescriptions are delayed or not filled.

Table 1. Problems and Solutions for Physicians, Pharmacists and Patients
Related to PBMs.

Dimensions	Physicians	Pharmacists	Patients	Solutions
Effects of the PBM as third party payor	Loss of authority in making medical decisions.	PBMs may refuse to share necessary information.	May not obtain the advocacy of the physician or pharmacist when an appeal would improve outcomes.	PBM is responsible to contact the physician, and to cooperate with the pharmacist when a prescription is denied to improve outcomes.
Effects of switching formularies	May be required to prescribe from multiple health plan formularies rather than base prescribing on experience.	Physicians may be slow or uncooperative in helping to negotiate denied prescriptions.	Delays in the most effective drug treatment and non-compliance related to out-of-pocket costs or side effects may result in undesired outcomes, serious complications and death.	Utilize computer technology to reduce formulary problems, speed the approval of prescriptions and improve outcomes.
Added work and risk	Increased workload to handle denied prescriptions, and poorer patient outcomes.	Increased workload to handle denied prescriptions, and poorer patient outcomes.	PBM policies may restrict or delay obtaining an adequate supply of drugs, drugs prescribed by non-physicians, payment for previously covered drugs, or the most effective drugs.	Group staff model of HMO operating its own formulary so physicians know the formulary and can efficiently bypass formulary restrictions to improve outcomes.

Physicians are pressured to order drugs that the patient's insurance plan will cover that can result in them prescribing drugs they know little about. Each brand name drug in a drug class is chemically different from others in that class and operates somewhat differently, and side effects may differ. Patients may be harmed from either not receiving timely treatment (due to delays) or not getting optimum benefit where the switched drug is less beneficial than the one originally prescribed. Physicians who refuse to switch to PBM requested drugs may fare badly when patients who cannot afford to self pay consequently switch to more cooperative physicians. Some patients may be forced to switch when they change health plans. Schauffler et al. (2001) report 5.2% enrolled in California managed care plans had been forced to change drugs for continued reimbursement in the prior 12 months.

Clinical concerns have been heightened by studies on outcomes and restrictive formularies provides some evidence that drug switching can actually increase healthcare costs in the form of increased hospital admissions and physician visits. Horn, Sharkey and Phillips-Harris (1998) studied nearly 13,000 patients in 6 HMOs in New England, Mid and South-Atlantic, Rocky Mountains, and Southwest U.S. Each patient had at least one of the following five diseases: asthma, otitis media (middle ear infection), arthritis, gastric pain or ulcers, and hypertension. Most of the time, all of these require medication.

The authors ranked each HMO's formulary on its degree of restrictiveness. Beginning in 1992 they collected data on patients' use of the following healthcare services: physician office visits, hospital admissions, and prescriptions. They found positive, significant associations between the restrictiveness of the formulary and the use of these healthcare services. The more restrictive the formulary, the higher the costs (Horn et al., 1998).

These associations were particularly strong for the elderly portion of the sample and remained positive for non-elderly patients. These findings indicate that some patients are being harmed by restrictive formularies in the form of extra hospitalizations and physician visits caused by drug side effects (Horn et al., 1998). Limiting the formulary and requiring drug switching may be "penny-wise and pound-foolish" for HMO executives trying to increase profits. If these findings are confirmed in future studies, perhaps HMOs will reduce restrictiveness and financial penalties for patients on non-formulary, brand name drugs. Huskamp et al. (2003) found increasing out of pocket drug costs resulted in fewer patients filling their prescriptions, a strategy used to discourage high cost drugs that may also result in poor outcomes.

In 2003, Congress enacted a Medicare drug benefit for implementation in 2006. It prohibits the federal government from directly bargaining with drug companies to negotiate prices with the benefit provided via private insurance plans offering coverage for non-drug costs not covered by Medicare or as part of a Medicare HMO or PPO (Harris, 2003). The law forbids coverage for drug deductibles and co-payments. It also requires coverage for only 2 comparable drugs in a drug class. No single health plan is likely to capture a majority of the Medicare market, but each will use its market power to gain substantial rebates on drugs that are little differentiated from others in its drug class. With a dozen or more large PBMs negotiating with manufacturers for deep price cuts for their health plans, the largest rebates are most likely to come from the lowest selling drugs in that class. As a result, Medicare formularies may significantly differ between plans.

By February 2004, 106 PBMs, health plans, and retail pharmacy associations had submitted applications to provide Medicare discount cards that is a 2005 interim benefit under the new law. Freudenheim (2004) reports their motivation is to position themselves for providing the full benefit program that begins in 2006. For 2005 they are negotiating with drug companies for their own unique set of rebates (Freudenheim, 2004) that lends support for likely variation between each plan's formulary. In brief, there may be little overlap in formulary preferred or required, brand name drugs. As a result, many primary care physicians will be pressured to prescribe drugs they do not know well.

Given these problems, it is unfortunate that the nation missed an opportunity to reduce the confusion from multiple formularies through a redesigned Medicare drug benefit that would require the federal government to establish a single Medicare formulary, after using its market power to set lower prices and reduce confusion, delays, and work (Hernandez & Pear, 2003). A single Medicare formulary might reduce formulary variation for other health insurance plans.

In addition, incentives are needed to encourage physicians and pharmacists to implement sophisticated computer technology to reduce formulary problems and delays in filling prescriptions. The large medical group practice experience discussed earlier in this paper shows that computer technology can reduce the negative effects of multiple formularies. Medicare policies should be structured to encourage the adoption of better technology.

An important solution to incorporate in Medicare policy is requiring PBMs to assume responsibility to work with the physician and pharmacist to manage denied prescriptions more efficiently, thus reducing the risk to the patient caused by delays or unsuitable drug substitutes. Quality standards are commonplace for HMOs and other managed care providers, and should be developed and reviewed for PBMs. Requiring the PBM to contact the physician and to release necessary information to the pharmacist upon denial of a prescription is an example of a quality standard that would improve outcomes while controlling costs.

Future research should include studying the health effects of PBM-influenced prescribing and delays in patients receiving drugs as a result. How many prescriptions are delayed for 24 hours or more? How many delayed prescriptions are never filled? What are the patient outcomes for delayed or unfilled prescriptions?

The costs for pharmacy and medical office administration deserve careful study, if nothing else to document the costs resulting from this benefit management system for drug store business decisions and physician office procedures, and estimating the amount of patient care resources diverted for this effort. For example, a physician might delegate routine switching approvals to a nurse practitioner or physician assistant. Physician time spent on reviewing suggested substitutions to some extent takes time away from patient visits, and pharmacist time from patient education.

CONCLUSION

This exploratory research shows that current efforts at pharmaceutical benefit management frequently result in a considerable amount of additional work for pharmacies and physician offices. Patients and health plans may benefit from lower drug costs, but patients may not receive the best or most timely drug treatment for their conditions. Physician and pharmacist advocacy appears to be reduced by conflicting time and cost incentives from PBMs. This multiple formulary approach of private health plans is the structure that will be used to provide Medicare's drug benefit. We can expect to see the problems identified in this paper affecting the treatment of chronically ill patients in the Medicare population, and having a greater impact on physician and pharmacist workload and autonomy.

REFERENCES

Anonymous (2003). Clients, covered lives for selected pharmacy benefit management firms. *Managed Healthcare Executive, 13*, 52.

Avorn, J. (2002). Balancing the cost and value of medications: The dilemma facing clinicians. *Pharmacoeconomics, 20*(Suppl. 3), 67–72.

Freudenheim, M. (2004). Drug discount for elderly may confuse as well as help. *The New York Times,* February 6, pp. C-1, C-4.

Harris, G. (2003). Medicare law might limit drug discounts for insurers. *The New York Times,* December 24, pp. C-1, C-6.

Hernandez, R., & Pear, R. (2004). State officials are cautious on Medicare drug benefit. *The New York Times,* January 4, p. A-15.

Horn, S. D., Sharkey, P. D., & Phillips-Harris, C. (1998). Formulary limitations and the elderly: Results from the managed care outcomes project. *American Journal of Managed Care, 4,* 1105–1113.

Huskamp, H. A., Deverka, P. A., Epstein, A. M., Epstein, R. S., McGuigan, K. A., & Frank, R. G. (2003). The effect of incentive-based formularies on prescription-drug utilization and spending. *New England Journal of Medicine, 349,* 2224–2232.

Schauffler, H. H., McMenamin, S., Cubanski, J., & Hanley, H. S. (2001). Differences in the kinds of problems consumers report in staff/group health maintenance organizations, independent practice association/network health maintenance organizations, and preferred provider organizations in California. *Medical Care, 39,* 15–25.

Smith, C. (2004). Retail prescription drug spending in the national health accounts. *Health Affairs, 23,* 160–167.

SECTION II:
HOME AND COMMUNITY BASED CARE AND SYSTEMS OF CARE: THE ELDERLY AND CHRONIC CARE POPULATIONS

OLDER PERSONS' EXPECTATIONS AND SATISFACTION WITH HOME CARE: THEORETICAL ORIGINS AND UNCHARTED REALMS

Eileen J. Porter

ABSTRACT

Despite the long-term interest of medical sociologists in persons' expectations of care, there is little known about older persons' expectations of home care. Because satisfaction with home care is important to older persons, the construct of home-care satisfaction (H-CS) is an important concern of practitioners and researchers. Influenced by theories of expectations and satisfaction, researchers have characterized expectations of home care as pre-existing variables in relation to which persons appraise satisfaction. Although theorists have emphasized the importance of obtaining data about expectations when measuring satisfaction, there are few data about expectations of home care. This narrative review points out the gaps between the current research and related theories. The frameworks and methods of studies designed to measure HC-S are reviewed with particular attention to expectations. The need to add to the knowledge base about expectations (and thereby to increase the validity of the HC-S construct) is emphasized. Definitions and categories of expectations from various disciplines are presented as untapped realms for exploring expectancies and expectations in descriptive studies. An interface between the principle of individual

Chronic Care, Health Care Systems and Services Integration
Research in the Sociology of Health Care, Volume 22, 101–119
© 2004 Published by Elsevier Ltd.
ISSN: 0275-4959/doi:10.1016/S0275-4959(04)22006-3

*differences and the parameter of personal importance of home-care issues is
highlighted as a framework for descriptive research.*

INTRODUCTION

The topic of persons' expectations of health care has long been of interest
to medical sociologists from a macro-level perspective (Mechanic, 1972) and
a micro-level bent (Friedson, 1961; Stimson & Webb, 1975; Tagliacozzo &
Mauksch, 1972). However, there have been few efforts to reflect upon the
early theoretical work about expectations in medical sociology, relative to more
recent theoretical developments in the field and in other relevant disciplines. In spite
of the early theoretical interest in expectations, researchers have concentrated on
the measurement of satisfaction relative to expectations, slighting the description of
the nature of expectations. Recent research reviews have focused upon expectations
of medical care (Kravitz, 1996). Appraisals of theory and research relevant to
clients' expectations in specialized areas of health care, such as home health care,
are particularly warranted. In view of the dearth of such work, a narrative review
of the literature about clients' expectations of home care was undertaken.

The rationale for addressing the knowledge base about clients' expectations of
home care is grounded in the nature of health care delivery for older persons in
the United States. Within the long-term care system, the importance of home care
services has grown markedly over the past several decades; the use of such services
is likely to increase substantially as the number of older persons increases and as
greater numbers of older persons elect to continue living at home (Wiener et al.,
2002). Frail persons who live alone, particularly unmarried women (Jenkins &
Laditka, 2003), are likely to need assistance from home care agencies (O'Keeffe
et al., 2001). Creating a more balanced system of long-term care delivery, in which
home-based services are emphasized over institutional services, has become a goal
of policy-makers across the United States (Wiener et al., 2002)

In concert with the expanding focus upon home-care at the macro-level, the
satisfaction of older persons with home care is an important concern on the
micro-level, for both practitioners (Milone-Nuzzo et al., 1997) and scholars
(Hawes & Kane, 1991). Some researchers in home-care satisfaction (H-CS) have
characterized expectations of home care as pre-existing entities in relation to
which persons appraise satisfaction. To develop theoretical frameworks, H-CS
researchers drew from the works of scholars who, in turn, had been influenced
by sociological theories of satisfaction. Theorists have emphasized the need to
obtain data about persons' expectations when satisfaction is measured, but few
researchers in H-CS have done so.

This narrative review has three purposes. The first aim is to review the theoretical frameworks of studies designed to measure H-CS, paying particular attention to the concept of expectations. The second goal is to reconsider theories from several disciplines that are relevant to expectations, comparing them to the views espoused by researchers who have measured H-CS. The final aim is to present the rationale for drawing upon those theories to enrich the scope of descriptive research about older persons' expectations of home care.

THE LINEAGE OF THEORY BASIC TO RESEARCH ON SATISFACTION WITH HOME CARE

In the small set of studies reporting the development of tools to measure H-CS, researchers have treated the relationship between expectations and satisfaction in a myriad of ways. Reeder and Chen (1990), who developed the Client Satisfaction Survey (CSS), simply noted that differences in satisfaction "reflect personal preferences as well as expectations" (p. 37). Like other researchers who reported small, agency-based studies of satisfaction (Gray & Sedhom, 1997; Twardon & Gartner, 1991), Laferriere (1993), who modified the CSS, did not refer to expectations. However, in reports about the development of instruments to measure H-CS, Westra et al. (1995) and Geron et al. (2000) mentioned expectations of home care relative to a theory of satisfaction. Because they placed the relationship between expectations and H-CS in a theoretical context, Westra et al. (1995) and Geron et al. (2000) are referred to here as *third-generation scholars*. Westra (1995), a home care nurse, and her colleagues, developed and tested the Home Care Client Satisfaction Instrument (HCCSI). The Home Care Satisfaction Measure (HCSM) was created and tested by Geron (2000), a social worker, and his colleagues.

The term *second-generation scholars* is a reference to researchers who synthesized either the theoretical literature, the empirical literature, or both relevant to satisfaction with health care. In presenting the HCSM, Geron et al. (2000) credited several second-generation scholars (Davies & Ware, 1988; Linder-Pelz, 1982; Locker & Dunt, 1978; Pascoe, 1983), and Westra et al. (1995) cited one such synthesis (Ware et al., 1983).

To designate authors who proposed theories about satisfaction, expectations, or both from the perspective of a particular discipline, the phrase *first-generation scholars* is used. Like some second-generation scholars (Linder-Pelz, 1982; Pascoe, 1983), Geron et al. (2000) cited first-generation scholars who had addressed job satisfaction (Lawler, 1973) or consumer satisfaction (Miller, 1977; Rust & Oliver, 1994a,b; Yi, 1990). Unlike some second-generation scholars (Oberst, 1984; Pascoe, 1983), neither Westra et al. (1995) nor Geron et al. (2000)

cited first-generation scholars of medical sociology (Mechanic, 1972; Stimson & Webb, 1975; Tagliacozzo & Mauksch, 1972) or social psychology (Thibault & Kelley, 1958).

Certain theories of satisfaction were influences upon the theoretical frameworks of the HCCSI (Westra et al., 1995) and the HCSM (Geron et al., 2000); these theories are reviewed next. Later, neglected insights about expectations from first- and second-generation scholars are discussed; those ideas are renewable sources of energy in research relative to H-CS.

Theoretical Influences upon the Framework of the HCCSI

In the framework of the HCCSI, Westra et al. (1995) did not cite a specific theory of satisfaction, but they referenced two influential studies with ties to discrepancy theory (Oberst, 1984; Risser, 1975). In discrepancy theory, which had been developed in job satisfaction research (Pascoe, 1983), satisfaction is generally defined as the perceived difference between an ideal outcome and the actual outcome (Pascoe, 1983), or in the case of health care, as the difference between expectations of care and perceptions of actual care (Locker & Dunt, 1978). The treatment of discrepancy theory by Risser (1975) and Oberst (1984) sets the stage for that of Westra et al. (1995).

Although Risser (1975) did not mention an underlying theory when reporting the development of an instrument to measure satisfaction with nursing care, Pascoe (1983) stated that Risser's (1975) tool was based on discrepancy theory. Pascoe's (1983) conclusion was credible; Risser (1975) defined satisfaction as "the degree of congruency between a patient's expectations of ideal nursing care and his perception of the real nursing care he receives" (p. 46). Risser (1975) did not cite a source for that definition of satisfaction, but there is some evidence as to its possible origin. Risser (1975) credited Tagliacozzo (1965) as one source of the "descriptions and definitions of nursing characteristics and behaviors" (p. 46) featured in items of the satisfaction tool. Working with Mauksch, Tagliacozzo (1965) interviewed hospitalized persons about what they "ideally expected" (p. 219) from a nurse. In an expanded report of Tagliacozzo's (1965) work, published several years before Risser's (1975) paper, Tagliacozzo and Mauksch (1972) stated: "The relative discrepancy between "realistic" and "ideal" experiences is a significant variable in the patients' responses to actual experiences" (p. 197). Thus, Risser's (1975) definition of satisfaction might have been influenced by the concept of expectations and the realistic-ideal discrepancy (Tagliacozzo, 1965; Tagliacozzo & Mauksch, 1972).

Oberst (1984) was one of many scholars who referred to Risser's (1975) definition of satisfaction and the accompanying view of expectations. In a study of ambulatory chemotherapy patients' judgments of satisfaction with care, Oberst (1984) cited Risser (1975) as a source for a "framework of expectations" (p. 2367). Oberst (1984) did not mention discrepancy theory, but its influence is evident in the thesis that expectations of the care environment and health professionals "form the context within which satisfaction and dissatisfaction must be assessed" (p. 2367). Oberst (1984) envisioned a linear relationship between expectations and satisfaction, noting that expectations "form the standard against which care actually received is judged to be satisfactory or not satisfactory" (p. 2367). Oberst (1984) did not cite other scholars on those statements. However, Oberst (1984) cited Tagliacozzo and Mauksch (1972) concerning the distinction between "ideal expectations which can rarely be met and more realistic anticipations which take into account the more obvious limitations" (p. 2367). Although Oberst (1984) did not define the term expectations, Oberst (1984) said that expectations emerged from clients' knowledge, characteristics, experiences, and attitudes.

Like Oberst (1984), Westra et al. (1995) were influenced substantially by Risser's (1975) work. However, when reporting about the development of the HCCSI, Westra et al. (1995) did not explain why they modified Risser's (1975) focus on the "*degree* [emphasis added] of congruency" (p. 46). Westra et al. (1995) elected to define satisfaction as the "evaluation of congruency between client expectations of care and perceptions of the care received" (p. 394). Westra et al. (1995) also leaned upon Oberst's (1984) framework of expectations, using it as a basis for obtaining pilot data, but they expanded its scope. Westra et al. (1995) asserted that in addition to client-related attributes, attributes and behaviors of providers were also influential relative to expectations.

Finally, Westra et al. (1995) defined the term expectations as "cognitive beliefs shaped by client characteristics and experiences in interaction with health care providers' characteristics and behaviors" (p. 394). In so doing, Westra et al. (1995) cited researchers who had studied satisfaction in other health-care settings (e.g. Zastowny et al., 1989) as well as Cleary and McNeil (1988), who are considered here as second-generation scholars. In a research review, Cleary and McNeil (1988) noted that expectations were related to satisfaction with health care, but they did not define expectations. The precise origin of the definition of expectations by Westra et al. (1995) is not certain, but their assertion that expectations were cognitive beliefs is consistent with the view of Oliver and Winer (1987), two scholars of marketing. Oliver and Winer (1987) had noted that expectations were beliefs because they had a cognitive basis, rather than an emotional origin.

Theoretical Influences Upon the Framework of the HCSM

Geron et al. (2000) did not reference a specific theory as basic to the HCSM, and they did not define expectations. However, in an earlier paper, Geron (1998) had described the model of *disconfirmation of expectations* as the predominant approach in health care satisfaction research, citing a book edited by Rust and Oliver (1994b). Geron et al. (2000) also cited that book in a definition of satisfaction as arising in part from a "cognitive evaluation of the actual experience of the service compared to expectations about the service" (p. S260). The precise source of the definition is uncertain because Geron et al. (2000) did not cite a chapter within the book.

However, in the first chapter of the book edited by Rust and Oliver (1994b), the "process theory of 'expectancy disconfirmation'" (Rust & Oliver, 1994a, p. 4) was reviewed; this is likely the theory to which Geron et al. (2000) referred. Expectancy disconfirmation is a theory of consumer satisfaction, in which a judgment of satisfaction is based on meeting or exceeding expectations (Oliver, 1977). Two sequential processes are involved: (a) Expectations are formed based upon external and internal cues; and (b) expectations are compared against the outcome (Rust & Oliver, 1994a). If performance (of a product) exceeds expectations, a positive disconfirmation of expectations arises, and satisfaction increases. Increases in dissatisfaction are anticipated if the performance is less than expected. Thus, expectations function as standards (Rust & Oliver, 1994a; Yi, 1990), just as in the discrepancy model. Several second-generation scholars (Davies & Ware, 1988; Pascoe, 1983; Strasser et al., 1993) had suggested that a cognitive evaluation of satisfaction was insufficient without an affective component. Addressing that issue, Geron et al. (2000) noted that a judgment of satisfaction arises in part from both a comparative evaluation of actual service to expectations (as mentioned earlier) and "an affective response to the evaluation" (p. S260).

Summary: Theory and Definitions in H-CS Research
In 1978 Ware, Davies-Avery, and Stewart found inconsistencies in definitions of constructs in research on health care satisfaction. More than a decade later, Yi (1990) made a similar comment about definitions of the term expectations in the consumer satisfaction literature. At present a comparable situation exists in relation to research on satisfaction with home care. Geron et al. (2000) and Westra et al. (1995) said that expectations were directly related to satisfaction. Westra et al. (1995) defined the term of expectations from an atheoretical perspective. Geron et al. (2000) referred tangentially to a theory of satisfaction linked to expectations, but they did not define expectations. Thus, in the study of H-CS, there is a gap

between scholars' allegiance to the theoretical relationship between expectations and satisfaction and scholars' attention to defining expectations. Ideas for research to address this gap are evident in earlier theoretical works about expectations, and those ideas are discussed in the next section.

THEORETICAL DEVELOPMENT ACROSS THE GENERATIONS: CATEGORIZATIONS OF EXPECTATIONS

To highlight the wealth of topics about expectations that could be explored in the study of H-CS, the works of some first- and second-generation scholars about expectations are reviewed. The facets of the concept of expectations that are similar (either within or across generations) share the same row within Table 1.

First-Generation Scholars

Friedson (1961) was among the first medical sociologists to contrast a patient's ideal expectations (preferred outcomes) with practical expectations (anticipated outcomes based on past experience or knowledge of the experiences of others). As noted earlier, Tagliacozzo and Mauksch (1972) referenced a similar dichotomy of ideal versus realistic expectations. In contrast, Stimson and Webb (1975) identified three categories of persons' expectations of medical care, all of which can be viewed as specific cases of practical or anticipated expectations (Friedson, 1961; Tagliacozzo & Mauksch, 1972). Background expectations were characterized as emerging over time as a person learned about the process of having medical care. Interaction expectations were ideas about what was likely to occur during contacts with the physician, whereas action expectations were ideas about what the physician would likely do to be of aid.

Miller (1977) espoused the view that the two chief determinants of consumer satisfaction were "expected performance" and an evaluation of "perceived actual performance" (p. 74). Although Miller (1977) did not define the term expectations, he referred to them as "comparison standards for performance evaluations" (p. 72). Drawing upon theories from social psychology (Lewin et al., 1944; Thibault & Kelley, 1958), Miller (1977) described these categories of expectations: (a) ideal (the "can be"); (b) expected (the "probably will be"); (c) minimum tolerable (the "must be"); and (d) deserved (the "ought to be" or "should be") (pp. 74–75). Miller (1977) emphasized that the categories might not be mutually exclusive.

Table 1. A Comparison of Categorizations of Expectations.

First-Generation Scholars			Second-Generation Scholars		
Friedson; Tagliacozzo & Mauksch	Stimson & Webb	Miller	Pascoe	Thompson & Suñol	Kravitz
Ideal	Background, interaction, and action	Ideal	Subjective ideal	Ideal	Wants (expectations)
Practical or realistic		Expected	Subjective sense of the past average	Predicted	Expectancies
		Minimum tolerable	Minimally acceptable level		Normative (expectations)
		Deserved	Sense of the deserved	Normative	Entitlement (expectations)
					Necessity (expectations)
		Combination	Combination		
				Unformed	Importance (expectations)

Second-Generation Scholars

Some second-generation scholars were quite influenced by Miller's (1977) schema of expectations. In 1983 Pascoe wrote a classic synthesis of the health care satisfaction literature, in which he suggested that the term of expectations was too broad. As Miller (1977) had done relative to consumer satisfaction, Pascoe (1983) challenged researchers to state an interest in particular types of expectations when measuring health care satisfaction. However, in creating his own schema, he did not retain a focus upon expectations. Instead, invoking terms similar to Miller's (1977) categories of expectations or "comparison standards" (Miller, p. 72), Pascoe (1983) listed the following types of standards for evaluating a health care experience: "a subjective ideal, a subjective sense of what one deserves, a subjective average of past experience in similar situations, or some minimally acceptable level" (p. 189). In asserting that standards were subjective, Pascoe (1983) expanded Miller's (1977) contention that different persons might have different standards.

Other second-generation scholars also used Miller's (1977) categorization as a template for detailed typologies of expectations. Thompson and Suñol (1995) proposed some working definitions of types of expectations as determinants of satisfaction with health care. Citing Miller (1977) among others, they expanded the *ideal* category to include desires, wants, preferences, and hopes. They referred to the *predicted* category as a practical, realistic, or anticipated outcome, similar to Miller's (1977) expected category. Thompson and Suñol (1995) designated a normative category, akin to Miller's (1977) deserved category, to specify a subjective appraisal of what is deserved in a health care situation – "what should or ought to happen" (Thompson & Suñol, 1995, p. 130). Finally, Thompson and Suñol (1995) emphasized the need for an *unformed* category, noting that some persons were unwilling or unable to state expectations of care.

In contrast to Pascoe (1983) and Thompson and Suñol (1995), Kravitz (1996) distinguished expectancies (beliefs about probabilities of particular occurrences relative to the health care experience) from expectations (standards) of medical care. As shown in Table 1, the notion of expectancies is similar to that of anticipated or predicted outcomes. Kravitz (1996) remarked that few scholars had addressed expectancies, but he did not present sub-categories of expectancies, as Stimson and Webb (1975) had done. In contrast to Westra et al. (1995), who defined expectations as cognitive beliefs, Kravitz (1996) added the possibility of an affective dimension. Kravitz (1996) defined expectations as values, attitudes, or "cognitive or affective orientations toward events or phenomena" (p. 16).

On the topic of expectations as values, Kravitz (1996) presented contradictory views. After defining expectations simply as "expressions of what the patient wants" (p. 15), Kravitz (1996) stated that wants were only one type of expectations.

The set of expectations also included expressions of "necessity, entitlement (that which is owed or to which one has a right), [and] normative standards (that which should be)" (Kravitz, 1996, p. 16). Kravitz (1996) also included "importance" (p. 16) as a category, noting that persons could be asked to rate elements of care from that perspective.

TRENDS IN THE RESEARCH ON H-CS

Researchers in H-CS have referred to second-generation scholars of health care satisfaction, but they have not drawn sufficiently upon their methodological suggestions. Furthermore, they have not tapped the first-generation theoretical works from relevant disciplines that suggest the possibility of a diversified perspective about expectations. To date the research in H-CS has been characterized by three inter-related trends, which are discussed below. First, researchers have relied upon the dichotomy between ideal and practical expectations as a framework. Second, researchers have not differentiated expectancies from expectations. Finally, insufficient empirical data have been obtained about expectations. To progress in understanding older persons' expectations of home care, researchers must purposefully buck each trend in turn.

The Dichotomy as a Framework

The dichotomy of ideal versus realistic expectations (Friedson, 1961; Oberst, 1984; Risser, 1975; Tagliacozzo & Mauksch, 1972) has been a pervasive influence upon research on health care satisfaction and in satisfaction with home care (Geron et al., 2000; Westra et al., 1995). This perspective has functioned as a silent partner even in the theoretical frameworks of the rare qualitative studies. For instance, to clarify the dimensions of satisfaction and dissatisfaction, Forbes (1996) interviewed 10 older home care recipients. Forbes did not mention the concept of expectations in the conceptual framework, but an aim was to learn what clients expected from home care workers. Therefore, clients were asked to rate certain characteristics of care in importance, "reflecting on the ideal rather than their experience" (Forbes, 1996, p. 379).

Differentiating Between Expectancies and Expectations

In line with Pascoe's (1983) remark that researchers should specify their interests relative to expectations, Kravitz (1996) emphasized that scholars should differentiate between expectancies and expectations to enhance the clarity of theoretical frameworks and research findings. Specifying a focus relative to expectations has implications for methodological decisions in the study of H-CS, as illustrated below in a review of the congruence of theory and method in the studies of Geron et al. (2000) and Westra et al. (1995).

Theory-Method Congruence of the HCSM

In formulating items for the tool, Geron et al. asked pilot group participants what they liked and disliked about home care services. This thrust is somewhat similar to a "preferred outcome" (Thompson & Suñol, 1995, p. 130) or a preference for care (Locker & Dunt, 1978). Data about likes and dislikes might pertain to an ideal dimension of expectations, but such data are not likely to tap the dimensions of expectations relative to necessity or entitlement. Furthermore, what people like about a service might have little to do with how satisfied they are (Owens & Batchelor, 1996; Williams, 1994).

In the theory of expectancy disconfirmation (Oliver, 1977), which Geron et al. (2000) referenced secondarily (Rust & Oliver, 1994a) as the framework of the HCSM, expectations are conceptualized as probabilities (Oliver & Winer, 1987) or "beliefs about the range of likely outcomes of a service provision" (Folkes, 1994, p. 109). As a probabilistic theory, expectancy disconfirmation is suited to testing hypotheses about anticipated satisfaction with products, such as a prospective client's anticipated satisfaction with home care. Thus, the theory is more compatible with a prospective design rather than the post-hoc approach used by Geron et al. (2000), in which persons who received care were asked to rate their satisfaction with it.

Theory-Method Congruence of the HCCSI

Westra et al. (1995) did not have access to Kravitz's (1996) paper, but Westra et al. (1995) might find Kravitz's (1996) distinction between expectancies and expectations useful in refining the framework of the HCCSI. Concerning the cognitive beliefs that they characterized as expectations, Westra et al. (1995) did not specify whether they were interested in beliefs about: (a) the likelihood of occurrences (expectancies); or (b) orientations toward events or phenomena (expectations). However, Westra et al. (1995) stated that expectations are related to "the type of care provided, the number and types of care providers, the kinds of interactions encountered, and the setting in which the care was provided" (p. 394). These foci are examples of orientations to events and phenomena rather than likelihood or probability, so Westra et al. (1995) might have been more interested in tapping expectations than expectancies. If Westra et al.

(1995) elected to state a specific focus on expectations in further work, that approach would be consistent with the post-hoc design used to test and refine the HCCSI.

Thus, researchers in H-CS might find it useful to specify the focus of the research problem (and the findings) relative to the distinction between expectancies and expectations (Kravitz, 1996). Of the work in H-CS, Forbes' (1996) paper is the best example of the potential inherent in that differentiation. Forbes (1996) probably did not have access to Kravitz's (1996) work, but Forbes' (1996) definition of expectations featured both facets of Kravitz's (1996) definition. That is, Forbes (1996) stated: "Expectations are defined as events or attributes that are considered to be probable, reasonable, and/or necessary, and may be different from the actual experience" (p. 379). The reference to the "probable" (Forbes, 1996, p. 379) addresses the concept of expectancies, whereas the references to the "reasonable" and the "necessary" (Forbes, 1996, p. 379) are relevant to expectations. In the study of HC-S, researchers should consider refining their definitions of expectations to embrace the expectancy-expectation distinction, supporting those enhanced definitions with literature and empirical evidence.

Insufficient Empirical Data

Across the generations, scholars have emphasized the dearth of data about the nature of persons' expectations of health care (Fitzpatrick, 1984; Forbes, 1996; Geron et al., 2000; Kravitz, 1996; Linder-Pelz, 1982; Locker & Dunt, 1978; Owens & Batchelor, 1996; Pascoe, 1983; Sitzia & Wood, 1997; Stimson & Webb, 1975; Thompson & Suñol, 1995; Uhlmann et al., 1984; Williams, 1994). Researchers have often cited Risser (1975) relative to expectations (Laferriere, 1993; Oberst, 1984; Twardon & Gartner, 1991; Westra et al., 1995), but Risser (1975) simply stated that patients had expectations of ideal care. Risser (1975) did not cite empirical evidence to support that assertion.

Notwithstanding the proposals of categorization schemes for expectations (Oberst, 1984) or the lists of matters to which home-care expectations might be related (Westra et al., 1995), no exploratory studies of the expectations of home care have been reported. In Forbes' (1996) qualitative study of HC-S, the term of expectations was defined in the findings; there was no explanation about whether the definition was data-based or drawn from the literature. Forbes (1996) did not report data about expectations; Forbes (1996) simply noted that most of the clients' expectations had been met. Because researchers in H-CS have not differentiated between expectancies and expectations, few studies have been designed to describe those two realms.

DRAWING UPON THE LINEAGE: IDEAS FOR FURTHER RESEARCH ON H-CS

To develop a richer knowledge of expectations of home care, researchers must move beyond the dichotomy of ideal versus realistic expectations (Friedson, 1961; Oberst, 1984; Risser, 1975; Tagliacozzo & Mauksch, 1972). Having articulated more precise definitions expectancies and expectations, researchers would then be poised to state a rationale for focusing data-collection on expectancies, expectations, or both (Kravitz, 1996). Home-care clients could voice expectancies about what might occur vis-à-vis their health in conjunction with a home visit from a provider. Clients also could hold expectations or standards about matters such as the nature of the interaction or the number and types of providers (Westra et al., 1995). These standards could be either cognitive or affective in nature (Kravitz, 1996); therefore, the universe of such standards could embrace both cognitive and affective realms.

Descriptive research that assays the nature of both expectancies and expectations of home care is essential to enable the development of definitive sub-categories for both concepts. Specific topics for such descriptive research are evident in the ideas of first- and second-generation scholars, as shown in Table 1. After these ideas are sketched, the interface between the "principle of individual differences" (Strasser et al., 1993, p. 227) and the parameter of importance (Kravitz, 1996) is addressed as a theoretical basis for further research.

Expectancies Concerning Home Care

Researchers need to interview older persons to learn about their "speculations" (Fitzpatrick, 1984, p. 173) concerning home care. Home-care clients might have anticipations relative to both interactions with providers and the actions of providers (Stimson & Webb, 1975), but some anticipations might be more relevant in certain situations. Clients with relatively acute needs might have expectancies about their health and the provider's actions. For instance, such clients might consider the likelihood that daily dressing changes would bring about the healing of a wound. However, in a long-term care model of home care, expectancies might be more basic to interaction; for instance, an older woman might speculate as to whether the home-care nurses upon whom she relies will continue to visit her (Porter, 2001).

Expectations of Home Care

"Expectations which define a role are normally attributed to the social system surrounding a status" (Tagliacozzo & Mauksch, 1972, p. 200). That assertion conjures up the possibility of wide-ranging studies of the normative dimension of expectations (Larsen & Rootman, 1976). Although home care providers represent various professional disciplines as well as various non-professionals, there has been little research to discern clients' normative expectations related to those various roles. It would be important to learn whether clients differentiate home-care workers along the normative dimension.

Another focus of interest is akin to Miller's (1977) category of expectations – "the deserved" (p. 75). Lawler's (1973) discussion of the equity theory of satisfaction is relevant to expectations as well as satisfaction with health care (Linder-Pelz, 1982; Yi, 1990). If equity is viewed as a balance between inputs and outputs, then social comparison processes could be at work if one evaluates satisfaction with care by comparing one's balance with that of other persons (Linder-Pelz, 1982). Few scholars have explored empirical linkages between discrepancy theories and equity theories of satisfaction in home care. For instance, it is not known whether older persons hold expectations related to the equitable provision of home care relative to: (a) oneself and other persons in a provider's caseload; or (b) sub-groups of their contemporaries differentiated along lines of class, ethnicity, gender, or age.

THE INTERFACE OF EXPECTANCIES AND EXPECTATIONS: INDIVIDUAL DIFFERENCES AND IMPORTANCE

To obtain data about either expectancies or expectations relative to home care, researchers must start by delineating the incident of interest. Third-generation scholars have used global terms to refer to the focus of interest, such as satisfaction with care (Westra et al., 1995). Geron et al. (2000) spoke of satisfaction in relation to "a service" (p. S260), citing Rust and Oliver (1994b). However, Rust and Oliver (1994a) actually highlighted "a service incident (or sometimes . . . a long-term service relationship) (p. 3). Similarly, Pascoe (1983) referred to the "salient characteristics of the individual's health care experience" (p. 189) as the focal point of expectations and satisfaction.

Compared to the foci of third-generation scholars on satisfaction with care (Westra et al., 1995) or with a service (Geron et al., 2000), an interest in either incidents (Rust & Oliver, 1994a) or the nature of clients' experiences (Pascoe, 1983) is more attuned to the theory of aged heterogeneity (Dannefer, 1988). If it is held that each older person becomes more distinct from other older persons with time (Dannefer, 1988), then the related "principle of individual differences" (Strasser et al., 1993, p. 227) is critical in descriptive studies about older persons' expectations of and satisfaction with home care. Persons might formulate expectancies and expectations using similar cognitive or affective processes, but the manifestations of those processes are likely unique to an individual (Strasser et al., 1993). Indeed, expectations are likely to vary due to factors such as personality (Cleary & McNeil, 1988), prior contact with providers (Cleary & McNeil, 1988; Pascoe, 1983), and cultural and social values (Cleary & McNeil, 1988).

Although third-generation scholars of H-CS (Geron et al., 2000; Westra et al., 1995) did not refer to the principle of individual differences (Strasser et al., 1993), concepts underlying that principle are evident in the works of some first- and second-generation scholars. For instance, Miller (1977) noted that: (a) Each type of expectation could produce different responses; and that (b) certain persons might be more inclined to use one type of expectation rather than another as a comparison standard. Such inclinations vary across situations as well as individuals. Similarly, Pascoe (1983) emphasized the subjective nature of the standard against which the client compares the characteristics of the health care experience.

Alongside the principle of individual differences, the parameter of importance (Kravitz, 1996) of a care issue is very basic to exploratory research about expectancies and expectations. Thompson and Suñol (1995) argued that when appraising any criterion of satisfaction, the evaluator's interest lies in the perceptual realm rather than in the absolute realm. For instance, the duration of time spent waiting for a practitioner is not as relevant as the person's appraisal of that time as short or long. Thompson and Suñol (1995) reiterated, then, that expectations (and therefore, satisfaction) "will always be subjective, dependent upon the evaluator" (p. 134).

This subjectivity also is a factor in the larger arena of importance across the gamut of possible standards that the individual could select as critical. However, if they are simply asked to rate elements of care based on perceived importance, respondents will select their own parameter upon which to base a response, such as entitlement to care (Kravitz, 1996).This possibility would engender concerns about the validity of data obtained with standardized questionnaires. In qualitative studies, however, the parameter of perceived importance can be tapped spontaneously by asking persons to share perceptions of their experiences. Working from data about what a person perceives to be important, the interviewer could devise probe questions to clarify the parameter of concern to the person, such as need for care or entitlement to care.

Thus, when viewed from a qualitative perspective, a focus on the personal importance (Kravitz, 1996) of issues associated with home care is conceptually consistent with the principle of individual differences (Strasser et al., 1993). The interface of the two foci is an appropriate and necessary basis for obtaining qualitative data about expectancies and expectations of home care. Research in H-CS could take a new, compelling direction based on the interface between the principles of importance and individual differences. Researchers could use the interface as a framework to assay each person's expectations relative to a personal appraisal of satisfaction and to consider those expectations within a broader social context.

Indeed, moving the study of expectancies and expectations across the socio-cultural horizon is a critical step. The normative parameter of expectations merely affords a tangential reference to those contextual facets; they remain unexplored. A warrant for exploring those contexts relative to home care is to be found in the work of the social psychologists Thibault and Kelley (1958), who influenced Linder-Pelz (1982) and Miller (1977). Thibault and Kelley (1958) asserted that ratings of satisfaction are a function of social influence processes. From that perspective, expectancies and expectations have a social dimension as well as intra-personal dimensions. Researchers need to explore the social dimensions that might be inherent in older clients' creation of expectancies about home care. For instance, certain expectancies could arise in the mind of a potential consumer of home care while in conversation with a neighbor who suddenly has someone "coming in to help." Different expectancies might arise in conversations with various neighbors and friends, adding to the complexity of a complex experience.

Furthermore, social comparison theory (Thibault & Kelley, 1958) holds that people in dyadic relationships evaluate those relationships against a standard comparison level. Such standards could be influenced by criteria grounded in cultural perspectives. Relative to expectations, clients might compare one provider to another over the course of home care experiences. These notions have not been explored in H-CS studies; researchers have sought data at their convenience rather than in concert with natural rhythms of the experience of home care.

To capture the nuances of expectancies and expectations of home care that emerge in an older person's daily life, a greater spontaneity is needed in methods. Alongside colleagues who continue to refine the theoretical frameworks basic to standardized measurement of home-care satisfaction, qualitative researchers must focus on describing older persons' broader experiences with home care in socio-cultural context. In studies of that experience, data relevant to expectancies and expectations will emerge, leading to new insights, new questions, and possibly, to new theories about the linkages between expectations and satisfaction with home care.

ACKNOWLEDGMENTS

This work was funded by NIH/NINR 5 R29 NR04364-02, awarded to Dr. Eileen J. Porter.

REFERENCES

Cleary, P. D., & McNeil, B. J. (1988). Patient satisfaction as an indicator of quality care. *Inquiry*, *25*(Spring), 25–36.

Dannefer, D. (1988). What's in a name: An account of the neglect of variability in the study of aging. In: J. E. Birren & V. L. Bengtson (Eds), *Emergent Theories of Aging* (pp. 356–384). New York: Springer.

Davies, A. R., & Ware, J. E., Jr. (1988). Involving consumers in quality of care assessment. *Health Affair* (Spring), 33–48.

Fitzpatrick, R. (1984). Satisfaction with health care. In: F. Fitzpatrick, J. Hinton, S. Newman, G. Scambler & J. Thompson (Eds), *The Experience of Illness* (pp. 154–175). London: Tavistock.

Folkes, V. S. (1994). How consumers predict service quality: What do they expect? In: R. T. Rust & R. L. Oliver (Eds), *Service Quality: New Directions in Theory and Practice* (pp. 108–122). Thousand Oaks, CA: Sage.

Forbes, D. A. (1996). Clarification of the constructs of satisfaction and dissatisfaction with home care. *Public Health Nursing, 13*, 377–385.

Friedson, E. (1961). *Patient views of medical practice*. New York: Russell Sage.

Geron, S. M. (1998). Assessing the satisfaction of older adults with long-term care services: Measurement and design challenges for social work. *Research on Social Work Practice, 8*(1), 103–119.

Geron, S. M., Smith, K., Tennstedt, S., Jette, A., Chassler, D., & Kasten, L. (2000). The home care satisfaction measure: A client-centered approach to assessing the satisfaction of frail older adults with home care services. *Journal of Gerontology: Social Sciences, 55B*, S259–S270.

Gray, Y. L., & Sedhom, L. (1997). Client satisfaction: Traditional care versus cluster care. *Journal of Professional Nursing, 13*(1), 56–61.

Hawes, C., & Kane, R. L. (1991). Issues related to assuring quality in home health care. In: P. R. Katz, R. L. Kane & M. D. Mezey (Eds), *Advances in Long-Term Care* (Vol. 1, pp. 200–251). New York: Springer.

Jenkins, C. L., & Laditka, S. B. (2003). A comparative analysis of disability measures and their relation to home health care use. *Home Health Care Services Quarterly, 22*(1), 21–37.

Kravitz, R. L. (1996). Patients' expectations for medical care: An expanded formulation based on review of the literature. *Medical Care Research and Review, 53*(1), 3–27.

Laferriere, R. (1993). Client satisfaction with home health care nursing. *Journal of Community Health Nursing, 10*(2), 67–76.

Larsen, D. E., & Rootman, I. (1976). Physician role performance and patient satisfaction. *Social Science and Medicine, 10*, 29–32.

Lawler, E. E. (1973). *Motivation in work organizations*. Belmont, CA: Wadsworth.

Lewin, K., Dembo, T., Festinger, L., & Sears, P. S. (1944). Level of aspiration. In: J. M. Hunt (Ed.), *Personality and the Behavior Disorders: A Handbook of Experimental and Clinical Research* (Vol. 1, pp. 340–367). New York: Ronald Press.

Linder-Pelz, S. (1982). Toward a theory of patient satisfaction. *Social Science and Medicine, 16*, 577.

Locker, D., & Dunt, D. (1978). Theoretical and methodological issues in sociological studies of consumer satisfaction with medical care. *Social Science and Medicine, 12*, 283–292.

Mechanic, D. (1972). *Public expectations and health care.* New York: Wiley-Interscience.

Miller, J. A. (1977). Studying satisfaction, modifying models, eliciting expectations, posing problems, and making meaningful measurements. In: H. K. Hunt (Ed.), *Conceptualization and Measurement of Consumer Satisfaction and Dissatisfaction* (pp. 72–91). Cambridge, MA: Marketing Science Institute.

Milone-Nuzzo, P., Brink, S., Huang, J., Levine, K., & O'Neill, M. (1997). Measurement of outcomes in home care: An overview. In: C. E. Adams & A. L. Anthony (Eds), *Home Health Outcomes and Resource Utilization: Integrating Today's Critical Priorities* (pp. 1–18). New York: National League for Nursing.

Oberst, M. T. (1984). Patients' perceptions of care: Measurement of quality and satisfaction. *Cancer, 53*(suppl.), 2366–2373.

O'Keeffe, J., Long, S. K., Liu, K., & Kerr, M. (2001). How do they manage? Disabled elderly persons in the community who are not receiving Medicaid long-term care services. *Home Health Care Services Quarterly, 20*, 73–90.

Oliver, R. L. (1977). Effect of expectation and disconfirmation on post exposure product evaluations: An alternative interpretation. *Journal of Applied Psychology, 62*, 480–486.

Oliver, R. L., & Winer, R. S. (1987). A framework for the formation and structure of consumer expectations: Review and propositions. *Journal of Economic Psychology, 8*, 469–499.

Owens, D. J., & Batchelor, C. (1996). Patient satisfaction and the elderly. *Social Science and Medicine, 42*, 1483–1491.

Pascoe, G. C. (1983). Patient satisfaction in primary health care: A literature review and analysis. *Evaluation and Program Planning, 6*, 185–210.

Porter, E. J. (2001). An older rural widow's transition from home care to assisted living. *Care Management Journals, 3*(1), 25–32.

Reeder, P. J., & Chen, S. C. (1990). A client satisfaction survey in home care. *Journal of Nursing Quality Assurance, 5*(1), 16–24.

Risser, N. (1975). Development of an instrument to measure patient satisfaction with nurses and nursing care in primary care setting. *Nursing Research, 24*(1), 45–52.

Rust, R. T., & Oliver, R. L. (1994a). Service quality: Insights and managerial implications from the frontier. In: R. T. Rust & R. L. Oliver (Eds), *Service Quality: New Directions in Theory and Practice* (pp. 1–19). Thousand Oaks, CA: Sage.

Rust, R. T., & Oliver, R. L. (1994b). *Service quality: New directions in theory and practice.* Thousand Oaks, CA: Sage.

Sitzia, J., & Wood, N. (1997). Patient satisfaction: A review of issues and concepts. *Social Science and Medicine, 45*, 1829–1843.

Stimson, G., & Webb, B. (1975). *Going to see the doctor: The consultation process in general practice.* London: Routledge and Kegan Paul.

Strasser, S., Aharony, L., & Greenberger, D. (1993). The patient satisfaction process: Moving toward a comprehensive model. *Medical Care Review, 50*, 219–248.

Tagliacozzo, D. L. (1965). The nurse from the patient's point of view. In: J. K. Skipper & R. C. Leonard (Eds), *Social Interaction and Patient Care* (pp. 219–227). Philadelphia: J. B. Lippincott.

Tagliacozzo, D. L., & Mauksch, H. O. (1972). The patient's view of the patient's role. In: E. G. Jaco (Ed.), *Patients, Physicians, and Illness* (2nd ed., pp. 172–185). New York: Free Press.

Thibault, J. W., & Kelley, H. H. (1958). *The social psychology of groups.* New York: Wiley.

Thompson, A. G. H., & Suñol, R. (1995). Expectations as determinants of patient satisfaction: Concepts, theory, and evidence. *International Journal of Qualitative Health Care, 7*, 127–141.

Twardon, C. A., & Gartner, M. B. (1991). Patient satisfaction with primary nursing in home health. *Journal of Nursing Administration, 21*(11), 39–43.

Uhlmann, R. F., Inui, T. S., & Carter, W. B. (1984). Patient requests and expectations: Definitions and clinical applications. *Medical Care, 22*, 681–685.

Ware, J. E., Davies-Avery, A., & Stewart, A. L. (1978). The measurement and meaning of patient satisfaction. *Health & Medical Care Services Review, 1*(1), 3–13.

Ware, J. E., Snyder, M. K., Wright, R., & Davies, A. R. (1983). Defining and measuring patient satisfaction with medical care. *Evaluation and Program Planning, 6*, 247–263.

Westra, B. L., Cullen, L., Brody, D., Jump, P., Geanon, L., & Milad, E. (1995). Development of the Home Care Client Satisfaction Instrument. *Public Health Nursing, 12*, 393–399.

Wiener, J. M., Tilly, J., & Alecxih, L. M. B. (2002). Home and community-based services in seven states. *Health Care Financing Review, 23*(3), 89–114.

Williams, B. (1994). Patient satisfaction: A valid concept? *Social Science and Medicine, 38*, 509–516.

Yi, Y. (1990). A critical review of consumer satisfaction. In: V. A. Zeithaml (Ed.), *Review of Marketing 1990* (pp. 68–123). Chicago: American Marketing Association.

Zastowny, T. R., Roghmann, K. J., & Caffereta, G. L. (1989). Patient satisfaction and the use of health services: Explorations in causality. *Medical Care, 27*, 705–723.

THE EFFECTS OF RACE AND GENDER ON PREDICTING IN-HOME AND COMMUNITY-BASED SERVICE USE BY OLDER ADULTS

Man Wai A. Lun

ABSTRACT

The purpose of this study was to re-examine racial and gender differences in home and community-based services utilization. Using the 1999 National Long Term Care Survey, the Anderson-Newman (1995) health behavioral model, social supports and structural factors were used to examine predictors of service use among four in-home and two community-based services. The results showed that race did not have a significant main effect on service use, but gender had a significant main effect for housework, home delivered meals, and congregate meals. Using an interaction term, older white women reported higher usage of housework. Among the predictors, enabling factors had the strongest effect on the use of personal care/nursing, home delivered meals, transportation and senior centers' services. The results also indicated the importance of social supports and structural factors, particularly service awareness, in predicting service use. Implications for policies and practice to improve community outreach, access and utilization of services by different racial groups of elders are discussed.

Chronic Care, Health Care Systems and Services Integration
Research in the Sociology of Health Care, Volume 22, 121–139
© 2004 Published by Elsevier Ltd.
ISSN: 0275-4959/doi:10.1016/S0275-4959(04)22007-5

BACKGROUND

Long-term care in the U.S. refers to informal care, in-home and community-based care, and nursing home care services that are needed by individuals who are functionally or mentally impaired. The continuum of formal long-term care in the U.S. refers to medical, social, and personal care services provided in home or community-based settings and paid for from either private or public funds. As the size of the aging population in the U.S. increases, the frail oldest old among this cohort (elders over age 85) will require more long-term care services (Feder et al., 2000; Scanlon, 1998; Wiener & Stevenson, 1997). For non-institutionalized frail elderly persons, the use of the formal services may strengthen their quality of their life, maintain functions, and prevent decline. Despite this benefit, older non-Hispanic black elders, who tend to be in poorer health and to live in poverty, are also less likely to use institutional facilities (Federal Interagency Forum on Aging-related statistics, 2000; Mui & Burnette, 1994). While studies on formal in-home service use by older non-Hispanic blacks (blacks) and non-Hispanic whites (whites) have been long standing, study results are inconclusive. In addition, formal service use gender differences within race/ethnicity groups have not been examined.

The study reported here was undertaken in order to understand the effect of race/ethnicity and gender separately and jointly on formal service use among the frail elderly. Knowledge of the predictors of formal in-home service use and the impact of race/ethnicity and gender on these factors is important for developing culturally sensitive services and targeting services in future long-term care policies. The most recent National Long-Term Care Survey (1999) data was used to re-examine the predictors of different formal long term care services used by older blacks and whites. The study also examined the effect of barriers to service use based on social and economic structure and the impact of social support on formal service use. Lastly, this study expanded previous knowledge of service use by exploring gender differences within these two racial/ethnic groups.

LITERATURE ON ELDERS FORMAL SERVICE USE

The Andersen and Newman (1973) Health Behavior Model has been widely used by many studies to examine elders' utilization of long-term care services (Burnette & Mui, 1995; Calsyn & Roades, 1993; Calsyn & Winter, 2000; Jackson & Mittelmark, 1997; Mitchell, 1995; Mitchell & Krout, 1998; Mitchell et al., 1997; Mui & Burnette, 1994).

As demonstrated by the empirical studies, predictors of frail elders' formal service use are multi-faceted. Within the context of the Anderson-Newman

Health Behavior model, studies show that need factors contribute the most to the prediction of in-home service use. These studies demonstrate that more *ADL and IADL impairments* predict greater in-home service use (Burnette & Mui, 1995; Calsyn & Roades, 1993; Calsyn & Winter, 2000). Other predictors include having *less upper-body disability* (Johnson & Wolinsky, 1996) or *having been hospitalized* (Burnette & Mui, 1995; Cagney & Agree, 1999; Choi, 1994; Wallace et al., 1994). Elders who report *having other chronic diseases* (Wallace et al., 1998), *having poorer perceived health* (Calsyn & Roades, 1993), and/or *having less cognitive impairment* (Mui & Burnette, 1994) were also more likely to use in-home services.

The prediction power of the Health Behavior Model's predisposing and enabling factors has been mixed. In general, *old age* (Burnette & Mui, 1995; Calsyn & Winter, 2000; Mui & Burnette, 1994), *being female* (Calsyn & Roades, 1993; Wallace et al., 1998), and *living in poverty* (Wallace et al., 1994, 1998) are factors that increased the use of home services. Other studies found that having a higher income (Ettner, 1994) and being male (Calsyn & Winter, 2000) were associated with greater in-home service use.

Consistent with studies of in-home service use, need variables explain the most variance in prediction of community service use. Elderly who reported more *ADLs* or *IADLs* were more likely to use community-based services (Calsyn & Roades, 1993; Calsyn & Winter, 2000; Choi, 1994; Mitchell et al., 1997). However, other studies report contrasting results (Burnette & Mui, 1995; Mitchell & Krout, 1998; Mui & Burnette, 1994). Some suggest that there was an interaction effect between ADLs, IADLs and other factors (Calsyn & Winter, 2000; Mitchell, 1995; Mitchell & Krout, 1998; Mitchell et al., 1997). The few studies that included mental health factors (Mui & Burnette, 1994) found that elders with *less depressive symptoms* used community-based service more often. Predictors of community-based service use included the predisposing factors of *old age* (Burnette & Mui, 1995; Calsyn & Winter, 1999, 2000; Miner, 1995; Mitchell & Krout, 1998; Mitchell et al., 1997) and *being female* (Calsyn & Roades, 1993; Miner, 1995). Such service use was also predicted by the enabling factors of *living alone* (Burnette & Mui, 1995; Johnson & Wolinsky, 1996; Mitchell & Krout, 1998; Mitchell et al., 1997), *use of other services* (Burnette & Mui, 1995; Calsyn & Winter, 2000) and *lower education level* (Mitchell & Krout, 1998).

Structural Barriers and Elder Formal Service Use

Although the study of in-home and community-based service use has been long standing, how structural barriers are associated with formal home and community-based service use had not been tested prior the study reported here. This study used the Yeatts et al. (1992) practice-oriented perspective to examine the impact of structural barriers and unmet needs on service use. This perspective is concerned with the interface between service use and structural factors including knowledge or intent, accessibility, and availability. A number of studies found that older people who had *greater service awareness* were more likely to use community-based services (Calsyn & Roades, 1993; Calsyn & Winter, 1999; Mitchell, 1995). Jackson and Mittelmark (1997) found that old people who reported *transportation* as unavailable were more likely to report unmet service needs. Regional differences can also become a barrier to service access with studies finding that elders who live in *rural* areas were more likely to use community-based services (Calsyn & Winter, 1999; Miner, 1995; Miner et al., 1993; Mitchell & Krout, 1995).

Informal Support and Elder Formal Service Use

The influence of informal support on formal service use has been examined by two theories: "Linking/Bridging" (Ward et al., 1984) and "Compensatory/Substitution" (Cantor, 1979) theories. Linking/bridging theory addresses how the informal network links older people to services and at the same time continues to be highly involved even after initiation of the use of formal sources of support. As Ward et al. (1984) suggest, the informal network plays the role of "lay referral" in assisting older people to obtain formal services. Some studies confirm the positive relationship between informal support and formal service (Calsyn & Winter, 1999; Logan & Spitze, 1994; Miner, 1995). These studies also found that formal services may in turn link needy elderly persons to informal networks for support that go beyond the help provided by that agency. Compensatory/Substitution theory is based on Cantor's (1979) model that there is a negative association between informal and formal support. It is widely believed that the use of formal services is diminished by the availability of a supportive family and friendship circle. A number of studies confirmed that elders who had fewer informal supports were more likely to use formal in-home and community-based services (Miner, 1995).The number of children is an important indicator of formal service use with childless older adults (Choi, 1994) and elders with few adult children (Burnette & Mui, 1995; Ettner, 1994) reportedly using more formal home services.

Race/Ethnicity and Gender on Service Use

Previous studies indicate that race/ethnicity and gender always had an independent effect on service use. These are the predictors of greatest interest in this research project. A number of studies show that race/ethnicity was a significant predictor of in-home and community-based service use (Burnette & Mui, 1995; Cagney & Agree, 1999; Calsyn & Roades, 1993; Johnson & Wolinsky, 1996; Miner, 1995). However, there were also few studies that found that race/ethnicity was not a significant factor (Calsyn & Winter, 1999, 2000; Logan & Spitze, 1994). More studies showed that gender had no effect on in-home and community-based service use (Johnson & Wolinsky, 1996; Miner, 1995) than did the few studies that showed being female to associate with service use (Calsyn & Roades, 1993; Mitchell & Krout, 1998; Mitchell et al., 1997; Mui & Burnette, 1994). A few studies examined differences in in-home and community-based service use by black and white elders and found older blacks tended to use more community-based services. However, for in-home services use, the results were inconclusive. Common factors predicting the use of in-home and community services for both older blacks and whites include having fewer informal supports, being in old age, living alone, having more ADL/IADL needs, low perceived instrumental support, lacking transportation and having more chronic illnesses. However, different factors were associated with service use by different racial groups. Others report that different factors were associated with service use by race and gender. For instance, white female elders with high education, receiving Medicaid, less stable residence, living in Northeast, and certain chronic illnesses were more likely to use in-home services. But for black female elders, those who had no kin social support, having stroke, Alzheimer's disease and certain chronic illnesses were more likely to use in-home services (Johnson & Wolinsky, 1996).

Even though previous studies confirmed that there were different factors contributing to in-home and community based service use among older blacks and whites, differences on each service use was rarely examined. Indeed, some studies have suggested that different factors determine racial group differences in the services used and that race disparity exists in service use. Examining predicting factors by racial group differences for each service use separately is necessary so that it would provide a clear picture how racial disparity exists on each service.

FRAMEWORK AND METHODOLOGY

Recognizing that most previous elder service use studies only adopted the health behavioral model, this study added the Practice-oriented perspective in order to strengthen the understanding of elder's formal service use. The Practice-oriented conceptual framework supplemented the enabling factors in the health behavioral model framework with variables of service awareness, service accessibility, and service affordability. The impact of informal support on formal service use was

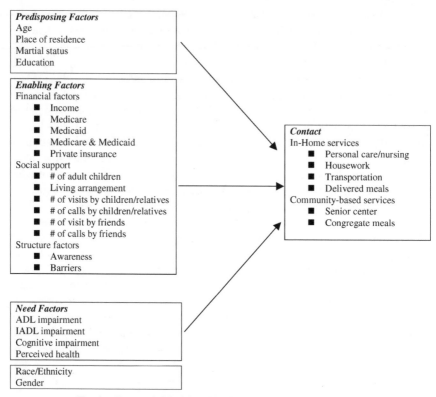

Fig. 1. Research Model: A Health-Behavior-Practice Model.

also tested. Using this unique conceptual model as shown in Fig. 1, this study examined the main effects of race and gender on each in-home and community-based service use. Moreover, the joint effects of race and gender on each service were also examined.

Sample and Date Source

This study conducted a secondary analysis of data gathered in the 1999 National Long-Term Care Survey (NLTCS). This data is the fifth wave (1982, 1984, 1989, 1994, 1999) of a national, longitudinal data collection of Medicare beneficiaries aged 65 or over with chronic functional disabilities living in the community and in nursing homes. It provides data on service use over time. The NLTCS is based on a list sample drawn from Medicare eligibility files. The 1999 NLTC survey is a cross-sectional study that has screened a total of 19,875 people aged 65 or over. This study included information from 2666 non-institutionalized frail older persons aged 65 or over with at least one ADL/IADL impairment for three months who completed a detailed community interview. 2487 (90.6%) were white elders and 179 (6.5%) were black elders.

Measures

Based on the Andersen-Newman model, three categories of independent variables were identified. These are the predisposing, enabling, and need factors. Predisposing factors measured individual demographic characteristics including age, gender, martial status, education, race/ethnicity, and place of residence. Enabling factors measured financial characteristics, social support, and structure factors. Need refered to the functioning of individual elders including ADLs, IADLs, cognitive impairment, and perceived health.

Predisposing factors measured individual demographic characteristics including age, martial status, education, and place of residence. Age was categorized into three interval groups: (1) 65–74 yrs old; (2) 75–84 yrs old; and (3) 85 or over. Martial status was also categorized into three nominal groups: (1) married; (2) not married; and (3) never married. For education, respondents were asked what the highest level of education they completed was. These levels were categorized into three ordinal groups as follows: (1) grade school or below; (2) high school; and (3) college. For place of residence, respondents were asked what type of area did they live in which was categorized into three nominal groups: (1) rural; (2) suburban; and (3) urban area.

Enabling factors measured financial factors, social support, and structural factors. Financial factors included income, Medicare, Medicaid, dual insurance receiver, and private insurance. Income was measured by asking respondents their monthly income and is categorized into three ordinal groups: (1) less than $599; (2) $600–999; and (3) $1000 or over. To measure Medicare coverage, respondents were asked whether they received Medicare or not which was coded into a dichotomous dummy code as (0) yes and (1) no. Medicaid, both Medicare and Medicaid, and private insurance were also coded in the same way. Social support include number of adult children, living arrangement, number of visits by children/relatives, number of calls by children/relatives, number of visits by friends, and number of calls by friends. The number of adult children was a continuous variable. Living arrangement was measured by asking the respondents whether they lived with their caregiver or not. Number of visits is measured by asking respondents how often their adult children or relatives' visited per month and is categorized into three ordinal groups: (1) 0–5 times; (2) 6–29 times; and (3) 30 times or more. Number of calls by children/relatives, number of visits by friends, and number of calls by friends were asked and categorized in the same way. To measure structural barriers, respondents were asked the types of structural barriers they had experienced. Responses were attributed to create an index of three groups: (1) no barriers; (2) not aware of service; and (3) other barriers.

Need refers to the functioning of individual elders including ADLs, IADLs, cognitive impairment, and perceive health. ADL impairment is measured by the composite score of yes responses on nine difficulties including eating, bedding, getting in or out of bed, getting in or out of chairs, getting around inside, dressing, bathing, toilet, and controlling bowel movement/urinating. For IADLs, it is measured by the composite score of yes responses on seven difficulties including heavy housework, light housework, laundry, meals, shopping, getting around outside, and walking. Cognitive impairment status is measured by the composite score of mini mental status exam where the items were found in the NLTCS data.

Race/Ethnicity and gender will be entered last into the regression model in order to examine their effect after controlling for temporal effects of all other independent variables. Race/Ethnicity will be dummy coded into either (0) white or (1) black. Since the sample size of other ethnic groups was too small for group comparisons, this study excluded these groups. Gender was also dummy coded into (0) male or (1) female.

Dependent variables included in-home and community-based service category. Personal care/nursing, housework, transportation, and delivered meals services were tested as in-home services; senior center and congregate meals were tested as community-based services. Each service was coded as dichotomous dummy variables and measured whether older person has ever used this service.

Data Analysis

Among the 2666 community-dwelling frail elders aged 65 and over in the data set, almost 12% (11.6%) had at least one ADL impairment and almost 17% (16.9%) had at least one IADL impairment. About 43.5% of the respondents were between 75–84 years old. The majority of respondents (56.8%) were not married and 38.8% were married. Most of these elders lived in urban areas (73.3%) and had a grade school level education (43.2%). About 45% of the respondents reported having a $600–$999 monthly income. Among these community-dwelling frail elders, whites were by far the largest group (93.3%) followed by black elderly (6.7%). Almost two thirds were female (64%).

Univariate analyses were conducted on all measures in the data set. First, simple frequencies were conducted to check for data errors, skewness, and outliers across all measures. With the exceptions of dichotomous and nominal variables (such as race/ethnicity), skewness for most variables was within $+1$ to -1 range indicating a normal distribution of scores. Since three independent variables, number of ADL impairments (skewness $= 4.56$), number of IADL impairments (skewness $= 2.48$), and number of adult children (skewness $= 2.86$) were positively skewed, the natural logs of these variables were used for multivariate analyses. Second, univariate statistics for measures were conducted to analyze measures of central tendency (mean, median, and mode) and variation (standard deviation, range, and variance). Where appropriate, data was re-coded and summed to create composite index scores (dummy coded, ordinal, interval, or scale measures) or collapsed into fewer groups to achieve normalcy for bivariate group analysis. These data condensing processes assisted in building the multivariate models of the study.

The zero-correlation analysis was conducted among the independent and dependent variables. In this study, significant correlation between independent and dependent variables ranged from $r = -0.209$ to $r = 0.207$. Among significant correlations between independent variables, correlation ranged from $r = -0.348$ to $r = 0.469$ indicating no multicollinearity.

MUILIVARIATE ANALYSIS

Hierarchical logistic regression analyses were conducted to test the hypotheses regarding any contacts the respondent had with each type of in-home (personal care/nursing, housework, delivered meals, and transportation) and community-based services (senior center and congregate meals).

Analyses were based on hierarchical analysis of predisposing, need, and enabling sets of predictors to test for the main effects of race/ethnicity and gender on in-home and community-based service use, and the interaction term of race/ethnicity by gender on service use. In the hierarchical model of this study, the set of predisposing variables was entered first, followed by the sets of enabling and need variables in hierarchical order of succession. This ordering was determined by the assumptions of time precedence in the behavioral model (Calsyn & Winter, 2000). Race/ethnicity, gender, or the interaction term of race/ethnicity by gender was entered last in order to examine their unique contribution after other variables were taken into account. The interaction term was entered last in order to measure whether it explained any additional variance in service use. Questions on structural barriers of congregate meals were not asked in the data set. As a result,

Table 1. Summary of Significant Predictors from Logistic Regression Models of In-Home and Community-based Service Use ($n = 2{,}666$).

Predictors (Reference Group in Parentheses)	In-Home Services			Community-Based Services		
	Personal Care/Nursing	Housework	Delivered Meals	Transportation	Senior Center	Congregate Meals
Predisposing						
Age	0.05****	0.06****	0.05****		0.04*	0.06****
Martial status (married)	0.70****	0.93****	0.55**	0.54*		–
Education level (<grade school)						
High school	−0.56****		−0.70**			−0.55**
College	0.34*	0.55**			0.78*	0.48**
Place of residence (Rural)						
Suburban	−0.34*	−0.48*				
Urban				1.11****	1.12*	0.58**
Enabling						
Income (<$599)						
$600–$999		−0.97**				
$1000>						
Medicare (No)						
Medicaid (No)						
Dual (No)						
Private insurance (No)		−0.53**				−0.33*
# of Adult children	0.12****	0.09**	0.08*	0.11**		0.07*
Living w/caregivers (No)	−2.77****	−1.30****	−1.54****	−2.29****	−2.75****	
Children/relative visit (0–5 times)						
6–29 times		−0.57**		−0.57*		−0.53**
30+ times	0.64*****		0.82**			
Children/relative calls (0–5 times)						
6–29 times						
30+ times		0.60*				
Friend visit (0–5 times)						
6–29 times						
30+ times	−0.73**					1.03****
Friend calls (0–5 times)						
6–29 times			−0.71**			−0.76****
30+ times						−0.56*
Structural barrier (No barrier)						
Not aware	−0.37****	−0.16****	−0.13****	−0.12****	−0.05****	
Other barriers	−0.37****	−0.17***	−0.13***	−0.11***	−0.05****	
Need						
# of ADLs	0.09**					
# of IADLs	0.17****	0.16***	0.13*		0.16*	
Cognitive impairment						
Perceived health (excellent)						
Good				−1.26**	−0.41*	

Table 1. *(Continued)*

Predictors (Reference Group in Parentheses)	In-Home Services			Community-Based Services		
	Personal Care/Nursing	Housework	Delivered Meals	Transportation	Senior Center	Congregate Meals
Fair	1.42****	0.89****	1.08***	0.96**		
Poor	2.05****	1.06****	1.36****	1.21***		
Race (white)						
Gender (Male)		0.70****	0.52*			0.30*
Race × Gender (white male)						
White female		0.66**				
Black male						
Black female						
χ^2	1705.38	658.80	498.47	513.52	265.39	579.17
Cox & Snell R^2	0.08	0.03	0.03	0.03	0.02	0.03

Note: Number is unstandardized regression coefficient.
*$p < 0.05$.
**$p < 0.01$.
***$p < 0.001$.
****$p < 0.0001$.

no structural barrier variable was included in the regression model of congregate meals.

Hierarchical logistics regression models for contacts with four in-home service use categories (personal care/nursing, housework, delivered meals, and transportation) and two community-based service use categories (senior center and congregate meals) are summarized in Table 1. The statistical significance level for all the models is two-tailed since the hypotheses being tested here were non-directional. The table contained the unstandardized regression coefficients and its *p*-value. R^2 value, the coefficient of determination, indicated the explanatory power of the regression model.

The effects of race/ethnicity and gender were inconsistent across various in-home and community-based service uses. In the multivariate analyses, the variance in explaining the full model by race/ethnicity and gender individually was small. This was also true for the variance in service use explained by the interaction of race/ethnicity and gender.

The findings showed that there were significant gender main effects but no race/ethnicity main effects. Gender had a significant main effect in three models of in-home and community-based service use including housework ($\gamma = 0.70$, $p = 0.000$), delivered meals ($\gamma = 6.04$, $p = 0.021$), and congregate meals ($\gamma = 3.97$, $p = 0.046$). There was one significant term of the interaction effect found for housework service use.

The Effects of Predisposing, Enabling and Needs Factors

In addition to race/ethnicity and gender, predisposing factors, enabling factors, and need factors were found to have varying statistical significance depending on the type of service. These results demonstrate the multi-faceted nature of service use predictors. Predisposing factors were found to have the strongest explanatory power for use of housework services and congregate meals. On the other hand, enabling factors were found to contribute the most to predicting the use of personal care/nursing, home delivered meals, transportation and senior centers. Need factors were found to contribute the least to predicting service use in all the regression models.

For *predisposing factors*, age was a significant predictor for use of personal care/nursing ($\gamma = 0.05$, $p = 0.000$), housework ($\gamma = 0.06$, $p = 0.000$), delivered meals ($\gamma = 0.05$, $p = 0.000$), senior centers ($\gamma = 0.04$, $p = 0.025$), and congregate meals ($\gamma = 0.06$, $p = 0.000$). Transportation was the only service where advanced age was not a predictor of more service use. Martial status was a significant predictor for use of personal care/nursing ($\gamma = 0.70$, $p = 0.000$), housework ($\gamma = 0.93$, $p = 0.000$), delivered meals ($\gamma = 0.55$, $p = 0.003$), and transportation ($\gamma = 0.54$, $p = 0.002$) services. Older people who were not married (separated/divorced, widowed, or never married) were more likely to use these services. Education level predicted variance in the use of personal care/nursing, housework, delivered meals, senior centers and congregate meal services. It did not predict variance in transportation service use. Place of residence was a significant predictor for using personal care/nursing ($\gamma = -0.34$, $p = 0.029$), housework ($\gamma = -0.48$, $p = 0.019$), transportation ($\gamma = 1.11$, $p = 0.000$), senior center ($\gamma = 1.12$, $p = 0.020$), and congregate meals ($\gamma = 0.58$, $p = 0.004$) except delivered meals. Compared with older people living in rural areas, people living in suburban areas were less likely to use personal care/nursing and housework. On the other hand, older people living in urban areas were more likely to use transportation, senior center, and congregate meals services.

Regarding the *enabling factors*, income was rarely found to be associated with service use except for using housework service. Here those with higher incomes used fewer services than those with lower incomes. This finding may be related to the means testing requirements for chore (housekeeping) service programs. Private insurance was another predictor rarely found to be significant in service use except for delivered meals and congregate meals with respondents who had private insurance less likely to use these two services. The number of adult children predicted four in-home services: personal care/nursing ($\gamma = 0.12$, $p = 0.000$), housework ($\gamma = 0.09$, $p = 0.006$), delivered meals ($\gamma = 0.08$, $p = 0.042$), and transportation ($\gamma = 0.11$, $p = 0.005$). Older people with more adult children were more likely to use these services. Living with a caregiver was an important predictor of all services except congregate meals. In each instance, older people living with a caregiver were less likely to use these services.

Social contacts with family and friends also exhibited mixed predictive power. Visits from children were found to be inconsistent across various services. Older people having 30 or more visits by their children/relatives monthly were more likely to use personal care/nursing ($\gamma = 0.64$, $p = 0.000$) and delivered meals ($\gamma = 0.82$, $p = 0.001$) compared to those having only 0–5 visits. Older people having 6–29 visits by their children were less likely to use housework ($\gamma = 0.57$, $p = 0.008$), transportation ($\gamma = -0.57$, $p = 0.015$) and congregate meals ($\gamma = -0.53$, $p = 0.003$). Visits by friends were found to have mixed results across services. Compared with elders having 0–5 visits from friend(s), older people having 30 or more visits were less likely to use personal care/nursing ($\gamma = -0.73$, $p = 0.011$) and more likely to use congregate meals ($\gamma = 1.03$, $p = 0.000$). Older people receiving 6–29 calls by friends were less likely to use delivered meals ($\gamma = -0.71$, $p = 0.004$) and congregate meals ($\gamma = -0.76$, $p = 0.000$) compared with those receiving 0–5 calls from their friends. Those receiving 30 or more calls from their friends were also less likely to use congregate meals ($\gamma = -0.56$, $p = 0.023$) than those receiving 0–5 calls from their friends.

Structural barriers were found to be predictors across both in-home and community-based services. Older people who reported being unaware of a service were less likely to use personal care/nursing ($\gamma = -0.37$, $p = 0.000$), housework ($\gamma = -0.16$, $p = 0.000$), delivered meals ($\gamma = 0.13$, $p = 0.000$), transportation ($\gamma = -0.12$, $p = 0.000$), and senior center ($\gamma = -0.05$, $p = 0.000$) (The regression model of congregate meals did not test structural barriers). In addition, older people who reported having other barriers were less likely to use all these services than were those who reported no barriers.

For the *need factors*, perceived health status was found to be a predictor for all services but the results were mixed. Compared to those reporting excellent health status, older people who reported fair or poor health status were more likely to use in-home services including personal care/nursing, housework, delivered meals and transportation. On the other hand, older people who reported good health were less likely to use two community-based services including senior center ($\gamma = -1.26$, $p = 0.005$) and congregate meals ($\gamma = -0.41$, $p = 0.028$). Number of ADL impairments was found to be associated with utilizing personal care/nursing ($\gamma = 0.09$, $p = 0.010$). Older people with more ADL impairment were more likely to use this service. Number of IADL impairment was found to be associated with utilizing personal care/nursing ($\gamma = 0.17$, $p = 0.000$), housework ($\gamma = 0.16$, $p = 0.001$), delivered meals ($\gamma = 0.13$, $p = 0.016$), and senior centers ($\gamma = 0.16$, $p = 0.021$). Once again, older people with more IADLs impairment were more likely to use these services. Certain predictors, such as Medicare, Medicaid, and cognitive impairment were found to have virtually no predictive significance.

STUDY LIMITATIONS

This study of service use among the U.S. elderly is the first known to this author to examine the interaction effect of race and gender on in-home and community based service use. There are limitations in this study. First, it is a secondary data analysis study. As a result, some variables cannot be tested. For example, even though cultural factors are believed to be important factors in service acceptance, the 1999 NLTCS contained very limited cultural variables. Moreover, no measures on duration of service use were found in the data set. As a result, this study is limited to a cross-sectional point in time. The issue of service utilization changing over times is not examined in this study. Second, analysis of patterns of service use among other ethnic/cultural group was not feasible because the size of other ethnic groups in the sample was too small for group comparisons. Third, this study excluded proxy interviews because the respondents were unable to finish the interview. It excluded the most impaired elders living in the community. Forth, the NLTCS data did not contain all variables which might be associated with race and gender. Within the constraints of this limitation, only one of the six regression models run had a statistically significant interaction effect. This was the model predicting housework service use where elder white women were more likely to use housework services than were their male counterparts. This result was similar to that of Miner's study (1995) which reported that older white women were more likely to use housework compared with older white men.

DISCUSSION

Race was not found to have a significant effect on service use in this study confirming the findings of earlier studies (Calsyn & Winter, 1999, 2000; Choi, 1994; Ettner, 1994; Logan & Spitze, 1994; Miner et al., 1993; Wallace et al., 1998) even though this finding contradicted other studies that have shown race to have an effect on service use (Calsyn & Roades, 1993; Mitchell, 1995; Mitchell et al., 1997; Mitchell & Krout, 1998). One possible explanation for this variation in effect is differences in national versus local samples (Miller et al., 1996). Another possible reason is samples drawn from different geographic areas of residence. For instance, black elders were more likely to live in urban areas than their white counterparts. As a result, an analysis of national data sets may not be able to capture the racial differences on community-based long-term care service use (Miller et al., 1996). In addition to these issues, race/ethnicity is a complex variable that it could be considered an indicator of cultural identity or socioeconomic status (Pan et al., 1999). As a result, Miller et al. (1994) have suggested that examining the effect race/ethnicity on service use should include contextual differences such as cultural norms, family traditions, and local community values. In future studies, these contextual differences should be considered as well as how individual behaviors, family structure, and policy requirements impact service accessibility, acceptability, and availability. The discrepancies in the effect of race on service use indicate that elder program planners are wise to take into account racial, cultural and geographic factors in determining program service needs.

In terms of in-home and community-based service use, the results of group comparisons varied more by gender than by race/ethnicity. The finding that women were more likely to use community based services may be due to the fact that older women are reported to be much frailer in general and to have a longer life expectancy (Parrott, 2002). These findings indicate that professionals working with the elderly need to be attuned to women possibly being at greater risk of needing these services than are older men. They also indicate that long-term care policy should review and re-think the present gender-neutral direction in order to avoid gender-specific outcomes that are harmful or inequitable due to the special needs of older women (Parrott, 2002). Policy and planning in long term care needs to address the impact of gender based roles on elderly women and how their financial and health status in old age impact their unique in-home and community based service needs. It is important that long-term care policies consider expanding publicly funded coverage of disability prevention and routine home care services. Expanded public and private sector coverage of in-home and community non-medical assistance with the activities of daily living for women as they age is another vital long-term care policy issue. Older women dwelling in the community have a higher need for non-medical assistance. The needs of maintaining and expanding the continuum of care, especially in-home and community-based services are necessary in order to maintain these women in their homes at a cost far less than in long-term care institutions.

In this study, enabling factors were found to have the strongest prediction power for three in home (personal care/nursing, home delivered meals, transportation) and one community-based service (senior centers). It is of interest that the financial factors were not found to be very significant in predicting the use of either in-home or community-based services. The variable that most often had the strongest Wald chi-square was whether the elder was living with their caregiver. These results indicated that older people living with a caregiver were less likely to use the in-home and the community based services. This indicates a substitution relationship.

This finding is consistent with other studies of social support and formal service use (Johnson & Wolinsky, 1996; Miner, 1995; Mitchell & Krout, 1998). It may well indicate that the presence of a lay caregiver provides the immediate help elderly people require so that they do not need to seek formal service help in the community. As a result, present policy and programs that support caregivers should be strengthened in order to keep them in the caregiving role and reduce the demands for formal services.

In contrast to previous studies (Burnette & Mui, 1995; Choi, 1994; Ettner, 1994), this study found older people with more adult children to have a positive association with service use across most of the services. This may be due to the fact that adult children play an advocate role for their elderly parents by gathering information and seeking different services in the community (Davitt et al., 2002). As a result, to improve both awareness of and access to formal services, providers need to promote their services to both elders and their caregivers.

Why inconsistent findings of the effect on service use of visits/calls from family/friends is unclear. What is uncertain from this study is whether these inconsistent associations by service category is due to the overall health of the elder resulting in both more family visits and the need for more nursing and personal care services. The frequency of friends' visits also showed a mixed effect on service use. The impact of contact with family and friends may well have different service use outcomes between health functional services (such as personal care/nursing) and services related to socialization (such as senior centers or congregate meals). Social support has been reported to maximize advocacy efforts with community-based services (Davitt et al., 2002). While it was beyond the ability of this data set to test if certain services were being accessed and/or provided for the elder by family or friends, the important relationship of family/friend social support and service use was confirmed. In the best interest of assisting older people who might be in need of, but do not receive, in-home and community based services, social workers and/or long-term care service providers need to reach out to both the older person and also to their informal support network. In this manner awareness and accessibility of services can be advanced. From a long-term care policy perspective, this raises the question of whether in-formal caregiver needs should be considered when targeting and reimbursing in home and community services (Houde, 1998). If family caregivers as an important social support can be reimbursed or supported, it would enhance their ability and interest in providing care to their older family members.

Another important aspect of this study was the examination of the impact of structural barriers on service use. In multivariate analysis, structural barriers including not being aware of services and other barriers (unavailability, unaffordable, and inaccessibility) were significantly associated with less service use across all services (note: congregate meals did not test this variable). This result was consistent with previous studies (Calsyn & Roades, 1993; Calsyn & Winter, 1999; Mitchell, 1995). The process of using a continuum of long-term care depends on obtaining the appropriate level of care. The presence of structural barriers can reduce the quality of care received at any point along this continuum (Wallace, 1990). If in-home and community-based services are an important part of long-term care, continued attention to reducing use barriers is necessary. Long-term care policies should evaluate the organizational adequacy of the in-home and community service system in order to eliminate structural barriers such as awareness, affordability and accessibility. At the community level, attention needs to be focused on outreach to clients who might lack knowledge of available services. In addition, elders and their families' needs to become familiar with when services are needed, service eligibility requirements and the procedures of enrollment (Yeatts et al., 1992). Service providers need to be sensitive to barriers that may exist among the elders in their catchments area and to develop strategies for overcoming these barriers. For instance, information on programs/services can easily be disseminated through the use of public media, the use of other providers across the health service continuum, the use of groups and social gatherings as well as the use of significant individuals in the community. Agency staff can also assist in overcoming the knowledge barriers through public education and outreach.

It is hoped that this study can provide a reference point for the place of race/ethnicity and gender in the utilization of in-home and community-based long term care services. Understanding the utilization of in-home and community-based services help policy makers and service providers assist elders with needs more effectively and efficiently.

ACKNOWLEDGMENTS

I thank Professor Ada Mui at Columbia University School of Social Work for her consultation and statistical advice. Special thanks to Center for Demographic Studies, Duke University for releasing the National Long-Term Care Survey Data.

REFERENCES

Andersen, R. M., & Newman, J. F. (1973). Societal and individual determinants of medical care utilization in the United States. *Milbank Memorial Fund Quarterly, 51*, 95–124.

Burnette, D., & Mui, A. C. (1995). In-home and community-based service utilization by three groups of elderly Hispanics: A national perspective. *Social Work Research, 19*, 197–206.

Cagney, K. A., & Agree, E. M. (1999). Racial differences in skilled nursing care and home health use: The mediating effects of family structure and social class. *Journal of Gerontology: Social Sciences, 54B*, 223–236.

Calsyn, R. J., & Roades, L. A. (1993). Predicting perceived service need, service awareness, and service utilization. *Journal of Gerontology Social Work, 21*, 59–76.

Calsyn, R. J., & Winter, J. P. (1999). Who attends senior centers? *Journal of Social Service Research, 26*, 53–69.

Calsyn, R. J., & Winter, J. P. (2000). Predicting different types of service use by the elderly: The strength of the behavioral model and the value of interaction terms. *The Journal of Applied Gerontology, 19*, 284–303.

Cantor, M. H. (1979). Neighbors and friends: An overlooked resource in the informal support system. *Research on Aging, 1*, 434–463.

Choi, N. G. (1994). Patterns and determinants of social service utilization: Comparison of the childless elderly and elderly parents living with or apart from their children. *The Gerontologist, 34*, 353–362.

Davitt, J. K., Kaye, L. W., Bagati, D., & Graub, P. (2002). Beneficiary profiles and service consumption patterns in an urban Medicaid home and community-based waiver program. *Care Management Journals, 3*, 84–90.

Ettner, S. L. (1994). The effect of the Medicaid home care benefit on long-term care choices of the elderly. *Economic Inquiry, 32*, 103–127.

Feder, J., Komisar, H. L., & Niefeld, M. (2000). Long-term care in the United States: An overview. *Health Affairs, 19*, 40–56.

Federal Interagency Forum on Aging-related statistics (2000). *Older Americans 2000: Key indicators of well-being.* Washington, DC: U.S. Government Printing Office.

Houde, S. C. (1998). Predictors of elders' and family caregivers' use of formal home services. *Research in Nursing and Health, 21*, 533–543.

Jackson, S. A., & Mittelmark, M. B. (1997). Unmet needs for formal home and community services among African American and White older adults: The Forsyth County Aging Study. *The Journal of Applied Gerontology, 16*, 298–316.

Johnson, R. J., & Wolinsky, F. D. (1996). Use of community-based long-term care services by older adults. *Journal of Aging and Health, 8*, 512–537.

Logan, J. R., & Spitze, G. (1994). Informal support and the use of formal services by older, Americans. *Journal of Gerontology: Social Sciences, 49*, 25–34.

Miller, B., Campbell, R. T., Davis, L., Furner, S., Giachello, A., Prohaska, T., Kaufman, J. E., Li, M., & Perez, C. (1996). Minority use of community long-term care services: A comparative analysis. *Journal of Gerontology: Social Sciences, 51b*, S70–S81.

Miller, V., McFall, S., & Campbell, R. T. (1994). Changes in sources of community long-term care among African American and white frail older persons. *Journal of Gerontology: Social Sciences, 49*, S14–S24.

Miner, S. (1995). Racial differences in family support and formal service utilization among older persons: A nonrecursive model. *Journal of Gerontology: Social Sciences, 50B*, 143–153.

Miner, S., Logan, J. R., & Spitze, G. (1993). Predicting the frequency of senior center attendance. *The Gerontologist, 33*, 650–657.

Mitchell, J. (1995). Service awareness and use among older North Carolinians. *The Journal of Applied Gerontology, 14*, 193–209.

Mitchell, J., & Krout, J. A. (1998). Discretion and service use among older adults: The behavioral model revisited. *The Gerontologist, 38*, 159–168.

Mitchell, J., Mathews, H. F., & Griffin, L. W. (1997). Health and community-based service use: Differences between elderly African Americans and White. *Research on Aging, 19,* 199–222.

Mui, A. C., & Burnette, D. (1994). Long-term care service use by frail elders: Is ethnicity a factor? *The Gerontologist, 34,* 190–198.

Pan, C. X., Glynn, R. J., Mogun, H., Choodnovskiy, I., & Avorn, J. (1999). Definition of race and ethnicity in older people in Medicare and Medicaid. *Journal of American Geriatrics Society, 47,* 730–733.

Parrott, T. M. (2002). Bringing gender into our discussion of policy issues. *Gerontology and Geriatrics Education, 22,* 57–67.

Scanlon, W. J. (1998). Future financing of long-term care. *Consumers' research,* June, 16–19.

Wallace, S. P. (1990). The no-care zone: Availability, accessibility, and acceptability in community-based long-term care. *The Gerontologist, 30,* 254–261.

Wallace, S. P., Campbell, K., & Lew-Ting, C. Y. (1994). Structural barriers to the use of formal in-home services by elderly Latinos. *Journal of Gerontology: Social Sciences, 49,* 253–263.

Wallace, S. P., Levy-Storm, L., Kington, R. S., & Andersen, R. M. (1998). The persistence of race and ethnicity in the use of long-term care. *Journal of Gerontology: Social Sciences, 53B,* 104–112.

Ward, R. A., Sherman, S. R., & LaGory, M. (1984). Informal networks and knowledge of services for older persons. *Journal of Gerontology, 39,* 216–223.

Wiener, J. M., & Stevenson, D. G. (1997). *Long-term care for the elderly and state health policy* (Vol. 2001). Urban Institute.

Yeatts, D., Crow, T., & Folts, E. (1992). Service use among low-income minority elderly: Strategies for overcoming barriers. *The Gerontologist, 32,* 24–32.

SERVICE SYSTEM INTEGRATION: PANACEA FOR CHRONIC CARE POPULATIONS?

Teresa L. Scheid

ABSTRACT

Chronic illnesses require long term, ongoing medical care as well as the provision of a variety of social support services. These diverse systems of care need to be integrated. However, under managed care, health care systems adhere to a disease model where emphasis is placed upon cure rather than care. While managed care can increase system coordination, the logic of cost containment favors acute services over the long term supportive services needed by chronic care clients. In this paper I describe efforts in one community which has received funding to integrate services for individuals with chronic mental illness as well as a planning grant to integrate multiple chronic care systems (HIV, mental health, and substance abuse) for minority clients. I describe various models of system integration and how diverse systems can be coordinated. In the conclusion I examine the barriers to system integration and argue that sociologists need to play a stronger role in understanding systems of care.

Chronic Care, Health Care Systems and Services Integration
Research in the Sociology of Health Care, Volume 22, 141–158
Copyright © 2004 by Elsevier Ltd.
All rights of reproduction in any form reserved
ISSN: 0275-4959/doi:10.1016/S0275-4959(04)22008-7

INTRODUCTION

Existing sociological research on chronic illness has focused on the experiences of the individual (Bury, 2000; Charmaz, 1991). By their nature, chronic illnesses require long term, ongoing medical care as well as the provision of a variety of social support services. Individuals with chronic are needs must access a number of diverse systems of care – formal and informal, medical and social. These diverse systems of care and support need to be integrated in order for the health care needs of those with chronic illnesses to be met (Schlesinger & Mechanic, 1993). According to the National Coalition for on Health Care (www.nchc.org), by 2030 one half of all Americans will have one or more chronic care conditions. Consequently, there has been a recent resurgence of concern with coordination of health care systems (see Health Affairs, 2001, Vol. 20(6) for a series of articles on chronic illness and coordination of care) with a particular focus on long term care populations and the elderly.

At the same time that the number of individuals with chronic care needs has increased, the health care sector has undergone profound organizational change in response to wider social forces promoting the corporatization and commodification of health care (Alexander & D'Aunno, 1990; Light, 1997; Scott et al., 2000). Managed care has been the organizational response in the U.S. to these larger forces, and has been propelled by an over-riding concern to control costs (Wholey & Burns, 2000). With managed care, decisions to reimburse health services are based upon external determinations of "medical necessity." A health condition must have a valid medical diagnosis, result in impaired functioning, and treatment must be effective and justified by the professional literature as efficacious. Treatment is expected to result in some measurable improvement, if not ultimately in "cure." Managed care is obviously designed for acute health problems which meet the condition of medical necessity. However, the experience of chronic illnesses has superceded acute health care problems (Mechanic, 1995) and chronic illness is now the primary reason that most people seek care (Anderson et al., 2001). Managed care imposes a medical model on care systems; however, sociologists have argued that the diagnostic disease model is not appropriate for the care of chronic illnesses (Kleinman, 1988; Mechanic, 1995; Strauss et al., 1985). While managed care has the potential to increase system coordination and efficiency (Feder & Moon, 1998), there is concern that integration will favor acute medical services over the long term supportive services needed by clients (Cohen, 1998).

Integration by itself is a "panacea" – it is offered as the cure to the problems of the healthcare system, without realistic understanding that the integration of inadequate and under-funded systems of care will not improve healthcare. In this paper I discuss a project which was funded to develop a plan to integrate multiple chronic care systems (HIV disease, mental health, and substance abuse) for minority clients. The community had prior experience with funded programs to integrate services for clients with mental illnesses, and I briefly describe these experiences before turning to a consideration of the integration of HIV, mental health (MH) and substance abuse (SA) systems. I will proceed by first presenting the case for integration (i.e. coordination of care and organizational efficiencies), and examining various ways that systems can be integrated.

THE THEORETICAL CASE FOR SYSTEM INTEGRATION

Service system integration is defined in terms of inter-organizational relationships or "network" ties between agencies in a given sector. Inter-organizational relationships help organizations manage their agencies' interdependencies (Longest, 1990). More critically for chronic care populations, integration enables individuals with diverse service needs to access needed services. Integration can occur at various levels: the client level with the coordination of clinical care; the organizational level with HMOs and other "one-stop shop" models of care and different types of vertical or horizontal integration between organizational units (such as networks of hospitals and community agencies); the system level with some kind of over-riding authority over the all the organizations in a given sector.

Most studies of integration focus on organizational integration, often with the hospital as the center of control. An example is Charns (1997) who describes four stages to the development of Healthcare Integrated Systems. There is first competition and little interdependence among hospitals. A system of pooled interdependencies results in horizontal integration, which is followed by sequential interdependencies (vertical integration). The final stage, community health care, involves reciprocal interdependencies which are achieved via integrated management. Scott et al. (2000) also identify medical groups and insurance companies as possible sources of control for integrated systems. While organizational units may be linked (and consolidation and privatization are producing a number of consolidated healthcare systems), they are not necessarily integrated such that the individual client is able to access different systems of care in order to meet diverse medical and supportive needs.

In contrast to integration, service system fragmentation occurs when there are categorical funding streams that pay for one type of service, but not another, and/or when service agencies focus on only one type of problem or illness (Provan & Sebastian, 1998). Individuals with chronic care conditions need integrated medical and social support services because they have multiple needs and are generally unable to navigate an unintegrated service system on their own (Provan & Sebastian, 1998). In a competitive environment, organizations with limited resources need to form inter-organizational ties with one another (D'Aunno & Zuckerman, 1987; Longest, 1990; Zuckerman & D'Aunno, 1990). Integrated systems also maximize organizational efficiencies by ensuring that services are not duplicated within a given system and enabling agencies to pool resources. Another advantage of inter-organizational linkages is enhanced opportunities for organizational learning and innovation (Goes & Park, 1997).

Leutz (1999) identifies three levels of integration:

(1) Linkage: Where providers are able to refer their clients to another provider to meet the diverse needs of clients.
(2) Coordination: Explicit organizational arrangements are used to coordinate care throughout the system.
(3) Full Integration: New programs or entities are created which allow for the pooling of resources.

More generally, linkages involve informal sharing and communication about programs, services, and clients between agencies while coordination involves formalized collaboration that operates informally via partnerships, written agreements, staff cross training, and shared information systems (Marquart & Konrad, 1996). Full integration can be achieved by either a consolidation of services where some services are centralized within an umbrella organization, but agencies retain authority over their services or via the development of a single authority which operates collectively (Marquart & Konrad, 1996).

In order to determine which level of integration is necessary, the client population must be analyzed in terms of the severity, stability, and duration of the illness, the urgency and scope of services required, and client's ability for self direction (Leutz, 1999). Informal linkages will work for populations with mild to moderate disabilities; coordination is best suited for those with moderate to severe conditions where care is routine; full integration is necessary for populations with long term disabilities.

The most familiar argument for system integration is Shortell et al. (1996) *Remaking Health Care in America*. The third element of the author's ideal health system is that care is coordinated and integrated across the continuum of care. Systems of care must be holistic in that the "whole" must exist before it can be embedded in each part. Integration will not occur by merely bringing together the parts of the system, rather integration is both a cause and effect of holistic care. Shortell et al. (1996, p. 30) identify three mechanisms by which care can be integrated in such a way as to produce holistic systems of care:

(1) Functional Integration: Where key support functions (information systems, financial management, planning, quality assurance) are coordinated across

all of the operating organizations in the system. Scott et al. (2000) identify functional with horizontal integration as well as diversification.

(2) Physician-system Integration: Where physicians are economically linked to the system and are active participants in planning, management, and governance. There are four types of physician system integration: physician-hospital organizations, management services organizations, medical foundations, and integrated healthcare organizations (Shortell et al., 1996; Scott et al., 2000).

(3) Clinical Integration: Where patient care services are coordinated across people, functions, and operating units so as to maximize the value of services delivered. Scott et al. (2000) note that clinical integration involves vertical integration.

For populations with chronic care conditions who see many providers (Anderson et al., 2001 found that individuals with one or more chronic conditions see eight different doctors during a year), physician and clinical integration is critical to receiving basic care. However, for care to be coordinated at the provider level (i.e. where services are received and from whom they are received) financial and functional integration is necessary. This is little more than repeated the oft cited bailiwick that "form follows financing." Clinical care cannot be integrated if organizations are separated by competition for scarce funding, different management structures, different client information systems, and specialization of function. Populations with long term disabilities and chronic health problems need a number of specialized interventions and coordination between knowledgeable professionals. Clearly the first obstacle to successful integration is determine whether the chicken – clinical integration, proceeds or follows the egg – functional integration (Leutz, 1999).

A second major barrier to integration is that efforts to coordinate care are not reimbursable (Anderson & Knickman, 2001). Consequently, managed care represents a major barrier to individual level integration (i.e. case management). At the organizational and systems level, integration must overcome the barriers of vested interests and categorical funding. Furthermore, diverse provider groups must agree on philosophies of care as well as standards of care (Cohen, 1998; Vladeck, 2001). Integration is best viewed as a process (rather than an outcome) which involves the sustained commitment of organizations, providers, and fiscal supports. Before I describe one systematic effort to develop a plan to integrate diverse chronic care systems, I describe efforts in the same community to integrate services for individuals with severe mental illnesses.

PUBLIC SECTOR MENTAL HEALTH

The public mental health system is the safety net, and serves those clients whose care is reimbursed by Medicaid and other forms of public support (Frank et al.,

1997; Institute of Medicine, 1997). Clients served by public mental health systems are often indigent, and consequently face a number of social problems related to poverty as well as their own mental illness. Clients in the public sector also face more serious, debilitating mental illness (for example in the public sector system described here, 58% of the clients are Black, 69% of all clients have schizophrenia, and 19% have bipolar or major depression).

Funding for mental health care has never been adequate to deal with the multiple needs of those with severe mental illness, and service system integration has been the solution to improve service delivery. Case management and multi-disciplinary treatment teams attempt to integrate services at the individual level, while Community Support Systems and Assertive Community Treatment programs seek to coordinate care among different agencies. Full integration was propelled by the Robert Wood Johnson Program on Chronic Mental Illness (PCMI) which established centralized authorities to provide coordinated care (Shore & Cohen, 1990, 1994). The Mecklenburg County Mental Health System was one of nine demonstration projects funded by the PCMI in 1986, and I have been conducting research at the mental health authority since 1991. The mental health system received five years of grants, low-interest lows, and federal rent subsidies (Section 8s) to develop an integrated, effective system of care for individuals with chronic mental illnesses. Local mental health authorities were to take clinical, fiscal, and administrative responsibility for services in order to coordinate and integrate diverse services (Morrissey, 1999). Local authorities are systems of integration imposed from above, rather than built from a negotiated consensus of agencies and participants.

Despite a number of complications, and different sets of problems faced by the other eight sites, local authorities were successfully implemented (Morrissey et al., 1994). However, changes in the community support systems were less apparent. In Mecklenburg County, there was a 23% increase in system performance as assessed by key stakeholders, but only a 15% increase in the community support system (Morrissey & Calloway, 1994). While there was noticeable improvement in service offerings at all the sites (due to increased funding), there was no appreciable effect of system integration on client outcomes as measured by psychosocial functioning, housing, continuity of care, and quality of life (Lehman et al., 1994).

What about 10 years after the end of the PCMI funding? Mecklenburg remains one of the most well funded mental health programs in North Carolina, and the system of care developed during the PCMI funding is largely intact. Treatment teams are still organized to provide coordinated care via case management, and housing and social supports are maintained by a system of contracts with both private and public agencies who provide the full continuum of care. However, Mecklenburg has moved to a managed care model (Scheid, 2003) and the data I have collected in 1998 and 2000 to analyze the effect of managed care on services indicates that providers are not able to provide the treatment or services that their clients need, there has been a declining organizational commitment to the fundamentals of community based care, and that providers have raised serious questions about the quality of care.

While in 1998 providers at the Area Authority felt that managed care had the potential to integrate delivery systems, increase accountability, and to widen access to under-served populations, two years later the only benefits of managed care were felt to be cost-containment and increased accountability. While some providers felt managed care affords an opportunity to develop a better system of mental health services (17.8%), a larger proportion disagreed with this statement (35.5%). Close to 80% disagreed that managed care had improved the quality of care; 64.4% disagreed that clinical outcomes had improved, and slightly over 50% felt that managed care inevitably results in under service to clients. Mental health providers believe that the institutional logic of cost containment (operationalized as the use of financial considerations to manage care) has resulted in reduced use of community based services, reduced duration of treatment, less intensive treatment, a greater reliance on psychiatric medication than providers would prefer, and reduced lengths of outpatient care for clients.

Change in the service orientation of the Area Authority (as measured by the Community Philosophy Program Scale) between 1998 and 2000 support provider's perceptions that managed care is having a negative effect on the services available to their clients (Scheid, 2003). On every dimension of the CPPS, there was less emphasis on the provision of community based care in 2000. In terms of integration, there was significantly less emphasis on outreach to clients in the community, housing assistance, referral advocacy, and emergency access.

A more recent effort to integrate services for Homeless Persons with Serious Mental Illness (the ACCESS project) was also conducted in Mecklenburg County within the Area Mental Health Authority (in fact, staff at ACCESS completed my questionnaire about managed mental health care). The ACCESS demonstration involved 18 communities in nine states (one site in each state was randomly assigned to services enhancement plus system integration and the other was assigned to the control group of services enhancement only). The sites were funded for four years (1994–1998).

In terms of approaches to system integration, 12 strategies were developed and were to be used by the sites to integration their services. These strategies include the development of an interagency coordinating body, co-location of services, systems integration coordination position, cross-training of providers, interagency agreements, interagency management information systems, pool/joint funding, uniform intake and eligibility, interagency delivery teams, flexible funding, use of special waivers, and consolidation of agencies. In order to measure whether system integration had improved, respondents were asked to evaluate client referrals, joint funding, and information exchanges with other agencies in the services network. While the ACCESS grantee organization did increase its inter-organizational linkages to other network organizations, overall the network had less integration (and Mecklenburg experienced a greater *loss* of total network integration than the other eight integration sites). However, system performance (as measured by stakeholders' evaluations of the accessibility, availability, and coordination of services) was greater at Mecklenburg than at the other sites.

In the final assessments of the ACCESS project, Morrissey et al. (2002) concludes that system level integration did not significantly change, although project integration (i.e. the integration of the ACCESS grantee organization with other agencies in the network) did improve. This was exactly the experience in Mecklenburg. Researchers also found that while service system integration can be improved, these efforts do not produce better client outcomes (Goldman et al., 2002). The ACCESS project was also a top-down strategy for improving system integration (as was the RWJPCMI), and Morrissey et al. (2002) suggest that a bottom-up approach may be more effective. For example, there was evidence that the use of community treatment teams increased integration and did not require system level interventions. I now turn to my own involvement with efforts to integrate services in Mecklenburg County for minority populations at risk for HIV/AIDS with co-occurring mental health and substance abuse problem; this time the integration effort was decidedly bottom-up.

INTEGRATING MULTIPLE CHRONIC CARE SYSTEMS FOR MINORITY CLIENTS

In October of 2000, the County Public Health Department (with whom I had been working to obtain funding for professional cross-training) obtained a planning grant to integrate services to minority populations at risk for HIV disease with co-occurring mental health and substance abuse problems. The planning grant provided $ 150,000 for $1\frac{1}{2}$ years and specifically targeted the active participation of consumers in the planning process. Only six sites were funded; Mecklenburg was the only single county system to be funded, but also the only urban SMSA.

As has been well documented, Blacks and Hispanics are at higher risk for new infections of HIV (www.niaid.nih.gov/factsheets?minor.htlm). As of June 2000, African Americans and Hispanics represented 62% of AIDS case reported among men and 81% among women. Infection drug use is a major factor in the spread of HIV in minority communities, accounting for 37% of all AIDS cases in both

African Americans and Hispanics through June 2000. Yet minority groups report significant barriers to care (Phillips et al., 2000), in large part due to a lack of cultural accessibility. Anderson et al. (2000), in analysis of a national probability sample of those in treatment for HIV, found that those vulnerable groups (i.e. women, injection drug users, African Americans, and those with lower educational levels) were last likely to gain early access to HAART medications.

Individuals with mental illness are also at risk for HIV (Carey et al., 1995; Cournos & Bakalar, 1996; IOM, 1994; NIMH, 1991) because of their risky behaviors, including multiple sex partners, use of alcohol or drugs, intravenous drug use, coercion into unwanted sexual activity, and unprotected sex (Coverdale, 1996; Knox et al., 1994; Rosenberg et al., 2001; Weinhardt et al., 1998). Rosenberg et al. (2001) reported higher rates of HIV infection (5.2–22.9%) among individuals with severe mental illness than the entire population (0.3–9.4%). This is because of the direct effects of severe mental illness (affective and cognitive) and the indirect effects (i.e. homelessness) as well as co-occurring substance abuse (Rosenberg et al., 2001). Consequently, individuals with mental illnesses are likely to be triply diagnosed with substance abuse and HIV infection.

Individuals with a positive HIV diagnosis are also at risk for mental health problems (Batki, 1990; Chyrstal & Schlosser, 1999; Simoni & Ng, 2000). In addition to anxiety and depression following a positive HIV diagnosis, HIV seropositivity strains social relationships and supports and results in a great deal of stress due to concern over work status and the experience of ongoing illnesses as well as adherence to complicated drug regimes. Many individuals consider HIV/AIDS to be a death sentence, and are at higher risk for suicide (Chyrstal & Schlosser, 1999).

There is a need for continuity of care and a comprehensive array of services for this target population; however HIV disease, substance abuse, and mental health services are delivered within independent service systems and organizations (Meyerson & Scofield, 1999). Providers generally have expertise in one, perhaps two, areas of disability and illness – either HIV/AIDS, mental health, or substance abuse. Because of the co-occurrence of mental illness and substance abuse, many mental health care providers do have training in substance abuse, although treatment orientations differ (Burton et al., 2001). Mental health and substance abuse providers often lack basic training in HIV/AIDS, and are unsure how to assess their client's risk. HIV/AIDS providers may have some background in either substance abuse or mental health, but may not be able to recognize or deal effectively with their client's substance abuse or mental health problems. Because of heavy caseloads and multiple demands, providers often work in isolation and have limited connections to other types of treatment providers and services.

In order to overcome the limitations of disciplinary isolation, the Charlotte based Regional HIV Consortium (serving a 13 county region in North and South Carolina) sponsored a cross training project referred to as Common Ground. The Common Ground resulted from a needs assessment conducted in 1996 where providers and consumers identified the need to integrate services and provider competencies in order to improve treatment outcomes and the quality of life of multiply diagnosed consumers. As noted earlier, the SAMSHA grant was a result of efforts to fund the Common Ground professional cross training.

I was the formative evaluator for the planning grant, and consequently played a critical role in the development of the integration plan. An Executive Advisory Board (EAB) consisting of representatives of various provider groups and consumers (86 people were on the EAB mailing list) was formed and met monthly to develop a plan. A continuing concern was to bring various minority groups (Black, Hispanic, and Asian) to the table and to elicit active consumer involvement. To this end, and inclusion committee was formed after the first EAB meeting. This committee went out into the community and "brought people to the table." While the majority of the members of the EAB were Black, leaders and consumers from the Hispanic, Asian, and Native American communities were present. There was also diversity in terms of sexual orientation, with consumers and providers who were homosexual, lesbian, or among the group of men who have sex with men. There was ongoing concern to reach out into the community and involve individuals who were not accessing services. Early on it was decided that 50% of the EAB members were to be consumers, a term which included advocates as well as clients. Grant monies were used to help cover consumer expenses to attend meetings, and to provide reimbursement for time spent working with the EAB. In addition, everyone helped with transportation. However, the majority attending the EAB meetings were providers and agency representatives.

Meetings were participatory and early efforts to define a common vision (and ultimately a mission statement) and objectives for attaining that vision were led by a facilitator who ensured the active involvement of everyone at each stage of the planning. In order to develop the mission statement, each of the 40 EAB members attending the workshop was asked to write down the key elements of a mission, their vision, and their beliefs about the EAB. A list of common beliefs was identified, and then individuals were placed into three groups to develop mission statements. All three statements were placed on large poster paper, and considered at length. The "best" one was selected by vote, and then another hour was spent making modifications. At each meeting, the mission statement was read, and time was given for any modifications (several occurred early on).

Following the development of the mission statement, the EAB clarified its role and responsibilities, and ways in which decisions based upon consensus would be made. There were several discussions that illustrated "turf" battles – for example key agencies asked how the EAB was different than the Regional HIV/AIDS Consortium, or from the Health Department. It was agreed that the EAB would work to develop an integration plan, would develop consumer involvement, would identify under-served populations, would recognize other partners and keep them informed, would provide a bridge between agencies and other initiatives, and would help break down "turf."

Before developing an integration plan, the EAB had to develop a map of services and identify gaps in services. Furthermore, there was a need to synthesize existing data and reports in order to identify what information needed to be collected. While data was being collected and assessed, the EAB defined the key elements of an integration plan: prevention, integration, cross-training, and cross cultural access. Subcommittees were developed, and work began on an integration plan that addressed each of these four areas. The process of collecting data, and developing a preliminary plan took most of the spring of 2001, during which the EAB also was planning a community forum. A community forum was one of the features specified in the grant as a means to elicit community participation in the planning process.

The community forum held in a church in a largely minority neighborhood with high rates of HIV/AIDs. The forum began with breakfast, provided lunch, and ended at 4:30. There were 47 participants who attended the morning session and worked in breakout groups. Only ten of these participants were EAB members, so the goal of obtaining increased community involvement was successful. Participation dwindled after lunch, although there were still over 30 participants in the afternoon sessions. 32 participants completed an evaluation instrument, from which we know that the majority of the participants were providers (81%), and that the majority of these providers represented HIV agencies (56.3%). 62% of the respondents were Black, and there were representatives of the Hispanic, Asian, and American Indian communities.

Rather than merely present the preliminary integration plan, the same facilitator who assisted with the development of a mission led the group in the development of its own plan to increase collaboration. The four priority areas (prevention, cross-cultural competence, cross training, and integration) were identified and participants self selected into one of these groups for the morning session. A facilitator was assigned to each group to keep track of the ideas developed and to present that group's "consensus" on gaps in the system and barriers to collaboration to the larger group before lunch. The groups ranged from 16 members (prevention) to 8 members (integration). In the afternoon the groups met again to develop specific strategies to improve the system in terms of their priority area. There was a great deal of overlap with ideas that had been generated and shared at

EAB meetings, and the results of the forum were integrated with the preliminary integration plan.

Following the forum, task groups consisting of consumers and providers were formed around each aspect of the integration plan. These task groups met weekly through the summer to work out the details of the integration plan and to apply for the SAMSHA implementation funding. Other sources of funding were also explored. I was a member of all of the task groups, and brought my understanding of system integration as well as barriers to such integration to the table. I drew heavily upon the guidelines developed by Joe Morrisssey (the Access project) for integrating service systems for homeless persons with severe mental illness and described various strategies for integrating service systems. I helped the group to determine current levels of system integration, and to determine what level of integration was ideal and which was feasible. The final plan specifies an overall objective of treating and educating as many HIV/SA/MH clients and potential clients as quickly as possible through a client centered holistic approach, and where the current system of cooperation (the existing level of integration) would move toward a more integrated state with an interagency coordinating body, multi-disciplinary, multi-agency case management teams, cross training of providers and consumers, culturally appropriate and sensitive materials, and an emphasis on prevention and outreach to minority populations at risk for HIV disease.

In terms of the level of integration desired, consumers actively sought the one-shop model where all of their health care needs could be met at one place. Providers found this system of care idealistic, and were also opposed to various types of consolidation where there was some centralization of authority. This opposition had two sources: conflict between the two obvious choices for an umbrella organization, and concern that organizational specialization and inefficiencies of either umbrella organization would be replicated. The model agreed upon by both providers and consumers as that of "no wrong door" in that whatever agency a consumer might turn to, they would be able to obtain the full array of services needed. Consequently, the integration plan reflects a more practical orientation toward collaboration which would be achieved by the development of a coordinator position, an inter agency multi-disciplinary treatment team, professional cross training, and common standards of care.

However, SAMSHA was not able to provide implementation monies (due to a change of political environment) and the integration plan was not funded. Consequently, formal integration has not occurred. Nor were the members of the EAB been able to arrive at consensus for local efforts to achieve integration beyond continued cross-training. Without additional funding, key agencies were not supportive of the multi-agency, multi-disciplinary treatment team as they did not want to give up ownership of their clients, nor could they afford to let key staff take time to work on an interagency treatment team. Stakeholders also feared a coordinator position would simply add on another layer of bureaucracy and raised questions about where such a position would be housed. Without additional funding, agencies could not take on any more work, although it is obvious that the existence of the EAB and the time spent planning improved system level coordination in a number of ways.

After the grant ended the EAB continued to meet, and it was decided this body should be a consumer run advisory board. However, consumers did not step up to the plate, and the board came to an end. Providers have continued to meet in a variety of ways, and recently spent a great deal of time preparing a strategic plan on HIV disease in Mecklenburg County that has been presented to the County Commissioners in an ongoing effort to confront the problems posed by HIV and the inability of the existing service system to deal with the growing need. Many of the same faces were at the table, and the process was once again inclusive and grass roots, with strong consumer representation and involvement. The key components of the integration plan were evident in the strategic plan: integrated service delivery with mental health and substance abuse, enhancement of existing levels of collaboration among providers, linguistic and cultural competency, an emphasis on prevention and outreach.

DISCUSSION

Was grass roots integration a failure? This is a difficult question to answer. It is clear that formal mechanisms for integration were not put into place, largely because of the lack of funding for the key components of the integration plan. However, had funding been available, there were key debates over who would have controlled these funds, and hence who would control the process of integration. While many assumed the Health Department was the logical place to house the coordinator position as well as the multi-agency, multi-disciplinary team, other agencies and many consumers were wary of the bureaucratic policies of the Health Department. Furthermore, providers were not willing to hand their clients over to a coordinator that did not operate within their agency or to another case management team. In short, while grass roots consensus was reached at a variety of levels, issues of governance and authority for system integration as identified by Konrad (1996) were not resolved. This failure was due to pre-existing domain disputes which were not resolved, largely because these disputes arise from functional specialization between providers which are maintained by inadequate categorical funding streams. Limited resources and inadequate funding was early recognized as a key problem, for which no easy solution exists.

Is system integration a panacea? If thought of as an outcome, it is clear that existing studies of system integration have not led to improved client level outcomes (Goldman et al., 2002; Rosenbeck et al., 2001). However, it is important to think about integration outcomes at the system level, rather than merely at the client level (Lohrmann et al., 1997). Furthermore, system integration may not lead to any noticeable improvements in client outcomes, if such outcomes are defined in terms of functional improvement or improved health. By their nature, chronic conditions often involve at best periods of respite followed by exacerbation or decline, rather than continued improvement. There are also multiple factors that affect individual outcomes, which cannot be controlled in evaluations of system integration.

It is probably more critical to determine whether integration makes the provision of care *better* for the provider. Does the HIV provider know who to call for a mental health referral, or for substance abuse treatment? Is the mental health provider comfortable discussing HIV disease, and does this person know where to send a client for testing? Does the infectious disease clinic know how to assess for mental illness, so that they do not prescribe medications that may interact with medications for schizophrenia or depression? Can the substance abuse provider overcome professional biases against harm reduction models and work with HIV providers to get their clients on HIV medication and treatment? This is the true measure of system integration, and it is providers who must recognize, and work to overcome, turf battles. As noted by one EAB member in the final evaluation, there is "naiveté about hidden agendas" among providers.

If thought of as a process (Hassett & Austin, 1997), integration is certainly *not* a panacea. Interagency teams and coordinating councils have been found to foster greater inter-organizational exchanges (Foster-Fishman et al., 2001), and community based programs lead to stronger inter-organizational relationships (McGuire et al., 2002). While the EAB disbanded, providers have continued to work collaboratively with consumers to improve the system. Continued engagement to achieve common purposes can potentially overcome domain disputes and open the door for more systematic efforts to integrate the diverse services needed by minority populations at risk for HIV disease. Any type of attempt to integrate services brings people to the table, where information and ideas can be exchanged, and it is this exchange of information that is the core element of an integrated system.

However, managed care also works against system integration and makes it harder, if not impossible, for providers to work effectively together. The Bazelon Center for Mental Health Law (2000) has found that managed care undermines system integration due to incentives to shift costs. The only way in which a managed care system can attain integration is with some form of centralized authority which manages the entire pool of resources for the diverse services needed by chronic care populations. Otherwise, categorical funding streams, different eligibility criteria, and diverse client information systems work against any form of clinical integration. More fundamentally, managed care is based upon a medical model with a focus on short term treatment for acute conditions, or else crises intervention. The future of the health care system is uncertain, and time will tell if managed care can meet the challenges of chronic illness and long term care.

Medical sociologists need to move beyond their focus on the individual's experience of illness, and examine the various ways in which systems of care are organized (or not) to meet the needs of chronic care patients. Flood & Fennell (1995) provide an excellent overview of the various theoretical approaches to organizational change, and Sofaer and Myrtle (1991) provide an overview of inter-organizational theory and research which can guide research and policy in healthcare. While there has been some sociological research on mergers and consolidations among health care organizations (Mohr, 1991; Zuckerman & D'Aunno, 1990), there is little in the sociological literature on how organizational and inter-organizational change can influence patient care or the experience of illness. Estes et al. (1993) provided an excellent model for the kind of systematic research on systems of care sociologists need to be engaged in if we are to have a voice in future policy debates over long term care.

REFERENCES

Alexander, J. A., & D'Aunno, T. A. (1990). Transformation of institutional environments: perspectives on the corporatization of U.S. health care. In: S. S. Mick et al. (Eds), *Innovations in Health Care Delivery* (pp. 53–85). San Francisco: Jossey-Bass.

Anderson, R., Boxette, S. et al. (2000). Access of vulnerable populations to antiretroviral therapy among persons with HIV disease in the U.S. *Health Services Research, 35*, 389–416.

Anderson, G., & Knickman, J. R. (2001). Changing the chronic care system to meet people's needs. *Health Affairs, 20*, 146–160.

Anderson, R., Smedby, B., & Vagero, D. (2001). Cost containment, solidarity, and cautious experimentation: Swedish dilemmas. *Social Science and Medicine, 52*, 1195–2004.

Batki, S. L. (1990). Substance abuse and AIDS: The need for mental health services. *New Directions in Mental Health Services, 48*, 66–67.

Bazelon Center for Mental Health Law (2000). *Effective public management of mental health care: Views from the states on Medicaid reforms that enhance service integration and accountability.* Washington, DC: Bazelon Center for Mental Health Law.

Burton, D. L., Cox, A. J., & Fleisher-Bond, M. (2001). *Cross training for dual disorders: A comprehensive guide to co-occurring substance use and psychiatric disorders.* New York: Vintage Press.

Bury, M. (2000). On chronic illness and disability. In: C. E. Bird, P. Conrad & A. M. Fremont (Eds), *Handbook of Medical Sociology* (5th ed., pp. 173–199). Upper Saddle River, NJ: Prentice-Hall.

Carey, M. P., Weinhardt, L. S., & Carey, K. B. (1995). Prevalence of HIV infection with HIV among the seriously mentally ill: A review of research and implications for practice. *Professional Psychology: Research and Practice, 26*, 262–268.

Charmaz, K. (1991). *Good days, bad days: The self in chronic illness and time*. New Brunswick, NJ: Rutgers University Press.

Charns, M. P. (1997). Organizational design of integrated delivery systems. *Hospital Health Services Administration, 42*, 411–432.

Chyrstal, S., & Schlosser, L. R. (1999). The HIV-mental health challenge. In: A. V. Horwitz & T. L. Scheid (Eds), *A Handbook for the Study of Mental Health* (pp. 526–549). Cambridge: Cambridge University Press.

Cohen, M. A. (1998). Emerging trends in the finance and delivery of long-term care: Public and private opportunities and challenges. *The Gerontologist, 38*, 80–89.

Cournos, F., & Bakalar, N. (Eds) (1996). *Aids and people with serious mental illness*. New Haven, CT: Yale University Press.

Coverdale, J. (1996). HIV risk behavior in the chronically mentally ill. *International Review of Psychiatry, 8*, 149–157.

D'Aunno, T. A., & Zuckerman, H. S. (1987). The emergence of hospital federations: An integration of perspectives from organization theory. *Medical Care Review, 44*, 323–342.

Estes, C. L., Swan, J. H., & Associates (1993). *The long term care crisis: Elders trapped in the no-care zone*. Newbury Park: Sage.

Flood, A. B., & Fennell, M. L. (1995). Through the lens of organizational sociology: The role of organizational theory and research in conceptualizing and examining our health care system. *Journal of Health and Social Behavior, Extra Issue*, 154–169.

Foster-Fishman, P. G., Salem, D. A., Allen, N. A., & Fahrbach, K. (2001). Facilitating interorganizational collaborations: The contributions of interorganizational alliances. *American Journal of Community Psychology, 29*, 875–905.

Frank, R. G., Koyanagi, C., & McGuire, T. G. (1997). The politics and economics of mental health "parity" laws. *Health Affairs, 16*, 108–120.

Goes, J. B., & Park, S. H. (1997). Interorganizational links and innovation: The case of hospital services. *Academy of Management Journal, 40*, 673–696.

Goldman, H. H., Morrissey, J. P., Rosenbeck, R. A., Cocossa, J., Blasinsky, M., & Randolph, F. (2002). Lessons from the evaluation of the ACCESS program. *Psychiatric Services, 53*, 967–969.

Hassett, S., & Austin, M. J. (1997). Service integration: Something old and something new. *Administration in Social Work, 21*, 9–12.

Institute of Medicine (1997). *Managing managed care: Quality improvement in behavioral health*. Washington, DC: National Academy Press.

Institute of Medicine (1994). *AIDS and behavior: An integrated approach*. Washington, DC: National Academy Press.

Kleinman, A. (1988). *The illness narratives: Suffering, healing and the human condition*. New York: Basic Books.

Knox, M. D., Boaz, T. L., Friedrich, M. A., & Dow, M. G. (1994). HIV risk factors for persons with serious mental illness. *Community Mental Health Journal, 26*, 559–563.

Konrad, E. L. (1996). A multidimensional framework for conceptualizing human services integration initiatives. In: *Evaluating Initiatives to Integrate Human Services* (pp. 5–34). San Francisco, CA: Jossey-Bass.

Lehman, A., Rostrado, L., Roth, D., McNary, S., & Goldman, H. (1994). An evaluation of the continuity of care, case management, and client outcomes in the RWJ program on chronic mental illness. *The Milibank Quarterly, 72*, 105–122.

Leutz, W. N. (1999). Five laws for integrating medical and social services: Lessons from the U.S. and the U.K. *The Milibank Quarterly, 77*, 77–110.

Light, D. W. (1997). The rhetoric and realities of community health care: The limits of countervailing powers to meet the health care needs of the twenty-first century. *Journal of Health Politics, Policy and Law, 22*, 106–145.

Lohrmann, G., Keyte, B., & LaFalce, M. B. (1997). Achieving functional integration: A continuum case study. *Healthcare Finance Management, 51*, 35–39.

Longest, B. B. (1990). Inter-organizational linkages in the health sector. *Health Care Management Review, 15*, 17–28.

Marquart, J. M., & Konrad, E. L. (1996). *Evaluating initiatives to integrate human services.* San Francisco, CA: Jossey-Bass.

McGuire, J., Rosenheck, R., & Burnette, C. (2002). Expanding service delivery: Does it improve relationships among agencies serving homeless people with mental illness? *Administrative Policy in Mental Health, 29*, 243–256.

Mechanic, D. (1995). Sociological dimensions of illness behavior, Social Science. *Social Science & Medicine, 41*, 1207–1216.

Meyerson, B., & Scofield, J. (1999). Getting it together: State agency activity to coordinate substance abuse, mental health, and hiv prevention and treatment services. Abstract 165, 1999 National HIV Prevention Conference.

Morrissey, J. P. (1999). Integrating service delivery systems for persons with severe mental illness. In: A. V. Horwitz & T. L. Scheid (Eds), *A Handbook for the Study of Mental Health* (pp. 449–466). Cambridge: Cambridge University Press.

Morrissey, J. P., & Calloway, M. O. (1994). Local mental health authorities and service system change: Evidence from the Robert Wood Johnson Foundation program on chronic mental illness. *Milibank Quarterly, 72*, 49–80.

Morrissey, J. P., Calloway, M. O., Thakur, N., Cocoza, J., & Steadman, H. J. (2002). Integration of service systems for homeless persons with serious mental illness through the ACCESS program. *Psychiatric Services, 53*, 949–957.

National Institute of Mental Health (1991). *Caring for people with severe mental disorder.* DHHS Pub. No. (ADM) 91-1762. Washington, DC: Superintendent of Documents. U.S. Government Printing Office.

Phillips, K. A., Mayer, M. L., & Aday, L. A. (2000). Barriers to care among racial/ethnic groups under managed care. *Health Affairs, 19*, 65–75.

Provan, K. G., & Sebastian, J. G. (1998). Networks within networks: Service link overlap, organizational cliques, and network effectiveness. *The Academy of Management Journal, 41*, 453–483.

Rosenbeck, R., Morrissey, J., Lam, J., Calloway, M., Stolar, M., Johnsen, M., Randolph, F., Blasinksy, M., & Goldman, H. (2001). Service delivery and community: Social capital, service systems integration, and outcomes among homeless persons with severe mental illness. *Health Services Research, 36*, 691–710.

Rosenberg, S. D., Goodman, L. A., Osher, F. C., Swartz, M. S., Essock, S. M., Butterfield, M. I., Wolford, N. T., & Salyers, M. P. (2001). Prevalence of HIV, Hepatitis B, and Hepatitis C in people with severe mental illness. *American Journal of Public Health, 81*, 31–36.

Scheid, T. L. (2003). Managed care and the rationalization of mental health services. *Journal of Health and Social Behavior, 44*, 142–161.

Schlesinger, M., & Mechanic, D. (1993). Challenges for managed competition from chronic illness. *Health Affairs, 12,* 123–137.

Scott, R. W., Ruef, M., Mendel, P., & Caroneer, C. A. (2000). *Institutional change and organizational transformation of the healthcare field.* Chicago: University of Chicago Press.

Shore, M. F., & Cohen, M. C. (1990). The Robert Wood Johnson Foundation program on chronic mental illness: An overview. *Hospital and Community Psychiatry, 41,* 1212–1229.

Shore, M. F., & Cohen, M. C. (1994). Observations from the program on chronic mental illness. *Health Affairs, 11,* 227–233.

Shortell, S. M., Gilles, R. R., Anderson, D., & Associates (1996). *Remaking health care in America.* San Francisco, CA: Jossey-Bass.

Simoni, J. M., & Ng, M. T. (2000). Trauma, coping, and depression among women with HIV/AIDS in New York City. *AIDS Care, 12,* 567–570.

Sofaer, S., & Myrtle, R. C. (1991). Interorganizational theory and research: Implications for health care management, policy, and research. *Medical Care Review, 48,* 371–409.

Strauss, A., Fagerhaugh, S., Suczek, B., & Wiene, C. (1985). *Social organization of medical work.* Chicago: University of Chicago Press.

Vladeck, B. C. (2001). You can't get there from here: Obstacles to improving care of the chronically ill. *Health Affairs, 20,* 175–179.

Weinhardt, L. S., Carey, M. P., & Carey, K. B. (1998). HIV-Risk behavior and the public health context of HIV/AIDS among women living with severe and persistent mental illness. *Journal of Nervous and Mental Disorder, 186,* 276–282.

Wholey, D. R., & Burns, L. R. (2000). Tides of change: The evolution of managed care in the United States. In: C. E. Bird, P. Conrad & A. M. Fremont (Eds), *Handbook of Medical Sociology* (5th ed., pp. 217–237). Upper Saddle River, NJ: Prentice-Hall.

Zuckerman, H. S., & D'Aunno, T. A. (1990). Hospital alliances: Cooperative strategy in competitive environment. *Health Care Management Review, 15,* 21–30.

SENSE OF COHERENCE AND MENTAL HEALTH SERVICE UTILIZATION: THE CASE OF FAMILY CAREGIVERS OF COMMUNITY-DWELLING COGNITIVELY-IMPAIRED SENIORS

Neale R. Chumbler, John Fortney, Marisue Cody and Cornelia Beck

ABSTRACT

The purpose of the present study is to investigate whether family caregivers with a stronger sense of coherence (SOC) who are caring for community dwelling older adults with cognitive impairment are less likely to use mental health services. An adaptation of the Anderson behavioral model of access to health care was employed as a conceptual framework. Data were collected for 304 impaired older adult/family caregiver dyads. Caregiver mental health service use and sense of coherence were measures as well as predisposing factors (age, gender, race, education, type of familial relationship, family size, and co-residence with impaired family member), enabling factors (self-reported awareness of services, travel times to mental health services, social support, and insurance), and need factors (chronic health conditions and distress). The impaired elder's age, level of physical impairment, and level of memory impairment were also examined. Logistic regression results indicated

Chronic Care, Health Care Systems and Services Integration
Research in the Sociology of Health Care, Volume 22, 159–173
Copyright © 2004 by Elsevier Ltd.
All rights of reproduction in any form reserved
ISSN: 0275-4959/doi:10.1016/S0275-4959(04)22009-9

that caregivers who have a stronger SOC were less likely to use mental health services (OR = 0.91, p = 0.006). Other significant independent predictors of mental health service use were social support (OR = 0.34, p = 0.032) and caregivers aiding family members with higher levels of physical impairment (OR = 1.14, p = 0.033). The results of this study support clinicians and planners developing mental health services that use SOC to mitigate the detrimental effects of caregiving. Future research is needed to target effective measures to positively manipulate this variable.

INTRODUCTION

A growing number of individuals are assuming the responsibility of caring for their older family members with memory impairment (Gonzalez-Salvador et al., 1999). It is well documented that this type of caregiving is a demanding experience that causes severe stress among family caregivers due to the intense amount of work that is needed to provide help with activities of daily living (Cochrane et al., 1997; Dunkin & Anderson Hanley, 1998; Gallagher et al., 1994). Policy makers in mental health systems have recognized a necessity to accommodate the needs of family caregivers by providing them with accessible mental health services. Thus, it is imperative to identify factors associated with caregivers' use of mental health services because it has consequences for service planning and health promotion. The health of the caregiver is a contributing factor in ensuring the well-being of the individual with memory impairment (Mockler et al., 1998).

Family caregivers to those with memory impairment experience a great deal of stress. However, people respond quite differently to the same stress, with some individuals living highly stressed lives and others remaining healthy (Antonovsky, 1987). Individuals have the capacity to select from various courses of action to deal with stress (Mockler et al., 1998). One is able to appraise various stressful events into an ongoing life plan that leads to a reduction in the effects of stress or an augmentation in the effects of stress (Antonovsky, 1987; Forbes, 2001; Mockler et al., 1998). The term sense of coherence (SOC), created by Antonovsky (1987), can be viewed as an important resource that may influence family caregivers' response to stress and use of mental health services.

SOC is defined as the self-perception of one's ability to cope with stressful events. It considers the extent to which one has a pervasive and enduring feeling of confidence, that in the course of life, demands are viewed as reasonable, resources are accessible to meet the burden imposed, and that these are worthy of investment and engagement (Antonovsky, 1987; Forbes, 2001). In other words, an individual is able to understand, appraise, and integrate various types of stressful events into a continuing plan of action which leads to a decline in their consequences and a diverse collection of reactions to stress across all circumstances (Mockler et al., 1998). SOC is a global and reasonably stable orientation to one's world (Antonovsky, 1987; Kivimaki et al., 2000), though it has been found to be adaptable (Schnyder et al., 2000). Previous research found that SOC was inversely associated with distress among family caregivers to cognitively impaired individuals (Chumbler et al., 2003; Gallagher et al., 1994). Less is known about the extent to which SOC is associated with mental health service use by family caregivers.

One study investigated the relationship between SOC and mental health service utilization in family caregivers to cognitively impaired elders (Mockler et al., 1998). This study, which consisted of a convenient sample of 50 caregivers, found that non-users of mental health services scored significantly higher on the SOC than the group of users. No multivariate analyses were performed in this study, leaving important concerns of whether or not SOC would still be associated with mental health service use even after controlling for key characteristics of the impaired elder and their family caregiver. It also leaves one to contemplate other predictors of mental health service use, such as geographic access characteristics or the extent to which caregiver social support is associated with mental health service use. A large body of research emphasized the importance of social support for family caregivers (Mockler et al., 1998).

In sum, we have little solid evidence on the predictors of mental health service use for family caregivers to cognitively impaired elders. Even less is known on how the SOC may impact mental health service utilization. Therefore, the purpose of this paper is to investigate whether family caregivers of community dwelling older adults with memory impairment and a stronger SOC are less likely to use mental health services. Also, past research has rarely examined the relationship between geographic access and service use for family caregivers. The present study controlled for three different measures of geographic access (rural-urban residence, self-reported awareness of mental health services, and travel time). One study of cognitively impaired elders found that perceived awareness significantly predicted a greater likelihood of mental health service utilization (Fortney et al., 2002).

Conceptual Framework

The original behavioral model, initially developed in the late 1960s (Andersen, 1968) and updated in the mid 1990s (Andersen) suggests that service use is a function of three main types of factors, classified as predisposing, enabling and need factors, which predict use of health care services. Predisposing factors describe the proclivity of people to use services and exist prior to the onset of illness. Enabling variables provide the means to use services for members of society. Need factors include health characteristics of the patient, such as their health status and chronic disease impairments. The behavioral model for vulnerable populations was employed as the conceptual framework (Gelberg et al., 2000). This model represents a revision of the original Behavioral Model (Andersen, 1968, 1995) that strives to be applicable to studying the use of health services of vulnerable populations. Gelberg et al. (2000) noted a wide range of vulnerable groups, such as the homeless, minorities and the elderly, but indicated that it could be tailored and applied to other groups. Following this recommendation, we use family members caring for community-dwelling seniors with cognitive impairment as a vulnerable population group for at least two reasons. First, as earlier indicated, the health of the family caregiver is highly associated with the well-being of the individual with memory impairment (Mockler et al., 1998). Second, in addition to the insufficient number of services (including mental health services), many family caregivers lack plenty of financial resources, social resources and other methods to access them (Anderson et al., 2000). The original model did not conceptually consider a response to stress variable like SOC. However, in the adapted model for vulnerable populations, psychological resources (e.g. mastery, coping) are included in the predisposing domain. For the purposes of the present study, SOC is conceptually categorized as a predisposing factor.

METHODS

This community-based cross-sectional study screened non-institutionalized Arkansas residents age 70 years or older for cognitive impairment. Eligibility criteria for the study included not being institutionalized in long-term care at the time of the study, being age 70 years or older, able to communicate in English, and having a family caregiver. For this study, we defined family caregivers as family members who either lived with or checked on the individual 70 years of age and older. Elder respondents were administered a brief telephone-screening interview for cognitive impairment (Chumbler & Zhang, 1998). The study was solely designed to collect information on older adults with mild to moderate cognitive impairment from a random sample of non-institutionalized seniors. Those who screened positive for suspected cognitive impairment were asked to complete a survey on health status and health service utilization. Family caregivers were identified and were then administered a corresponding survey. At the time of the initial telephone contact, each potential caregiver was confirmed to be the family member that either lived with or checked on the person with cognitive impairment. Caregivers also had to be able to communicate in English and were at least 18 years of age.

A total of 9100 Arkansas non-institutionalized residents age 70 years or older, with a family caregiver were considered to be eligible respondents. One half of the eligible respondents agreed to participate in the screening. Another 4.8% of the eligible respondents who originally agreed to participate in the screening interview were unable to complete the cognitive screening because of hearing difficulties. After considering these reasons for not completing, 3726 individuals age 70+ with a family caregiver responded. Of these respondents, 730 (19.6%) met screening criteria for cognitive impairment. Of those who screened positive for cognitive impairment, 73% ($n = 532$) completed the telephone survey. The non-completers were either verbally or hearing impaired and could not finish the interview or refused to participate. The 532 cognitively impaired participants were not significantly different from the general population of Arkansans age 70+ captured by the 1990 census (Chumbler et al., 2000). Interviewers administered corresponding interviews to 370 (69.5%) family caregivers who were originally identified by the impaired older adult and were willing to respond. Complete data were available on 304 older adult/family caregiver dyads (57%) of the 532 impaired elders. More extensive details regarding the study procedures and methods are described elsewhere (Chumbler et al., 2000; Fortney et al., 2002).

MEASURES

Use of mental health services, our dependent variable, was operationalized to include any visit to a psychiatrist, psychologist, social worker, counselor, or community mental health center in a medical care setting in the previous 12 months.

The Sense of Coherence was measured by the short-form version (13 items) developed by Antonovsky (1987). These 13 items are measured on a 7-point Likert scale on which the interviewer articulated the extreme responses (1 and 7) for each question. The SOC score can range from 13 to 91. The coefficient alpha was 0.75.

We chose the following variables as potential confounders because they are either established correlates of mental health service use or have been theorized and/or found to be important access variables that may explain some barriers to accessing mental health services. Predisposing factors operationalized as sociodemographic information included the family caregivers' age, gender, race (White vs. non-white), relationship to impaired family member (spouse vs. non-spouse), co-residence with impaired family member, and number of family members in household (excluding impaired family member). Enabling factors of the family caregiver included measures of access including financial access and geographic access to mental health services based on an earlier study on access to mental health services for cognitively impaired seniors (Fortney et al., 2002). Financial access or affordability was measured by a single self-reported item referring to whether or not family caregivers had some form of private insurance. Because participants were sampled from rural areas, three measures of access were considered. The first indicated whether or not a family caregiver lived in a county that was not a part of a Metropolitan Statistical Area. A second measure pertained to the perceived availability of mental health services that was based on the family caregiver's self-reported awareness of available mental health services. The survey items asked "Within a 30-mile radius of where you live, are any of the following services available?" A 30-mile cutoff was chosen based on the Graduate Medical Education National Advisory Committee (GMENAC) suggested time-to-service standards (Ricketts et al., 1994). The numbers of affirmative responses for: (1) community mental health center; or (2) psychiatrist, psychologist, or social worker; or (3) counseling or mental health services were summed to create an awareness scale from 0 to 3 for mental health services.

The third measure of geographic access, travel time of the family caregiver to the temporally closest provider, was calculated using a Geographic Information System (GIS) in conjunction with data about the residential locations of caregivers and the practice locations of providers in each sector. The geographic locations of mental health services in Arkansas were obtained from American Business Lists. The practice addresses of mental health services were geocoded at the street level. Because a large proportion of residential addresses in rural Arkansas are not geocodable at the street level (e.g. rural routes and P.O. Boxes) (Fortney et al., 2000), all caregivers were geocoded at the zip code level and assigned to the closest street segment. The travel time from the caregiver's residence to the temporally closest service location was calculated by determining the quickest route from the patient to the service location along the digital road network (see Fortney et al., 2000 for details).

The concept of social support, which is defined as assets provided by a network of individuals, was measured by a single item that asked the family caregiver whether or not they had a friend or relative who assisted in caring for their impaired family member (Lee et al., 2004). This item was categorized as an access indicator for two reasons. First, previous research involving caregivers to individuals categorized it accordingly (Mockler et al., 1998). Second, prior research indicates that when family caregivers receive additional assistance from family and friends, their burden is ameliorated (Aneshensel et al., 1995; Pearlin et al., 1990).

The need factors of family caregivers were operationalized by chronic health conditions and subjective caregiver burden. Family caregiver respondents were asked whether or not in the past 12 months they experienced 13 chronic health conditions (high blood pressure, heart and circulations problems, arthritis or rheumatism, eye trouble, ear trouble, dental problems, chest problems, stomach or digestive problems, kidney trouble, diabetes, trouble with feet and ankles, trouble with nerves, and skin problems). Responses ranged from 0 to 13.

Pearlin et al. (1990) Role Overload scale was employed to measure subjective caregiver burden. Specifically, it measured the caregivers' energy level, satisfaction with the level of care provided, and having enough time to do everything necessary, including time for oneself (Pearlin et al., 1990). The frequency related with each question (where 1 = not at all, 2 = somewhat, 3 = quite a bit, and 4 = completely) was summed across each of the four items to generate a role overload score. Higher scores indicated more caregiver burden. The coefficient alpha was 0.73.

We also controlled for three characteristics of the impaired elder – age (in years), level of physical disability, and level of cognitive impairment. In concert with numerous researchers (see Gallagher et al., 1994), we measured the degree to which the impaired family member was unable to perform various activities of daily living, using a variation of the activities of daily living (ADL) (Katz et al., 1963) and Instrumental Activities of Daily Living (IADL) (Lawton & Brody, 1969) developed by Pearlin et al. (1990). For each of the ADLs (dressing, bathing, toileting, getting in/out of bed, eating, walking, grooming) and IADLs (using the telephone, getting to places out of walking distance, shopping, preparing meals, doing housework, taking medicine, handling money), the interviewer coded the impaired elder respondents with 1 if they indicated they required assistance to complete the activity or 0 if they were able to complete the activity without assistance. The disability index was the sum of the seven ADL and seven IADL scores.

Pearlin et al.'s (1990) Cognitive Status measure was used to assess the family caregivers' evaluation of the elder's cognitive functioning. The measure represents memory functioning across eight items (e.g. remembering recent events; recognizing people). The degree of trouble in performing each item (0 = not difficult at all to 4 = can't do at all) was summed across each of the eight items to produce a score representing the impaired elder's memory impairment. The coefficient alpha was 0.90.

In addition to simple univariate and bivariate results, we employed multiple logistic regression procedures to determine the odds that a family caregiver would report one or more visits to mental health services during the 12 months prior to the interview. In particular, this analytic procedure was used to determine whether SOC was associated with mental health service use, net the effects of the predisposing, enabling and need factors discussed above.

RESULTS

Table 1 provides descriptive statistics as well as bivariate associations with 12-month use of mental health services. Ten percent (29 of 304) of the family caregiver respondents made at least one visit to mental health service providers in the past 12 months. As shown in the third column of Table 1, the family caregivers who completed the interviews were on average 54.87 years old (S.D. = 13.59). The sample of caregivers was 69% female and 19% non-white (almost exclusively black). Over seven-in-ten (72%) had at least a high school (or equivalent) education. About three-quarters (76%) were non-spouses, with most of them being adult children. Excluding the impaired family member, caregiver respondents reported, on average, 1.6 additional family members in their household. About one-half (49%) co-resided with their impaired family member.

In terms of the enabling factors and, in particular, geographic access measures, two-thirds of the caregiver respondents (67%) resided in a non-MSA (i.e. rural) county. The perceived awareness for mental health services within 30 miles of the caregivers' residence was relatively high (2.2 on a 0–3 scale). The average travel time to the temporally closest mental health service location was 22.4 minutes (range 1–88). Note the standard deviation was rather large comparative to the mean, indicating a large amount of variation in geographic access among the family caregiver participants. Slightly less than one-half (48%) of the caregiver respondents indicated that they had social support (i.e. an additional family member or friend that assisted them in caring for their impaired family member), while just over one-half (51%) reported that they had private insurance.

With reference to the need factors of the family caregivers, the average number of self-reported chronic health conditions was 2.2 (range 0–10). The mean caregiver distress score was 7.9 (range 4–16).

In terms of the impaired elder's characteristics, the average age was 78.3 years (S.D. = 5.84). The mean physical impairment and cognitive impairment scores were 2.97 (range 0–14) and 4.55 (range 0–30), respectively. Thus, according to these scores, the elders in the present study have fairly good physical functioning and would be classified as having mild cognitive impairment. However, since the standard deviations are greater than the means for these two measures, there is a wide range of physical impairment and memory impairment within the sample of elders.

Next, we performed bivariate comparisons for the mental health services summary variable on the measures to be used in the multivariate logistic regression model (the first and second columns of Table 1). As can be seen in Table 1, those who did not visit mental health services had a stronger SOC (69.88 vs. 57.48). There was no significant variation by caregiver predisposing factors in using mental

Table 1. Bivariate Associations with 12-Month Use of Mental Health Services ($N = 304$).

Variable	Any 12-Month Mental Health (MH) Services		
	Yes ($n = 29$)	No ($n = 275$)	Total
Sense of coherence (mean ± S.D.)	57.48 ± 16.73	69.88 ± 11.67	68.69 ± 12.71[***]
Predisposing factors			
Age (years, mean ± S.D.)	53.62 ± 13.88	54.00 ± 13.58	54.87 ± 13.59
Gender (% female)	58.6	70.5	69.4
Race (% non-white)	17.8	27.6	18.8
Education (% high school & beyond)	79.3	71.3	72.0
Family relationship (% non-spouse)	69.0	76.7	76.0
Family size (mean ± S.D.)	1.52 ± 1.40	1.6 ± 1.45	1.61 ± 1.44
Co-residence (% yes)	62.1	47.6	49.0
Enabling factors			
Rural residence (% rural)	58.6	68.0	67.1
Perceived awareness of MH services (mean ± S.D.)	2.52 ± 0.91	2.16 ± 1.10	2.19 ± 1.08
Travel Time (minutes) to MH services (mean ± S.D.)	19.80 ± 19.07	22.65 ± 17.00	22.38 ± 17.20
Social support (% Yes)	24.1	50.5	48.0[**]
Private insurance (% yes)	44.8	52.0	51.3
Need factors			
Chronic health conditions (mean ± S.D.)	3.24 ± 2.23	2.07 ± 2.09	2.18 ± 2.13[*]
Distress (mean ± S.D.)	9.38 ± 3.23	7.79 ± 2.99	7.94 ± 3.04[**]
Imparied elder's factors			
Age (years, mean ± S.D.)	78.38 ± 5.84	77.55 ± 5.88	78.30 ± 5.84
Level of physical impairment (mean ± S.D.)	4.69 ± 4.49	2.79 ± 3.52	2.97 ± 3.66[*]
Level of memory impairment (mean ± S.D.)	6.79 ± 7.09	4.31 ± 5.85	4.55 ± 6.01[*]

Note: S.D. = Standard Deviation; MH = mental health. For self-rated health status, higher scores indicate better health status. For the remaining health status measures (both the family caregiver and impaired elder), higher scores indicate worse health.

[*] $p < 0.05$.
[**] $p < 0.01$.
[***] $p < 0.001$.

health services. Only one of the enabling factor variables differed by proportion of mental health specialty service use. Those who did not receive social support are less likely to use mental health services (50.5% vs. 24.1%). All three-need factors of the caregiver were independently associated with use of mental health services. Those who did use services had more chronic health conditions and had more distress than those who did not (chronic health conditions: 3.24 vs. 2.07; distress: 9.38 vs. 7.79). Two of the three impaired elder characteristics were also associated with use of mental health services. Caregivers who used services were caring for family members who had higher levels of physical impairment (4.69 vs. 2.79) and memory impairment (6.79 vs. 4.31) than those who did not. After applying the Bonferroni correction of the overall Type I error, the bivariate differences involving SOC remained significant.

The multivariate logistic regression model for 12-month mental health service use was performed to calculate the effects of each independent variable while statistically adjusting for the influence of others in the equation. The odds ratios generated from these analyses are shown in Table 2. The odds ratios indicate that SOC was independently associated with use of mental health services, after controlling for the other predisposing, enabling, and need factors (OR = 0.91; $p = 0.006$). Specifically, caregivers who have a stronger SOC had a lower propensity to use mental health services. Caregivers who have social support had a lower likelihood of using mental health services (OR = 0.34; $p = 0.032$). Additionally, caregivers assisting family members with higher levels of physical impairment were significantly more likely to use mental health services (OR = 1.14; $p = 0.033$). None of the other caregiver predisposing and need factors were significantly associated with mental health service use. Likewise, measures of financial and geographic access were not correlated with service use.

DISCUSSION

The primary purpose of this study was to examine whether family caregivers with a stronger SOC who are caring for non-institutionalized, cognitively impaired older adults were less likely to use mental health services. In contrast to most previous studies, the present study was able to control for key geographic access variables, such as travel time from caregiver to the mental health service and perceived awareness of services. In both the bivariate and multivariate analyses, we found a significant, inverse association between SOC and mental health service use. Specifically, in terms of the multivariate analyses, caregivers who had greater SOC scores were significantly less likely to have reported use of mental health services. These findings support the only study that found an inverse association between

Table 2. Logistic Regression Model of Family Caregivers Use of Mental Health Services ($N = 304$).

Variable	Any Use of Mental Health Services in Last 12 Months	
	Odds Ratio (95% CI)	*p* Value
Sense of coherence	0.91 (0.91 − 0.98)	0.006
Predisposing factors		
Age	1.00 (0.95 − 1.05)	0.994
Gender: Male	0.47 (0.18 − 1.24)	0.127
Race: Non-White	1.72 (0.57 − 5.11)	0.330
Education: High school and beyond	2.02 (0.65 − 6.26)	0.221
Type of familial		
Relationship: Non-spouse	0.43 (0.08 − 2.47)	0.347
Family size	0.91 (0.65 − 1.30)	0.640
Co-resident	0.97 (0.32 − 2.96)	0.605
Enabling factors		
Rural residence	0.61 (0.24 − 1.56)	0.303
Self-reported awareness of services	1.39 (0.83 − 2.31)	0.212
Travel times to mental health services	1.34 (0.07 − 26.47)	0.848
Social support	0.34 (0.13 − 0.91)	0.032
Private insurance	0.65 (0.25 − 1.68)	0.376
Need factors		
Chronic health conditions	1.13 (0.91 − 1.41)	0.267
Distress	1.01 (0.84 − 1.21)	0.933
Imparied elder's factors		
Age	0.95 (0.87 − 1.04)	0.226
Level of physical impairment	1.14 (1.01 − 1.30)	0.033
Level of memory impairment	0.98 (0.91 − 1.06)	0.553

Note: Odds ratios and *p* values are highlighted only for significant regression coefficients ($p < 0.05$). For the health status measures (both for the family caregiver and the impaired elder), higher scores indicate worse health status.

high SOC and less mental health service use among family caregivers to older adults with dementia (Mockler et al., 1998). In order for SOC to be an effective framework for interventions, SOC should be composed of behaviors and attitudes that can be modified. Some recent research has found that SOC can be changed when individuals face stressful life events (Schnyder et al., 2000). However, this study did not involve caregivers and it did not examine the extent to which SOC varied beyond 12 months. More research is needed to provide more definitive data that SOC represents factors that can be changed over a longer period of time.

The present study also found that caregivers with social support were less likely to have used mental health services. This finding supports previous studies that the lack of social support is associated with negative emotional outcomes (e.g. depression) and a greater likelihood of formal service use (Williams & Dilworth-Anderson, 2002). We should emphasize that we employed only a single measure of social support. Further research is needed to know whether interventions that employ other measures of social support, such as social network size and family cohesion, may help bring family caregivers to mental health specialty providers (Booth et al., 2000).

In the multivariate results, we found that family caregivers caring for those with greater levels of physical impairment were more likely to have used mental health services. This finding is in accordance with a previous study which found that family caregivers for persons with more ADL and IADL impairments have more need for assistance and are more likely to have their needs unmet (Anderson et al., 2000). As described earlier, the sample impaired of elders were not very disabled according to the physical impairment measures, but there was a great deal of variability. Future research should examine in great detail how services can be planned for caregivers before the person they are caring for becomes even more impaired.

We found that neither the family caregivers' perceived awareness of mental health services nor their travel time (in minutes) to mental health services was associated with service use. These non-findings were inconsistent with a past study, which found that perceived awareness significantly predicted a greater likelihood of mental health service utilization (Fortney et al., 2002). However, more research is needed to test the extent to which geographic access is a significant predictor of service utilization for family caregivers to community-residing elders with mild to moderate levels of cognitive impairment.

A small number of studies have indicated the lower rate of mental health service use among family caregivers to impaired elders (Caserta et al., 1987; Golimbet & Trubnikov, 2001). As expected, we found a small proportion (10%) of the family caregiver respondents in our study used any mental health services at all during the 12-month study period, and as the multivariate analysis found this can not be contributed geographic access issues. The low rate of mental health service use in this sample of family caregivers signifies a missed chance to enhance outcomes in this population. Contact with mental health providers could possibly enrich quality of life by screening for and treating widespread comorbid illnesses such as depression (Fortney et al., 2002). Family caregivers to cognitively impaired seniors could benefit from the integration of mental health services into primary care settings (Fortney et al., 2002).

The present study had some limitations that need to be addressed. First, we do not know how closely the family caregivers in the present study are representative of all caregivers of individuals with other severe mental health conditions afflicting older people. In fact, due to the methods employed here, we cannot say that the sample of cognitively impaired elders in our study approximates a clinical, dementia sample. Bear in mind that our study was designed to collect information in elders with mild to moderate impairment. In fact, based on descriptive statistics, the sample can be depicted as having mild cognitive impairment. In short, the most severely impaired elders who were cared for in the home, and their family caregivers may have not been able to participate in the survey (Chumbler et al., 2003; Fortney et al., 2002). Second, our study was limited to the state of Arkansas, and we are unable to project how well our findings would generalize outside the state of Arkansas.

Third, we were unable to control for the number of years that respondents had spent caring for their impaired family member. Future research should control for this important variable when examining service use among family caregivers to cognitively impaired elders. It is possible that the longer the duration of caregiving, the better adjusted a person becomes to the demands of caregiving by having had sufficient time to adopt a lifestyle that renders caregiving as routine. This is in contrast to when they initially began caregiving and it was a huge lifestyle transition. Therefore, under this assumption, if one began caregiving recently, perhaps his or her use of mental health services is inflated because he or she is still struggling to work it into his or her daily life. On the other hand, after many years of being a caregiver a person's adjustment level may not progress but instead began to increase their level of stress. Fourth, caregivers reflected back on their reported use of mental health services. This situation could have lead to a recall bias. As past research indicated, a longitudinal study that observes the decision-making process as it develops is warranted (Yamamoto & Wallhagen, 1998).

While American policy has increasingly emphasized informal care for older adults with cognitive-impairment (with the expectation of controlling health care costs) an unintended impact of this strategy has been the psychological and physical morbidity that family caregivers have endured by assuming such a demanding task (Cochrane et al., 1997). Findings from the present study have connotations for planning of service provision, caregiver education and support. Future research should examine in greater detail caregivers with high SOC and their coping strategies in various caregiving situations for caregiver education and support groups (Mockler et al., 1998).

REFERENCES

Andersen, R. (1968). Behavior models of families' use of health services. Research series No. 15. Center for Health Administration Studies, University of Chicago.

Andersen, R. (1995). Revisiting the behavioral model and access to care: Does it matter? *Journal of Health and Social Behavior, 36*, 1–10.

Anderson, R. T., Bradham, D. D., Jackson, S., Heuser, M. D., Wofford, J. L., & Colombo, K. A. (2000). Caregivers' unmet needs for support in caring for functionally impaired elderly persons: A community sample. *Journal of Health Care for the Poor and Underserved, 11*, 412–429.

Aneshensel, C. S., Pearlin, L., Mullan, J. T., Zarit, S., & Whitlach, C. J. (1995). *Profiles in caregiving: The unexpected career.* San Diego: Academic Press.

Antonovsky, A. (1987). *Unraveling the mystery of health: How people manage stress and stay well.* San Francisco: Jossey-Bass.

Booth, B. M., Kirchner, J., Fortney, J., Ross, R., & Rost, K. (2000). Rural at-risk drinkers: Correlates and one-year use of alcoholism treatment services. *Journal of Studies on Alcohol, 61*, 267–277.

Caserta, M. S., Lund, D. A., Wright, S. D., & Redburn, D. E. (1987). Caregivers to dementia patients: The utilization of community services. *The Gerontologist, 27*, 209–214.

Chumbler, N. R., Grimm, J. W., Cody, M., & Beck, C. (2003). Gender, kinship and caregiver burden: The case of community-dwelling memory impaired seniors. *International Journal of Geriatric Psychiatry, 18*, 722–732.

Chumbler, N. R., Hartmann, D., & Beck, C. K. (2000). Appropriateness in acquiring a family caregiver interview from older adults with suspected cognitive impairment. *Aging & Mental Health, 4*(2), 158–165.

Chumbler, N. R., & Zhang, M. (1998). A telephone screening to classify demented older adults. *Clinical Gerontologist, 19*(3), 79–84.

Cochrane, J. J., Goering, P. N., & Rogers, J. M. (1997). The mental health of informal caregivers in Ontario: An epidemiological survey. *American Journal of Public Health, 87*(12), 2002–2007.

Dunkin, J. J., & Anderson Hanley, C. (1998). Dementia caregiver burden: A review of the literature and guidelines for assessment and intervention. *Neurology, 51*(Suppl. 1), S53–S60.

Forbes, D. A. (2001). Enhancing mastery and sense of coherence: Important determinants of health in older adults. *Geriatric Nursing, 22*(1), 29–32.

Fortney, J., Chumbler, N., Cody, M., & Beck, C. (2002). Geographic access and service use in a community-based sample of cognitively impaired elders. *The Journal of Applied Gerontology, 21*(3), 352–367.

Fortney, J., Rost, K., & Warren, J. (2000). Comparing alternative methods of measuring geographic access to health services. *Health Services and Outcomes Research Methodology, 1*(2), 173–184.

Gallagher, T. J., Wagenfeld, M. O., Baro, F., & Haepers, K. (1994). Sense of coherence, coping, and caregiver overload. *Social Science Medicine, 39*(12), 1615–1622.

Gelberg, L., Anderson, R. M., & Leake, B. D. (2000). The behavioral model for vulnerable populations: Application to medical care use and outcomes for homeless people. *Health Services Research, 34*, 1273–1301.

Golimbet, V., & Trubnikov, V. (2001). Evaluation of the dementia carers situation in Russia. *International Journal of Geriatric Psychiatry, 16*, 94–99.

Gonzalez-Salvador, M. T., Arango, C., Lyketsos, C. G., & Barba, A. C. (1999). The stress and psychological morbidity of the Alzheimer patient caregiver. *International Journal of Geriatric Psychiatry, 14*, 701–710.

Katz, S., Ford, A. B., Moskowitz, R. W., Jackson, B. A., & Jaffe, M. A. (1963). Studies of illness in the aged: The index of ADL-A standardized measure of biological and social function. *Journal of the American Medical Association, 185*, 914–919.

Kivimaki, M., Feldt, T., Vahtera, J., & Nurmi, J. (2000). Sense of coherence and health: Evidence from two cross-lagged longitudinal samples. *Social Science and Medicine, 50*, 583–597.

Lawton, M. P., & Brody, E. M. (1969). Assessment of older people: Self-maintaining and instrumental activities of daily living. *Gerontologist, 9,* 179–186.

Lee, S. D., Arozullah, A. M., & Cho, Y. I. (2004). Health literacy, social support, and health: A research agenda. *Social Science & Medicine, 58,* 1309–1321.

Mockler, D., Riordan, J., & Murphy, M. (1998). Psychosocial factors associated with the use/non-use of mental health services by primary carers of individuals with dementia. *International Journal of Geriatric Psychiatry, 13,* 310–314.

Pearlin, L. I., Mullan, J. T., Semple, S. J., & Skaff, M. M. (1990). Caregiving and the stress process: An overview of concepts and their measures. *Gerontologist, 30,* 583–594.

Schnyder, U., Buchi, S., Sensky, T., & Klaghofer, R. (2000). Antonovosky's sense of coherence: Trait or state? *Psychotherapy and Psychosomatics, 69,* 296–302.

Williams, S. W., & Dilworth-Anderson, P. (2002). Systems of social support in families who care for dependent African American elders. *The Geronologist, 42,* 224–236.

Yamamoto, N., & Wallhagen, M. I. (1998). Service use by family caregivers in Japan. *Social Science & Medicine, 47,* 677–691.

SECTION III:
LESSONS FROM BEYOND
THE UNITED STATES

THE EMERGENCE OF SELF-MANAGED ATTENDANT SERVICES IN ONTARIO: DIRECT FUNDING PILOT PROJECT – AN INDEPENDENT LIVING MODEL FOR CANADIANS REQUIRING ATTENDANT SERVICES

Karen Yoshida, Vic Willi, Ian Parker and David Locker

ABSTRACT

We identify the key social and political forces that brought about the Self Managed Attendant Service Direct Funding Pilot (SMAS-DFP). Attendant Services are services for people with physical disabilities (PWD) to assist with daily activities. Direct Funding means that individuals obtain funds through direct funding mechanisms and/or through third parties. Self-direction refers to consumers who know their attendant service needs and can instruct workers to meet these needs. Self-management refers to (PWD) who are employers under the law and are legally responsible for hiring, training, scheduling and paying their attendants. Our analysis of the success of the SMAS-DFP is based on pre-conditions and facilitating elements. The pre-conditions were the: (1) existence of social movements; (2) precedents to direct funding programs; (3) prior experience with the

Chronic Care, Health Care Systems and Services Integration
Research in the Sociology of Health Care, Volume 22, 177–204
Copyright © 2004 by Elsevier Ltd.
ISSN: 0275-4959/doi:10.1016/S0275-4959(04)22010-5

governance of attendant services; and (4) government health reform. Five
elements facilitated the SMASD-FP: (1) a clear vision by the community;
(2) a core group of leaders; (3) supporters of the SMAS-DFP came from
inside and outside of the community; and (4) supporters provided key
resources to be used and to deal with barriers. PWD successfully led the pilot
(1994–1997) and continue to administer the expanded government program
(began 1998).

INTRODUCTION

For many people living with disabilities, personal assistance or attendant services are essential services for their quality of life (Nosek, 1993). In fact, many people living with disabilities would be in institutions if attendant services did not exist. Over the past 30 years, adults with physical disabilities who use attendant services have shown their ability to live independently and take responsibility for all aspects of their daily lives (Working Group of the Direct Funding Pilot, 1993). However, these models of service had shortcomings in that they were not portable, there were no choice of attendants (e.g. some women had to accept male attendants) and the hours of service were not flexible. This lack of flexibility often meant social restrictions (e.g. no help at work). Many wanted to take more control of their support services by receiving the funds directly, managing and employing their own attendant workers.

The Ontario Self-Managed Attendant Service Direct Funding Pilot (SMAS-DFP) was a two-year pilot that began in 1994. The pilot objectives were to be responsive to the demands of Ontario consumers, (in Ontario, "consumer" is used to denote the recipient of attendant services), to have choice, flexibility, control and full responsibility as individual employers over their attendant services. This was achieved by testing the self-managed direct funding model with a group of 100 people. This pilot project was successful and an expanded government program was implemented in Ontario, Canada in 1998. The unique aspect to both the pilot and, later, the program has been the central role that people with disabilities have played in designing, administrating and operationizing the pilot and the full government program. To our knowledge, there is no other government program in the world that is fully administered by people with disabilities.

The purpose of this paper is to identify the key social and political forces between 1974 and 1994 that facilitated the emergence, development and achievement of the Ontario Self Managed Attendant Service Direct Funding Pilot (SMAS-DFP). In this paper, key definitions such as attendant services, consumer, individualized funding, self-direction and self-management are taken from the Direct Funding

Evaluation Report (1997b). Attendant Services consist of self-directed services for people with physical disabilities to assist them with routine activities of daily living. Assistance is provided by another person, and may include both house keeping and personal services. Consumer means people who receive attendant services. In the context of disability-related supports, individualized funding is an arrangement for allocating funds to individuals according to their disability-related needs. Individualized funding has been flowed to individuals through direct funding mechanisms and through third parties. In the context of attendant services, self-direction refers to consumers articulating their attendant service requirements and instructing workers to meet these needs. Finally, self-management refers to people with disabilities who are legally responsible for making their own arrangements for attendant services. Their attendants are their employees.

The drive or commitment of individuals to seek out more control and decision-making in their lives via alternate models of attendant services has relevance in the social movement literature. The literature on social movement theory is wide spread and varied. Given this, there are many different ways to define what is a social movement. The earlier literature on social movement theories can be categorized in two distinct ways. There are the social movement theories that viewed collective action as the response(s) to dis-equilibrium or dysfunction in the social system (Kornhauser, 1959; Smesler, 1962) and others which focus on collective action that works towards developing and sustaining an organization working towards a shared goal – resource mobilization theories. Gadacz (1994) believes that these two major types of theories of social movements can only partially explain the actions of contemporary social movements. She cites Melucci (1985, p. 792) critique of these two major orientations. That "older" theories of breakdowns in the system can explain why a movement develops but not how collective action is generated (the actors or actions). Alternatively, resource mobilization theories explain how actions are taken (i.e. what are the strategies) but not the why – the meaning which underpins the action. To Gadacz (1994), these models cannot explain the process of the definition of the action system and the process by which individuals and groups recreate their social order. While traditional approaches of social movement look at how social systems produce collective action, recent approaches to social movement examine how collective action reproduces or transforms society. Gadacz (1994) also believes that the new social movements are those in which the sources inequality and forms of domination are within the cultural realms of life – i.e. the time and place of everyday life and the dominant cultural and behavioral orientations of modernity.

In this paper, we use Melucci's (1985) orientation to contemporary social movements to analyze the emergence and development of the SMAS-DFP. Melucci

(1985) viewed collective action as an interplay of aim, resources and obstacles, as a purposive orientation that is set up within a system of opportunities and constraints. Mellucci believed (1988) that these movements be seen in the context of real or perceived threats to those public and private "spaces" which generate meaning and a sense of community for individuals.

The specific objectives of this paper are: (1) to illustrate an analytical framework of the important elements that facilitated the attainment of the SMAS-DFP during the 1990s; (2) to discuss the pre-existing conditions which promoted the emergence of the SMAS-DFP; and (3) to discuss the facilitating elements that allowed for the development and attainment of the SMAS-DFP. In addition, we provide an update on the status of the program in Ontario.

LITERATURE REVIEW

Direct Funding and Attendant Services: Applied Independent Living Movement/Disability Rights principles

The concept of living independently in the community has been a central impetus for the emergence of the Independent Living (IL) movements in the United States and Canada (Driedger, 1989; Shapiro, 1994).

Two "early" principles have remained fundamental to the IL movements. These are: first, that people with disabilities know best their needs and that second, that living in the community requires appropriate supports and services to meet those needs (Zukas, 1979). The concept of independence from an IL perspective, has also rejected traditional medical definitions of the term – that independence only means that someone is "physically capable" to do the activities of daily life. In Canada, the concepts of choice, flexibility and control are central to the ILM in Canada (CAILC, 2004). These elements must be in place for the person living with a disability to be able to participate in all aspects of his/her life. These concepts are central to the articulation and application of preferred models of service delivery related to attendant services.

Attendant Services: Managed Care or Self-Managed Services

Prior to this review of the literature on different models of funding attendant services are two essential differences in terminology. In Canada, Individualized Funding (IF) can be seen as a way of assessing service funding that "refers to service dollars that have been determined on the basis of an individual's needs" (Roeher Institute, 1993). Most forms of IF have funding mechanisms in which a consumer's dollars are sent to an agency on the person's behalf. The concept of direct funding (DF) refers to dollars sent *directly* to the recipient of the attendant services who then can use *the money* to employ attendants.

The term attendant services are used instead of personal assistance (Snow, 1993). The phrase attendant care has also been used. However, more recently, and specifically in Ontario, the term "attendant care" has also been rejected by the attendant service community as the word "care" has a medical connotation that is not in keeping with an IL perspective and is associated with helplessness, sickness and the inability to manage personal needs (Roeher Institute, 1997a).

In this literature review our focus in this paper is to illustrate differences in models of attendant service delivery based on a continuum ranging from least choice, flexibility and control of services to most choice, flexibility and control of services (by the consumer).

Managed Care Attendant Services
Traditionally attendant services have been delivered to consumers living in the community under a managed-care model. That is, a non-profit organization in the community run by a volunteer board of directors receives money from the government with a mandate to manage and provide attendant services. In managed care, a consumer's money goes to an organization and a consumer contracts with that organization for his/her services In Ontario, these services have been provided in two types of settings: (a) support service living units (SSLUs) – now called supportive living units – attendant care. Normally these units are leased by the tenant from the building management. Occasionally these units have a "shared living" component where, for example, a bathroom may be shared); and (b) outreach attendant services (attendants travel to your home or apartment). Both of these variations are managed care in that the designated service provider is responsible for all aspects of service from requesting and accounting for funds, selecting applicants and hiring, training and firing staff. Consumers may or may not be on the board of directors but in Ontario it is the norm that these organizations are controlled by non-disabled persons. The responsibility of a recipient of either of these two variants of attendant services is usually limited to self-directing, scheduling (negotiated with management) and some training, usually with an experienced attendant. Service recipients may also serve on their own board of directors. The services are not portable, there is sometimes no choice of the gender of attendants. Hours of services and time of services have to be negotiated. The consumer has little bargaining power. In addition, consumers must share the attendant with other users, hence there is no spontaneity; for example, one may

not be able to get up or go to bed whenever they want. Some attendant service providers in Ontario also do not always enforce the regulation that consumers must be able to self-direct their services. *Attendant Outreach Services: Policy Guidelines and Operational Standards* (Ministry of Health, 1996, p. 14) states that a person is ineligible to receive attendant services if "the individual is not capable of directing his/her own personal support and home making services . . .." This is important to note because there is considerable disagreement about the definition of attendant services. On one side, you have consumers and their advocates trying to limit the definition of attendant services as being something that is self-directed and non-institutional. On the other hand, health care providers and some service providers constantly work to expand the definition so as to switch the locus of control, choice and flexibility from the individual recipient over to the "attendant/service provider." This is a movement towards a "care-taking" model, it is disempowering and has been a prime reason for the development of the DF Model.

Returning to the continuum of choice, flexibility and control for attendant service delivery models, the managed care model with shared living and weak enforcement of self-direction would be the least empowering. At best, although managed-care is still a very valuable service and usually fairly flexible, key aspects of management sit with the community agency.

Self-Managed Direct Funding Model

The DF model of service is at the opposite end of the continuum. The applicant develops their own service plan based on experiential knowledge of their needs and negotiates the plan and budget with a panel of peers. Upon acceptance and being eligible, they are responsible for all aspects of managing their own services and must do a financial report quarterly based on generally accepted accounting principles. They register as an employer with Revenue Canada.

Self-management of funds that allow the consumer to hire whomever they want, train them in their lifestyle and dismiss them if they are unqualified, uncooperative or abusive. Now, risk and responsibility are accepted by the self manager who gains spontaneity and the ability to move throughout Ontario, pursue education, employment, even marriage – total control over ones life.

In Direct Funding, funds go directly to an individual who is fully responsible for all aspects of self-management. Examples of direct funds to consumers are in Utah (Centre for Research and Education in Human Services, 1993), the Manitoba Self Managed Care for Adults with Physical Disabilities and the Manitoba Pilot Project for People with Mental Handicaps (Roeher, 1997a). Internationally the Swedish STIL is also an example of direct funding (Ratzka, 1993).

STUDY METHODOLOGY

Philosophical Orientation

The approach we took to this research project was a participatory research approach. Traditionally, a participatory research approach stresses the participation of the "subjects" of the research in the development of all facets of the research process. This means that study participants develop research questions, methods of collecting data, participate in data analysis and interpretation and also be actively involved in the dissemination of the findings. Ultimately the "action" part of the research is that the findings will promote positive change in the lives of the participants (Oliver, 1990; Woodill, 1992). Our approach to participatory research is essentially the same with some modifications. We stressed the participation of people living with disabilities with regards to decision making, choice and control in developing the research questions and to the other aspects of the research process (Oliver, 1990; Woodill, 1992). Specifically, two of the research collaborators to this research project, and authors of this paper are people living with disabilities and they both were key members of the attendant service user community pushing for direct funding. They provided key directions for the research project. This orientation of our research project of the equality of the research members with respect to the direction of the project, analysis, dissemination and resources constitutes our "equitable partnerships" approach (Yoshida et al., 1998).

Case Study Approach

We used a qualitative case study methodology to achieve our objectives. A case study approach is appropriate when the focus is on a contemporary event within a real life context (Yin, 1994). Using a case study method, more than one source of evidence is used to answer the research questions. In our study, there were two sources of data – documents and key informant interviews. The documents collected and analyzed were key specific SMASDF movement materials (e.g. Attendant Care Action Coalition); key general movement materials (e.g. Independent Living Movement, normalization and consumer movement); relevant national and provincial government documents and conference proceedings. Key informants were interviewed who had a direct or an indirect role in the emergence of this movement. We used critical ethnography (Denzin, 1994) to analyze these data. Critical ethnography is a form of analyzing data that looks to understand the underlying elements or issues of an event. For the study, we wanted to know the "critical" factors that supported the appearance of the SMAS-DFP at this point in time.

STUDY FINDINGS

Overview of the Direct Funding Framework

Figure 1 illustrates the analytical framework for the SMAS-DFP. Based upon our analysis of the data, we believe that the emergence of the Ontario SMAS-DFP came about at this point in time due to pre-existing conditions and critical factors associated with the process of achieving the SMAS-DFP. Pre-existing conditions that created a social and political climate for the SMAS-DFP were: existing social movements and their similar ideological foci; precedents to self-managed direct funding in Ontario; prior experiences in the development and governance of attendant services and the changes in direction of the Ontario provincial

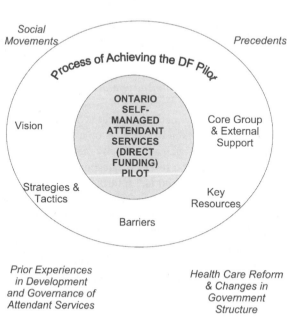

Fig. 1.   Direct Funding Framework.

government with respect to certain aspects of health care and the associated changes in government structure that supported the redirection at this time. These conditions allowed the SMAS-DFP to move forward with five critical factors that the attendant service user community developed and utilized to promote the pilot. These five main internal factors were: a strong and clearly stated vision; core group and external support; key resources; strategies and tactics and dealing effectively with barriers. The framework's overlapping circles reflects the interaction between the existing conditions and internal factors. These relationships will be more clearly articulated in the following sections.

Pre-existing Conditions

Pre-existing Social Movements and the Cumulative Vision
The emergence of the Ontario SMASDFP benefited from an evolving social environment in Ontario and Canada, which valued the rights of individuals to have control over their lives, to live "independently" in the community, and the equality of opportunity for all citizens. This social climate and vision on independent living evolved from the influence of four other social movements – the movements for de-institutionalization, normalization/community integration) consumerism and civil rights (Dejong, 1979; Shapiro, 1994). De-institutionalization and normalization have espoused the value of the individual and the right of the person to live outside of an institution in the community with appropriate supports. These social movements were primarily focused on people living with mental and intellectual disabilities. While consumerism has focused on the rights of consumers of goods and services, the civil rights movement has extended the notion of equal rights and opportunities to all citizens within a society.

The Independent Movements in the United States (Dejong, 1979) and in Canada (Driedger, 1989) were influenced by these social movements and have elaborated on the collective vision of individual rights and freedoms. The Canadian IL movement has strong civil and human rights principles as components of their philosophy and vision (CAILC, 2004). These principles stress the need for individuals with a disability to take responsibility for their lives, and to see themselves as citizens with rights and responsibilities. A guiding principle of the Independent Living movement is that disability has less to do with functional limitations and more to do with environmental barriers. The Independent Living Movement in Canada was supported initially by the federal government in the 1980s by the Department of the Secretary of State. There are now 25 centers (includes the national office) in Canada with 11 ILRCs (includes the national office) in Ontario (CAILC, 2004).

As discussed, the notion of individualized and direct funding payments for attendant services has been around for more than 20 years (Snow, 1993). The works of Adolf Ratzka of Stockholm, Sweden are most notable in this area. He started STIL, the Stockholm Cooperative for Independent Living, in 1984 (Ratzka, 1993). STIL functioned as a cooperative and the members were – and still are – able to receive payments directly to choose their own personal assistants. This Swedish initiative is an important catalyst for people with disabilities in Canada they began to examine mechanisms for personal support in the form of brokerage or individualized funding.

In 1987, a national symposium on brokerage and individualized funding was held in Ottawa. One of the reasons for this national conference was the need to clarify the use of the term "service brokerage" as professionals tended to use the term with respect to case management and co-ordination. In addition, federal/provincial governments were reviewing the Canada Assistance Plan and the Vocational Rehabilitation Disability Program with respect to increasing support and developing new ways of facilitating community living and employment for people with disabilities (Strachan & Tomlinson, 1987). This symposium created a Canadian context for further discussions on service brokerage/individualized funding.

Precedents to Self-Managed Direct Funding in Ontario
People with disabilities could draw upon existing programs in Ontario and Canada that also made direct payments for example, vocational rehabilitation, and worker's compensation occasionally allowed the person with a disability to purchase services of an attendant directly (Snow, 1993). While these programs were based on very specific criteria, such as, entitlement, they are examples in which people could receive money directly from the government to purchase goods and/or services. Another precedent to SMDF were Orders-in-Council (OIC). OIC's were exceptional provincial government arrangements to provide funding to a third party agency allowing a few individuals the opportunity to hire their own attendants. Orders-in-Council were implemented beginning in the late 1970s early 1980s.

Another precedent of direct funding that more closely resembled the direct funding model was the Ontario Special Services at Home Program (SSAH) which began in 1982. According to a senior government official, this program began after the closure of five institutions for children living with disabilities, between 1979 to 1984 as part of the de-institutionalization/normalization movement.

Prior Experience with the Development and Governance of Attendant Services
Another important pre-existing condition was that people with disabilities and their advocates in Ontario, had extensive prior experiences, individually and collectively,

in the development and governance of attendant services in the form of Support Service Living Units (SSLU). These were privately leased apartment units with 24 hour on site attendant services available within regular, integrated apartment units. The impetus for the creation of SSLU's was strongly advanced as a result of a conference in 1973 that was organized by the Ontario Federation for the Physically Handicapped. At this conference were representatives from Toronto and Ottawa where two of the four demonstration projects would be held. A representative from the provincial government's Ministry of Community and Social Services suggested that the services be without cost to consumers. The Toronto Mayor at the time, David Crombie, authorized a City of Toronto task force that examined various aspects of life (e.g. housing, transportation etc.) for people living with disabilities (Mayor's Task Force Report Regarding Disabled and Elderly, 1973). This task force with Cheshire Homes Foundation looked for alternatives to institutionalization in the form of four demonstration and support services housing projects (SSLU's). The success of these demonstration projects beginning in 1974, led to a working group of Cheshire Foundation representatives, service providers, consumers and government officials from the Ministry of Community and Social Services, to establish policies for the SSLU's in 1983 (Ministry of Community and Social Services, 1983). This partnership experience between the attendant service user community and the Ontario government provided the foundation for future interactions and collaborative work.

Health Care Reform and Changes in Provincial Government Structure
Another important pre-condition or contextual factor was the health care reform that occurred within the province of Ontario, starting the in late 1960s and 1970 and ending in 1995. The change in health care reform and the subsequent change in government structure of health would prove to be important to the achievement of the SMASDFP. Between the time-period of 1960 to the 1970s during the Progressive Conservative's leadership, there was a focus on long term care needs of seniors and persons with disabilities regarding living in the community. This interest continued during the Liberal Party's term as government (1985–1990) as they were examining new ways of viewing health. The Liberals position paper on long term care, "Redirection of Long-Term Care and Support Services in Ontario" (Ministries of Community and Social Services, Health and Citizenship, 1991), expressed the need to bring health and social services' related support programs together. The principles that provided the foundation for this reform were the right of the individual to self – determination; to promote racial equity and cultural diversity; the importance of family and community and equitable access to appropriate services. Given this policy framework, the potential for a SMASDF type pilot was now viable (Ministries of Community and Social Services, Health

and Citizenship, 1991). This potential was also realized in the form of an explicit verbal commitment in 1990 by the Liberal government to initiate a Direct Funding Pilot.

In 1990, under the Liberal government, the two ministries of Health and Community and Social Services amalgamated the Long-Term Care and Support Services into a single division entitled, the Community Health and Support Service Division. However, in September 1990, the New Democratic Party (NDP) won the provincial election. The NDP long term care report, "Partnerships in Long Term Care" (Ministries of Community and Social Services, Health and Citizenship, 1993) was more forceful on the issue of individual rights as "consumer empowerment" and the need for control of services. Most importantly, the issue of a SMAS-DF Pilot was explicitly stated in this document (Ministries of Community and Social Services, Health and Citizenship, 1993).

The Progressive Conservative Party became the government in 1995. Their view on Long-Term Care (LTC) was similar to the NDP government and there was no specific Progressive Conservative position paper on LTC. This evolving health care reform and the supporting policy frameworks and documents would be an important anchor upon which the attendant service user community would be able to lobby for DF in the face of changes in government leadership.

Critical Internal Factors in the Achievement of the SMASDFP

Based on our framework, there were a number of important factors that influenced the process of achieving the pilot. The factors will be discussed within this section.

Vision of Self-Managed Attendant Services: Competing Definitions and the Emergence of the Attendant Care Action Coalition (ACAC)

As discussed previously, Ontario-based Support Service Living Units (SSLUs) were set up first as demonstration projects, with the first SSLU established in 1974. Services are usually delivered by an agency that hires, and trains attendants. Usually these agencies are controlled by non-service users. In many cases, this works well and the consumers are happy with the arrangement. However, some consumers have begun to see this as limiting their life choices as the consumer has little or no control over who will come into their apartment, how much attendant time that might be available to them on short notice and that the service itself is not portable. Non-portable service means that the consumer can only receive attendant services in the SSLU. While these systems were originally designed with a great deal of input and lobbying from consumers (Ministry of Community and Social Services, 1983) – consumers that used attendants were coming forward asking for more responsibility and risk in return for greater choice, flexibility and control of their services.

In the early 1980s, due to these limitations, a number of consumers convinced government that they had the right to have individualized attendant services that were different from the SSLU program. Some people, whose needs went beyond the number of hours allocated in the SSLU, turned to Orders-In-Council (OIC) (individualized funding contracts with individuals administered through a third party) (ACAC, 1986).

The OIC became a catalyst to the ongoing movement toward direct funding as an option for Ontario consumers. In 1986, the government started the Outreach Attendant Care Program (OAC) which was an option not tied to dedicated housing units but rather a catchment area. Due to the high demand for OIC, many OIC recipients became concerned (although unsubstantiated), that the government was planning to transfer all OIC consumers to the new Outreach program (CILT, 1997). The Outreach program did have some advantages over OIC. OIC were subjected to yearly reviews and without the review there was no guarantee of monies (ACAC, 1986).

Some OIC users, together with consumers who wanted an alternative to Outreach or SSLUs, organized themselves into the Attendant Care Action Coalition (ACAC) to lobby for the continuation of the OIC mechanism. At that time, ACAC was a predominantly Southern Ontario based coalition with consumers from Toronto and London and parts between.

The Lord Report: Blue Print for Change
In 1988, the Ministry of Community and Social Services responded by contracting a consultant, John Lord, to write a report that would review attendant service programs; produce recommendations for program expansion; and seek a solution to the OIC mechanism. The findings from the Lord report "Independence and Control: Today's Dream, Tomorrow's Reality" (Centre for Research and Education in Human Services, 1988), showed the need to provide a direct funding option.

ACAC wanted to develop a service delivery model, which had as its foundation the independent living principles of choice, flexibility and control on the part of the consumer. The model would value the people who were the attendants and the relationship between a consumer and them. ACAC/CILT put forward a document (CILT, 1993) that was part of the vision for the development of the Direct Funding model in Ontario. The following principles were central to the vision for Direct Funding.

Principles to Guide the Development of Self-Managed Direct Funding Attendant Services in Ontario
- Self-directed attendant services are an essential support to some citizens, to enable full participation in society.
- The enhancement of full participation of the citizen with a physical disability in society must be an important part of the design and the operation of the self-directed attendant services.
- Recognizing there is a variety of individual capabilities, citizens with physical disabilities have the right to exercise the highest level of choice and control over services including the administration of resources.
- Recognizing individual lifestyles, citizens with physical disabilities have the right to exercise choice and control over all aspects of self-directed attendant services.
- Self-directed attendant services are a reasonable accommodation which allows the citizen with a physical disability to meet basic human needs and rights, and therefore should be provided free of cost to the person with a physical disability.
- Self-directed attendant services are different from other services, such as health care and welfare, in that the consumer is the center of expertise for his/her own services.
- Individuals who perform attendant services are engaged in valued and essential activities and should be paid accordingly.
- The level of resources for the self-directed attendant services must be sufficient to support full participation in society as determined by the citizen with a physical disability.
- Recognizing the citizen's right to freedom of movement, attendant services to individual persons, must be free from ties to specific physical locations, and must be fully portable.

These principles would guide the vision of SMASD-FP and provide the blueprint for lobbying to the government and other consumer and community groups.

Woodeden Conference 1990: Establishing Solidarity
ACAC's vision was supported by the Liberal government's Ministry of Community and Social Services' 1988 consultant report "Independence and Control: Today's Dream, Tomorrow's Reality." To solidify the success, in 1990, ACAC, together with London Cheshire Homes and the Centre for Independent Living in Toronto (CILT) Inc., organized a provincial Direct Funding conference called "Woodeden 90 – Flying On My Own" in London, Ontario. This was the first-ever provincial (Ontario) attendant services consumer conference. The conference brought together consumers and their attendants, researchers, ILRCs members, government

officials, service providers and even the Minister of Community and Social Services, the Honourable Charles Beer. The conference allowed government officials to see the strong support and hear directly from consumers about the need for direct funding. Following the conference, ACAC held a press conference stating that the government would announce a pilot using the Disability Network Television show during this time. This show was a partnership between the Centre for Independent Living in Toronto and the Canadian Broadcasting Corporation. The minister later announced that the government would pilot a project for Direct Individualized Funding for 500 people. A month later an election was called and the Liberal government lost the election and were replaced by the New Democratic Party (NDP) in the fall of 1990.

Resource Mobilization: CILT Joins the Cause

After the Woodeden conference, the Center for Independent Living in Toronto (CILT) staff and Board of Directors made an official commitment to support all activities surrounding the direct funding initiative. CILT, an established ILRC, was perfectly situated to act as support and later as the lead organization to the DF initiative. This was important as ACAC was a loosely knit group that did not have the resources to maintain and sustain lobbying efforts. CILT provided vital resources to ACAC in the way of organizational and resource support (i.e. receive grants, do mass mailings or hold meetings without seeking help from a supportive community agency) so that ACAC could mobilize and organize their efforts. Thus, ACAC became ACAC/CILT.

With the election of the New Democratic Party (NDP), ACAC was faced with having to re-educate and lobby a new government. CILT's resource base was vital during this time. CILT developed a database from the Woodeden conference list. This allowed for recruitment and communication to members for renewed lobbying efforts. ACAC could now mail DF information to over 400 individuals and organizations in Ontario. CILT began to write materials, and communicate with other ILRC's across the country for advice and support. For example, many discussions were held between ACAC and the Winnipeg ILRC and consumers there who had extensive experience lobbying for and administrating the supports and resources for a government – run DF program.

Developing a Broad Base of Support: Partnerships and Alliances

Between 1990 and 1993, CILT, ACAC, the seven members of the Ontario Network of Independent Living Centres (ONILC) and the Canadian Association of Independent Living Centres (CAILC) formed a partnership that eventually submitted a proposal for a DF pilot. ONIL came into being in 1993 as the executive Director of the Centre for Independent Living in Toronto needed partners to support the Direct Funding Pilot. During the 1990s there were four ILRC's in Ontario. This alliance submitted their proposal to the Ontario Minister of Health, Francis Lankin in February of 1992. The proposal outlined a 24-month pilot program that would be administered by CILT and run by the Ontario Network of Independent Living Centres. This proposal was endorsed by the Consumer Coalition on Long-Term Care Reform, which was established in April 1992. The Coalition consisted of consumer groups such as Persons United for Self-Help (PUSH), Advocacy Resource Centre for the Handicapped (ARCH) and the Association of Community Living. The Coalition was formed to give input into the LTC reform. ACAC/CILT sought their endorsement that was valuable at the negotiation table to show that Direct Funding had a broad cross disability base of support.

Support from Outside the Membership

Beside the support from ACAC members, ILRCs and other disability-related organizations, a few attendant service providers also supported this proposed new model of service delivery. Most notable of this group was Cheshire Homes, London who provided local consumers with both Outreach and SSLU attendants. The Executive Director, Judi Fisher, was instrumental in setting up both Woodeden conferences along with Jackie Rogers, a long time Cheshire Homes Foundation member and consultant. They, along with other key people in the London area used their time and government contacts to help the direct funding initiative. There were other key individuals from within and outside of government who also supported the project. Most notable were individuals from the Ontario Ministry of Health Policy Branch – Long Term Care Division and the Operations Branch. Their support was vital and the project would have failed without their tireless support. Government bureaucrats within the Ministry of Long Term Care understood the basic concept of attendant services and DF. Other key government officials either worked within the field or had relatives who were living with long term disabilities and the issues of control, choice and being able to live a life of dignity were important. These officials were able to champion the cause within the Ministry to senior levels of management. Officials there again had personal experience with the existing system so they understood the DF concept and its benefits. A senior service provider was also instrumental in facilitating the DF option. This individual used his/her contacts to let ACAC/CILT know when to ask for a meeting or when to set up a conference, and who to invite. These individuals were pivotal to achieving the DF pilot.

Strategies and Tactics

Lobby and Education

ACAC/CILT with support from their external supporters (i.e. government bureaucrats and community advocates) developed a number of strategies to maintain a "visible" profile and to educate government officials on the vision and goals of direct funding. The main strategy was to distribute detailed fact sheets aimed at government officials. These fact sheets stressed civil liberties, the consumer's right to portable, self-managed services that would allow freedom of movement throughout the province and similar, positive messages.

Over the next six months, this lobbying continued in a number of effective ways. One tactic was that ACAC/CILT devised a mock application for direct funding and sent copies of it out to almost 400 members of the now-growing database of ACAC members. More than 100 applications were returned to CILT which were then passed on to the Long Term Care Division of the Ontario Ministry of Health.

ACAC/CILT stayed away from demonstrating against the government, and avoided any type of negative advocacy. All of ACAC/CILT's activities promoted the message that directly funded attendant services would allow consumers to contribute to the community and carry out their social responsibilities. In addition, both ACAC and CILT presented at the Ontario Standing Committee on Social Development. Specifically, submissions were presented by both Mr. Ian Parker and Mr. Vic Willi to the Standing Committee regarding Bill 43 The Regulated Health Professions Act, August 8, 1991. The main reason for attending was to defend the concept of self-directed attendant services as non-medical. This also raised the profile of the Direct Funding initiative.

Defending the Concept

In carrying out these activities, ACAC/CILT constantly found itself relying on the previous experience of consumers – their knowledge of the development and governance of attendant services. ACAC/CILT realized that, consumers involved in the consultations had many years of daily experience (some as many as 25 years) with attendant services. ACAC/CILT had an extensive knowledge base and could offer common sense and workable solutions to the "What if . . ." type of questions that were often posed by government and community partners. For example, one question asked early on by government partners and the Minister's staff was related to what would happen if persons receiving direct funding were to "spend the money on beer."

ACAC/CILT pointed out to their government colleagues that there would be a large consequence to the individual if they choose to spend their direct funding monies in this way. For example, the individual recipient may not have the money to pay attendants and therefore, would have reduced service, e.g. having his/her food cooked, getting assistance in and out of bed, or receiving help using the washroom. ACAC/CILT pointed out that various government programs such as Vocational Rehabilitation Services and Workers Compensation (Snow, 1993) used various forms of direct funding without any similar issues. CILT also pointed out that individuals in society are generally allowed to make mistakes, take risks and even make stupid decisions so why shouldn't a few disabled persons have the right to benefit from that experience. This emphasis on responsibility and citizen rights were the important elements.

One of the most powerful tactics used was to point out that direct funding was happening in other Canadian provinces. These provinces had dealt with similar issues that the Ontario government partners were now raising. ACAC/CILT was able to connect with government officials in other provinces because of their collaborating relationship with the Independent Living Resource Centres (ILRC) across Canada. For example, in the case of Manitoba, the late Al Simpson of the Winnipeg ILRC, connected ACAC/CILT to the key government official of the Manitoba direct funding program. In turn, ACAC introduced one of their key government partners to speak with this individual and a province-to-province discussion was facilitated to discuss mutual government issues. This was a key point as provincial governments rarely "talk" to each other. It was important for a provincial jurisdiction to know that a proposed initiative is actually being done in another jurisdiction for validation purposes.

Development of a Proposed Model
These discussions were important because some of the issues surrounding direct payments to individuals could have powerful consequences. One such issue was the question of "income" versus "services," which had implications at a federal government level. In order for the federal department of Revenue Canada to allow cash payments to an individual to be considered something other than "income," the provincial ministries of Finance have to ask Revenue Canada for a special ruling. The payments to an individual on direct funding are usually explained by the provincial government to be "payments in lieu of service" that the individual would otherwise be entitled. Dealing with Revenue Canada was clearly beyond ACAC/CILT's ability but they were able to alert the Ontario government contacts to the fact that this had to be done and had been done successfully by Manitoba. In the Ontario case, Revenue Canada determined that Direct Funding payments to individuals would be considered to be similar to social assistance and the payments should not be reported as "income" as they are payments in replace of medical expenses. One other major strategy, was the preparation of a

comprehensive position paper called *Direct Individualized Funding for Attendant Services: Proposed Model* (June, 1991). A summary letter was prepared by the alliance consisting of ACAC, CILT and CAILC in 1992. As a result, the Ontario government set up a steering committee consisting of government policy people, political staff, and users of attendant services from the various consumer organizations involved (consumer partners). The Steering Committee worked on the government policy paper for the direct funding pilot. In October of 1992, a modest grant from the Ontario Ministry of Health was given to CILT to hire the ACAC spokesperson as a consumer-consultant to work fulltime on the initiative.

Between 1992 and 1994, the SMAS-DF Steering Committee met frequently to work through the policy paper and setting up of the SMAS-DF pilot. One of the major government requirements that had to be adhered to was the 180-hour per month cap on service. The cap at that time was 3 hours per day or 90 hours per month (4 hours with Ministry approval). SSLU's provided more than that with no cap. The Steering Committee was asking for 6 hours per day. It was felt that this limit might be restrictive in certain cases (i.e. ventilator users) however, it was a non-negotiable issue for the government at that time. Many drafts of the proposal were developed and circulated before a final proposal was accepted in August 1993. In 1994, a second Woodeden conference was held near London, Ontario. At this conference, the Minister of Health, Ruth Grier announced that the SMAS-DF pilot would begin in July 1994.

Barriers and Resolutions

As with any new vision, the proposal for a new model of service delivery was greeted with skepticism. Part of the reason for this initial caution was that the traditional models of service delivery for consumer were based on medical/rehabilitation principles that assume that recipients of attendant services are "sick people," in need of "care." Therefore, these recipients would not be responsible for making decisions and/or being in control.

Regulated Health Professions Act
The need to defend ACAC's original principles of self-directed attendant services and self-management, happened on a number of occasions. For example, the Ontario Medical Association (OMA) as well as the Ontario Nurses Association (ONA) were nearly successful in stopping some key activities of attendant services and in effect would have forced the role of the attendant to become more medical in nature. During the development of the Regulated Health Professions Act (RHPA) (government task force to regulated the practice of a number of health professions).

The authors of this draft regulations were not aware of the existence or concepts of attendant services/self direction, as they regulated certain acts such as requiring assistance to go to the washroom. In addition, the RPA assumed that, for example, catherization was a medical act performed by nurses. Thus, the OMA proposed draft legislation making it illegal and subject to a $25,000 fine for attendants to perform routine activities such as suctioning and catheterization. CILT/ACAC and ARC worked with the OMA (and later the ONA) and regulated an exemption written into the legislation for activities directly related to self-directed attendant services. CILT/ACAC and ARC did this in part to disconnect attendant services from traditional "health care" delivery.

Organized Labour
Another barrier to the Self-Managed Attendant Services Direct Funding was the case of organized labor. In prior years, there have been consumers who have complained about problems encountered with unionized workers, for example, refusing to lift or transfer them. Organized labor was concerned with the rights of the employee: employees working without a contract; not having wage parity, having no direct supervisor to lodge concerns; overall working environment safety and abuse of employees by the disabled employers. However, in meetings with labor representatives, CILT/ACAC clarified these concerns. Consumers are defined as "vulnerable employers," in this way, the consumer would be putting her/himself at risk if s/he abused the worker(s) that s/he was dependent on for her/his day-to-day existence. A mutually respectful, trusting and balanced relationship between the employer and the employee was vital in order for attendant services to work. ACAC/CILT believed that this relationship has always been at the heart of attendant services. As well, ACAC/CILT stressed the well being of attendants, ensuring that they were well treated and well paid.

The SMAS-DF Pilot moved ahead without a final resolution on these issues with organized labor. However, organized labor redirected their attention to the larger issues of long-term care reform and the provincial social contract (this was a government initiative for government workers to take unpaid days to help decrease the government deficit during that year. It was agreed that labor's issues would be examined during the pilot. ACAC/CILT continued to keep labour contacts informed of its progress.

Resistance to Change
Other barriers were in the form of the resistance to change by service providers and consumers. Some attendant service providers feared that the new model might result in the loss of current and future clients. To address their concern ACAC/CILT stressed that a large number of people were on waiting lists to receive attendant

services. Secondly, this self-managed option was not considered to be an answer to all attendant service needs. The self-management model was an option that was meant to complement the existing services. This model brings with it increased responsibility and risk, which is part of self-management. Also the SMAS-DF policy would not allow individuals to remain in an SSLU while on direct funding (Direct Funding Proposal, 1993). This allows access to SSLUs for people who are on attendant service waiting lists.

Self-managed direct funding was meant to be an additional option, not the only option for attendant services. However, for those individuals who prefer to be self-managers willing to take full responsibility, and receive a direct payment, DF may be an appropriate option.

Major Achievements in Pilot

There are two key areas with regards to this pilot that stand out as unique achievements among direct funded, self-managed attendant services programs anywhere in the world. The program is wholly administered by consumer-controlled organizations (an independent living resource centre in partnership with ILRCs in the province). Secondly, consumer management and administration extends down to the level of the Self Manager.

Administration by a Consumer-Controlled Organization (ILRC)

From the outset, consumer control was a prime goal. This consumer control would need to be central throughout the systems and processes used to govern and administer the pilot on a daily basis.

It was determined that having funds go from government to individuals would not be practical. The DF Steering Committee felt that CILT would likely be a stable funding distributor, and along with its partnership with the Ontario Network of Independent Living Centres (ONILC), could provide strong resource supports to participants across Ontario. CILT was contracted as Central Administration, which involved the sending of funds to participants, managing the individual agreements with each person, and reviewing financial reports.

This is the first example that we are aware of, where a consumer-controlled and operated organization has been given the responsibility to manage all the day-to-day administrative functions for a direct funded and self-managed attendant services program. This model allows for consistency of independent living principles throughout the operation of the pilot by establishing the credibility of consumer control in the overall process from top to bottom and allowing participants to deal with their peers in their own system.

Focus on Consumer Responsibility and Control

The concept of peer (consumer) validation (ACAC, 1991) was developed to reflect Independent Living (IL) principles within the application/selection process. The concept of peer validation process has philosophically underpinned the Direct Funding pilot application and selection. This means that the applicant is an active agent in becoming informed of the process and developing a proposal (the application), with the assistance of direct funding resource people. The peer validation process also means that the applicant presents and negotiates their application to a peer selection panel. This concept is new compared to the usual methods whereby professionals or other non-disabled persons control access to human services. A peer approach was put into effect in the pilot in two main ways: (i) focus on an informed consumer; and (ii) peer selection panels.

Informed Consumer. Consumers interested in self-managing their own attendant services were encouraged to become directly informed themselves about the expectations, criteria and responsibilities of the application/selection process. This approach reflects the IL principle that consumers are the ones who really need the information, if they are to make informed choices and decisions about their own services and lives. Other systems focus on educating the professional or other intermediary about the above details, and in many respects create dependency of recipients on these "experts." Since knowledge is power, our system of informing and targeting consumers directly led to their empowerment in this whole process, from start to finish.

Consumers were expected to start the process and complete their own individual applications with support from an ILRC resource person. The expectations of this process and the consumer's role in it are different to the many systems in which someone else fills out an application on the client's behalf, asking the client certain questions while offering "expert" advice about what is best for the client.

Our system demanded a great deal of ambition of applicants. In return, the applicants generally got to know their strengths based on past experiences, education, life/family roles and needs thoroughly, since it reflected their own work. This knowledge was extremely useful for the requirements that they would face if they were to self-manage their own attendants and act as independent employers.

Peer Selection Panels. The IL philosophy also was reflected in the establishment of selection panels, which took advantage of the life experience, and knowledge of using attendant services of consumers as panelists themselves. Panels typically consisted of three people, a consumer, such as, an experienced user of attendant services from the applicant's region, a representative of the ILRC (often a consumer him or herself) in the applicant's region, and a representative from the Project Administration (CILT) (again often a user of attendant services or a staff person educated and managed by a consumer administrator).

In the selection process, applicants attended an interview with the panel at a site outside of the individual's home, such as in the community and often at an ILRC. Applicants were required to present their application, explain and negotiate the hours and budget proposed, and come to an agreement with the panel. They were also asked questions concerning skills needed to self-manage. While some applicants felt the process was intensive, most applicants viewed it as an opportunity to put forth their own individual plans and strengths.

Final Evaluation Report

In early 1997, an external review of the Pilot Project for Self-Managed Attendant Services in Ontario was completed by The Roeher Institute. The evaluation of the Pilot Project was done over a two-year period between 1995 and 1996 with 100 participants chosen for the Pilot. The pilot achieved a number of outcomes which are summarized here (Final Evaluation Report of the Pilot Project for Self-Managed Attendant Services in Ontario, Roeher, 1997b).

(a) It established a consumer-driven partnership with CILT as the pilot administration and ONILC as a resource support network.

(b) The pilot achieved a diversity of participants with respect to the region of the province, rural/urban settings and living arrangements of participants.

(c) Self-managers stated that the pilot made a difference in terms of increased self-determination in all aspects of their lives, reducing their sense of vulnerability, greater independence, a stronger sense of self-esteem, more fulfilling personal relationships and greater social participation.

(d) A number of self-managers reported greater chances for paid employment and career advancement as a result of the pilot.

(e) The pilot created effective employer-employee relationships by enhancing the accountability of both employer and employee, which developed greater levels of mutual respect. As well, attendants who had worked in other service systems reported much higher degrees of job satisfaction in working directly for people with disabilities.

(f) Overall, the pilot provided appropriate supportive resources to consumers wishing to participate in the self-management pilot such as manuals and clear administrative and reporting procedures.

(g) The pilot was responsive to individual needs such as supporting the hiring of attendants where services were not previously available.

(h) Based on the findings from this pilot, direct funding for attendant services appears to be a cost-effective alternative to Outreach and SSLUs.

Labor's issues were addressed during the development of the self-manager training and in the Roeher Institute evaluation of the pilot. The final results of the evaluation suggest that labor's concerns were positively addressed. These issues continue to be addressed on an on-going basis through the DF program.

The success of this pilot was important in the government's announcement in July 1998 to make this a permanent program of the Ontario Ministry of Health. As a result, it was expanded to provide funding to an additional 600 people over the next few years.

The program currently has 691 participants, ranging in age from 17 to 93 years. The majority of the participants are between 45–64 years of age (46.5%) with the second largest group the 25–44 (35%). Sixty percent of the participants are females. The program also has participants with a diversity of health conditions. The largest groups of participants live with multiple sclerosis (24%) and the second largest group lives with spinal cord injuries (19%). The other participants live with other neuro-muscular conditions (e.g. cerebral palsy, polio, spinal muscular dystrophy, stroke and spinal bifida) or arthritis. Attrition to the program for the year 2003/2004 was 4% due to death or withdrawal. There are 300 applications pending for the program, which attests to the appeal of the program.

DISCUSSION

This case study analysis points to many elements that facilitated the emergence and development of the SMAS-DFP. These elements were internal factors related to the physical disability community, but also external factors such as, advocates outside of the community and changes in government philosophy on health reform and structure. All of these factors came together over a period of time, which allowed the SMAS-DFP to become a reality.

This vision was created and moved forward by a core group of people recognized for their leadership in the community. Supporters of the SMAS-DFP came from inside as well as outside of the core community/membership. These supporters provided key resources to be used toward the goal of the SMAS-DFP. The vision, leadership, broad-based support and resources were all important to deal with multiple barriers to the achievement of the SMAS-DFP. Proponents of the SMAS-DFP developed specific approaches and tactics to deal with barriers. We will briefly discuss these contextual and supporting factors to illustrate their importance in this process.

Setting the Stage: Existing Social Movements/Precedents to DF

In our analysis, specific social forces and existing examples created a positive environment for the emergence of the SMAS-DFP. As well, social movements lend themselves to the evolution and support of the ILRCs across Canada.

The network of ILRCs across the country became a resource to the Ontario ILRC's movement towards self-managed direct funding, as prior efforts in British Columbia, Alberta and Manitoba (not all were successful) were communicated to Ontario. The large number of ILRCs in Ontario also was an important resource to the Ontario Self-Managed Direct Funding (SMDF) initiative. This Ontario Network of Independent Living Resource Centres (ONILC) provided an Ontario wide infrastructure to distribute information and materials. Since all ILRCs are governed by criteria in that the centres must be controlled by consumer's (for example, key board and staff positions are held by consumer's), then this structure was an excellent way to help administer and deliver this new service model based on IL principles.

The international examples of various direct payment type programs for attendant services paved the way for discussions in Canada. The national symposium on brokerage/individualized funding provided a vision and knowledge base for consumers, advocates and government officials. These discussions paved the way for the Ontario Direct Funding Pilot as the principles and vision developed at this national symposium were carried forward into the 1990s by consumers, advocates and government. For example, a key Ontario government official during this time was able to promote the DF movement's ideas based on his/her knowledge of this brokerage/individualized funding movement. In addition, the international examples became an important guide and lobbying tool for direct funding in Ontario (Duncan & Brown, 1993).

Vision, Leadership and Internal and External Community Support

The vision for self managed direct funding provided a guide for the development of the SMAS-DFP. This vision, which consisted of many IL principles, gathered much support from the core community. Key partnerships with other disability organizations were formed at various times during the period towards the attainment of the SMAS-DFP, providing a broad base of support.

Resource support refers to support from the core community or membership but also to the significant support from outside of the community that would benefit from this initiative. Key government officials helped ACAC and the SMAS-DFP Steering Committee move through the bureaucratic process of government to gain increased acceptance of the DF model; to develop the proposal and policy framework; and to communicate with appropriate groups such as the Long Term Care area offices. Government representatives involved with the SMAS-DFP Committee were also important in gaining the necessary regulations and legislation to start up the pilot within the expected government requirements.

Government Discourse on Health Care Reform

Changes in government discussion regarding health care reform played a positive role in the appearance of the DF pilot. Despite changes in government, government talks on health reform were consistent with SMASDF. The SMASDF Pilot therefore had bi-partisan appeal – as its focus was to have individuals with physical disabilities take control over their lives. All three political parties could see the benefits of this initiative from their respective viewpoints.

The transition to Long-Term Care was uneven because of the changes in government between the period of 1987 to 1994. This created negative as well as positive consequences to the DF movement. Changes in government required the DF movement to "re-educate" the new government on its agenda. There were however, some positive consequences. The transition to Long-Term Care during the NDP government, provided additional resources by way of government official support for the SMASDF Steering Committee – the development of policy guidelines and implementation of the Pilot. While the SMASDFP could have been in danger of getting "lost in the shuffle," the LTC reform and its legislation, provided an avenue in which the DF pilot could be legislated and then implemented. According to key government officials at the time, the SMASDFP was a relatively small part of this larger reform, which allowed it to be put through as new legislation with larger issues. Thus, the Self-Managed Attendant Service Direct Funding passed through legislation, relatively uncontested. The challenge now in Ontario will be for the self managed attendant service user community to transform the concept of DF model into workable service models for the benefits of all people living with disabilities.

ACKNOWLEDGMENTS

We acknowledged the Social Science Humanities Research Council & Human Resource Development Canada in the form of a grant #817–95–0006 awarded to Dr. Karen Yoshida as principal investigator entitled, "A Case Study Analysis of the Ontario Self-Managed Attendant Services: Direct Funding Attendant Service

Pilot: Independent Living in Action." This project was funded within a Strategic Grant competition entitled, "Integration of Persons with Disabilities."

We also acknowledge the information and insights from our many key informants of the study.

REFERENCES

Attendant Care Action Coalition: Options for Independent Living Assistance (1986). Toronto, Ont.
Attendant Care Action Coalition – Principles to Guide the Development of Attendant Services in Ontario (1990). Reprinted in CILT in the Stream, Spring, 1993.
Canadian Association of Independent Living Centres (CAILC) (2004). Website: http://www.cailc.ca/CAILC/graphic/whatisil/intro_e.html.
Centre for Independent Living in Toronto (1997). Final evaluation report: Self-managed attendant services in Ontario: Direct funding pilot project.
Centre for Research and Education in Human Services (1988). *Independence and control: Today's dream, tomorrow's reality*. Toronto: Ontario Ministry of Community and Social Services.
Centre for Research and Education in Human Services (1993). *Review of individualized funding*. Kitchener, Ont.: Centre for Research and Education in Human Services.
Dejong, G. (1979). Independent living: From social movement to analytic paradigm. *Arch. Phys. Med. Rehabil., 60*, 435–446.
Denzin, N. (1994). The art and politics of interpretation. In: N. K. Denzin & Y. S. Lincoln (Eds), *Handbook of Qualitative Research*. Thousand Oaks, CA: Sage.
Driedger, D. (1989). *The last civil rights movement*. UK: C. Hurst & Co.
Duncan, B., & Brown, S. (Eds) (1993). *Personal assistance services in Europe and North America*. New York/Oakland: Rehabilitation International/World Institute on Disability.
Gadacz, R. (1994). *Rethinking disability*. Edmonton: University of Alberta Press.
Kornhauser, W. (1959). *The politics of mass society*. New York: Free Press.
Mayor's Task Force Report Regarding Disabled and Elderly (1973). Toronto, Ont.
Melucci, A. (1985). The symbolic challenge of contemporary movements. *Social Research, 52*(4), 789–816.
Melucci, A. (1988). Social movements and the democratization of everyday life. In: J. Keanne (Ed.), *Civil Society and the State: New European Perspectives* (pp. 245–260).
Ministries of Health, Community and Social Services and Citizenship (1993). Partnerships in long-term care: A new way to plan, manage and deliver services and community support – An implementation framework.
Ministry of Community and Social Services (1983). Support services for physically disabled adults.
Ministry of Community and Social Services, Ministry of Health, Ministry of Citizenship (1991). Redirection of long-term care and support services in Ontario: A public consultation paper. Ontario.
Ministry of Health (1996). *Attendant outreach services: Policy guidelines and operational standards* (p. 14). Ontario.
Nosek, M. (1993). Personal assistance: Its effect on the long-term health of a rehabilitation hospital population. *Arch. Phys. Med. Rehabil., 74*(2), 127–132.
Oliver, M. (1990). *The politics of disablement*. UK: Macmillan.

Ratzka, A. D. (1993). The user cooperative model in personal assistance: The example of STIL, the Stockholm Cooperative for Independent Living. In: B. Duncan & S. Brown (Eds), *Personal Assistance Services in Europe and North America*. New York/Oakland, CA: Rehabilitation International/World Institute on Disability.

The Roeher Institute (1993). *Direct dollars: A study of individualized funding in Canada*. North York: Author.

The Roeher Institute (1997a). *A literature review on individualized funding. Self-managed attendant services in Ontario: Direct Funding Pilot Project*. North York: Roeher Institute, Author.

The Roeher Institute (1997b). *Self-managed attendant services in Ontario: Direct Funding Pilot Project, Final evaluation report*. North York: Author.

Shapiro, J. (1994). *No pity: People with disabilities forging a new civil rights movement*. New York: Times Books, Random House.

Smesler, N. (1962). *The theory of collective behaviour*. New York: Free Press.

Snow, J. (1993). Advocating for personal assistance in Ontario and in Canada. In: B. Duncan & S. Brown (Eds), *Personal Assistance Services in Europe and North America*. New York/Oakland, CA: Rehabilitation International/World Institute on Disability.

Strachan, D., & Tomlinson, P. (1987, November 1–49). I am who I should be already. A report on the proceedings of the National Symposium on Brokerage/Individualized Funding, Ottawa, Ont.

Woodill, G. (1992). *Independent living and participation in research: A critical analysis*. A discussion paper. Toronto, Ont.: Centre for Independent Living in Toronto.

Working Group of the Direct Funding Pilot Project Self-Managed Attendant Services in Ontario (1993). *A proposal for self-managed attendant services in Ontario: Direct Funding Pilot Project*. Toronto: Working Group of the Direct Funding Pilot Project Self-managed Attendant Services in Ontario.

Yin, R. K. (1994). *Case study research: Design and methods*. Thousand Oaks, CA: Sage.

Yoshida, K. K., Willi, V., Parker, I., Self, H., Carpenter, S., & Pfeiffer, D. (1998). Disability partnerships in research and teaching in Canada and the United States. *Physiotherapy Canada*, 198–205.

Zukas, H. (1979). *CIL history*. Berkeley, CA: Centre for Independent Living.

WHO CRASHES ONTO DIALYSIS? HEALTH DETERMINANTS OF PATIENTS WHO ARE LATE REFERRED TO CHRONIC RENAL CARE IN CANADA

Nancy Blythe and Cecilia Benoit

ABSTRACT

Late nephrology referral, a problem currently identified across many high income countries, has been associated with reduced opportunities for delaying or halting the progression of chronic kidney disease (CKD), delayed dialysis initiation, reduced choice in treatment modality, increased morbidity and hospitalization, and premature death. Despite a recent finding that the progression of CKD nearly always presents warning signs, and despite the fact that all Canadians are entitled to receive medically necessary health care free at the point of patient entry, each year in the province of British Columbia (BC) a substantial number of people with CKD experience late or no referral to nephrology care prior to requiring renal replacement therapy. A subset of these CKD patients experience no referral and "crash" onto dialysis (experience an acute or emergent start). Existing research has not fully explored the range of potential health determinants that may affect the timing of nephrology referral. This paper adopts a "determinants of health" framework and assesses the impact of a variety of indicators

Chronic Care, Health Care Systems and Services Integration
Research in the Sociology of Health Care, Volume 22, 205–237
© 2004 Published by Elsevier Ltd.
ISSN: 0275-4959/doi:10.1016/S0275-4959(04)22011-7

on patients' physical health, demographics, socioeconomic status, social support, geographic and health system characteristics. Using a late referral definition of <3 months and data on BC patients who began dialysis between April 2000 and March 2003, multiple regression analysis indicates that the following determinants have an independent effect on the timing of referral: cause of end-stage renal disease ($p =< 0.0001$); age ($p = < 0.0001$); race/ethnicity ($p = 0.0019$); English ability ($p = 0.0158$); marital status ($p = 0.0202$); proximity to care ($p = 0.0118$); and, "age by first language" ($p = 0.0244$).

INTRODUCTION

The population health or "determinants of health" perspective is a relatively recent way to explain why some people are healthy and others are not. It has emerged in the last few decades as an additional sociological framework to build on and complement the dominant bio-medical model for explaining the health of individuals and populations by focusing on factors other than those determined by human genetics/biology. The health determinants perspective enables us to better understand disparities and inequalities in health outcomes by pointing to the range of social, economic, environmental, and health service factors that interact in complex ways with personal behaviors and predisposing biological pathways to positively or negatively influence health (Canadian Institute for Health Information, 2004; Evans et al., 1994; Marmot, 2003; Marmot & Wilkinson, 1999). Research exploring the complex interactions that determine health has practical implications for improving the health of individuals, communities and global populations by elucidating the multi-dimensional factors that affect the health of particular populations and are responsible for a differential prevalence in health concerns.

The determinants of health framework holds particular value for population occurrences of chronic illness and for determining why some patients fare better than others in regard to timely access to medical treatment. The chronic illness that is focused on in this paper is kidney disease, a condition prevalent across high-income countries today. We pose the research question of why some people with kidney disease fare better than others, by studying some of the main predictors of their referral to nephrology care. Late nephrology referral, a problem currently identified among particular populations in many high income countries (see, e.g. Cass et al., 2003; Curtis et al., 2002; Jungers et al., 1993; Roderick et al., 2002; Winkelmayer et al., 2001), has been associated with delayed dialysis initiation, reduced opportunities for choosing more ambulatory modes of renal replacement therapy or for delaying or halting disease progression, increased morbidity and hospitalization, and premature death (Iofel, 1998; Jungers, 2002; Levin, 2000). In addition to these health burdens for the patient (in terms of illness and reduced quality of life), there are also substantial financial and resource outlay costs for national health care systems. Yet, relatively little is known about the determinants of health of persons who are late-referred to nephrology assessment, and what is known is often in the form of conflicting evidence across studies.

Our research focuses on the case of people with chronic kidney disease (CKD) in the province of British Columbia (BC), Canada. Despite a recent Canadian finding that the progression of CKD nearly always presents observable warning signs (Curtis et al., 2002), and despite the fact that all Canadians are entitled to receive medically necessary health care (Benoit, 2003), each year in the province of BC a substantial number of persons with CKD experience late or no referral to a nephrologist prior to requiring renal replacement therapy (chronic dialysis or transplant). A subset of these patients reportedly "crash" or acute start[1] onto their initial dialysis treatment – that is, experience an emergent dialysis start. In contrast, early referred patients are able to participate in pre-dialysis programs designed to transition them to treatment and sustain their quality of life by minimizing the effect of their chronic illness on daily living.

Since existing late-referral research has not fully explored the range of potential health determinants, the purpose of our study was to broaden the scope of research by including available physical health data as well as potential demographic, economic, social, geographic and health system predictors available to us through existing BC provincial health datasets. Socio-demographic and clinical data on the total number of British Columbians with CKD who initiated dialysis during the period April 2000 to March 2003, as well as census income data by patients' geographic Enumeration or Dissemination Area (based on postal code), were accessed and subsequently analyzed to test the impact of particular health determinants on patients' type of referral to the renal care system. Type of referral was defined as: (1) early referral; (2) late referral without an acute start; and (3) late referral with an acute start. Late referral was defined and tested a number of ways given the various definitions used in prior studies (i.e. <1, <3, <4, <6 and <12 months referral) and the 12 month referral period proposed by the Canadian Society of Nephrology (Levin, 2000). The population under study included CKD patients only; i.e. those who experienced sudden temporary acute renal failure (ARF) due to an underlying disease/condition were not included. We hypothesized that persons with CKD who face certain social structural barriers in society are constrained in their ability to seek treatment before their chronic illness advances to an acute stage and they experience late referral to, and possibly crash onto, the renal care system. [2]

THEORETICAL BACKGROUND, RELEVANT LITERATURE & HYPOTHESES

The Population Health Framework

Our study adopted a population health perspective to investigate the impact of the determinants of health of persons who seek access to chronic renal care services. The population health perspective advanced by Canada's premier health data collection agency, the Canadian Institute for Health Information (CIHI), stipulates that "a range of factors interacting in complex ways determine health" (Canadian Population Health Initiative, CIHI, p. 1). The effects of the determinants of health (broadly categorized by CIHI as: social, economic, environmental, equity of access to health services, personal health practices and biological predisposition) have been repeatedly corroborated in sociological and other health-related research (see for example CIHI, 2004; Evans et al., 1994; Marmot, 2003; Marmot & Wilkinson, 1999; Williams, 2003). Although "access" is usually treated as one of the determinants of health status, the current research problem required that we treat access – in this instance defined as disparities in timing of nephrology referral – as the dependent variable of interest upon which other determinants act.

In order to make sense of what on the surface appears to be a surprising discrepancy in health care access, it is important to understand the strengths and weaknesses of the Canadian public health care system. The underlying assumption of the system is that individual need, not ability to pay, drives the utilization of publicly-funded health care services; therefore, all medically-necessary services are covered through the social insurance system at the point of patient entry (Benoit, 2003; Blomqvist & Brown, 1994). The evidence suggests that this is indeed the case: lower income groups have greater health care needs and use comparatively more services in the Canadian health care system (Broyles et al., 1983; Evans et al., 1994). Yet, the question remains whether those with poorer health status actually access health services *at the rate* that one would expect, given their level of morbidity. Researchers argue that even in relatively equitable public health care systems, such as that of Canada, "predisposing factors" and "enabling conditions" nevertheless mediate the relationship between sickness and the seeking of health services (Shortt & Shaw, 2003). Predisposing factors include demographic, socio-structural and attitudinal-belief variables, whereas enabling conditions include those conditions that facilitate use – such as access to social support and transportation, or the resources to pay for travel to health care facilities (Segall & Chappell, 2000). In short, although sickness determines health care need, the point at which someone identifies with the sick role and becomes motivated to seek treatment is likely to be influenced by their income and other social determinants, but also their geographical location (for a discussion on this topic as it relates to access to maternity care and morbidity for pregnant women in BC, see Benoit et al., 2002).

Relevant Research Literature

As will become clear below, it is probably useful to state upfront that the existing research on access to nephrology referral and/or dialysis has paid little attention to patients' health determinants, instead focusing largely on micro issues, such as the impact of physician attitudes/practices on whether persons with CKD are likely to be referred for nephrology assessment (see, e.g. Mendelssohn et al., 1995; Sekkarie et al., 2001; Wilson et al., 2001) and, once referred, offered the opportunity of dialysis (see, e.g. Hirsch et al., 1994; Kjellstrand & Moody, 1994; McKenzie et al., 1998; Wenger et al., 2000). These studies, as well as a growing number of others that deal specifically with the predictors of late referral (see, e.g. Arora et al., 1999; Cass et al., 2003; Curtis et al., 2002; Holland & Lam, 2000; Letourneau et al., 2003; Steel & Ellis, 2002; Winkelmayer et al., 2001) are important but nevertheless only partially answer the overarching question regarding the health determinants of persons who experience late or no referral to nephrology care prior to requiring treatment, and potentially an acute start onto dialysis. Instead, the determinants of health have been more thoroughly studied in research examining the predictors of developing renal disease (see, e.g. Cass et al., 2001; Fored et al., 2003; Kutner & Brogan, 2000; Nzerue et al., 2002; Perneger et al., 1995; Young et al., 1994), renal patient health status (see, e.g. Garg et al., 2001; Kriegsman et al., 1995; Kutner, 1987; Turner-Musa et al., 1999), and access as it relates to differences in dialysis treatment or kidney transplantation (see, e.g. Garg et al., 2001; Gordon, 2001; Kasiske et al., 2002; Kutner & Gray, 1981; McCauley et al., 997; Salvalaggio et al., 2003). Knowledge regarding the predictors of timing of access to this chronic care treatment remains largely untapped, despite the fact that renal patients represent one of the fastest growing groups utilizing health care services in Canada, at a cost that is rising exponentially (e.g. the total number of renal patients in BC has been growing at a rate of approximately 10% a year, with an estimated annual cost per patient of $50,000–$60,000 Cdn).

In preparation for the development of our hypotheses regarding the impact of renal patients' health determinants on their type of referral/access, we reviewed the relevant literature on the predictors of late referral to nephrology care, late initiation to dialysis and suboptimal pre-dialysis care. Literature on whether a person with CKD is ever likely to be referred to a nephrologist was largely excluded from our review, since it was beyond the scope of this study to ascertain the proportion and determinants of unmet need in the BC population.

The majority of late-referral studies are relatively recent, conducted during the late or early 1990s, presumably due to mounting interest in ways to stem the human costs and health system outlays associated with poor health outcomes for this growing chronic care population. The definition of late referral varies amongst studies, with the majority using a definition of <3 months referral (Cass et al., 2003; Curtis et al., 2002; Letourneau et al., 2003; Winkelmayer et al., 2001) or <1 month of referral (Jungers et al., 1993; Ratcliffe et al., 1984; Roderick et al., 2002; Schmidt et al., 1998). However, the following definitions have also been used: <4 months referral (Arora et al., 1999; Kinchen et al., 2002), <12 months referral (Ifudu et al., 1999), and the clinical marker "serum creatinine" (Holland & Lam, 2000; Ifudu et al., 1999). We located two studies on the predictors of late dialysis initiation and included these in our review due to an established link between delayed nephrology referral and late dialysis initiation (Arora et al., 1999; Iofel et al., 1998). These studies used the following definitions of late initiation: hematocrit of <22% (Iofel et al., 1998), and glomerular filtration rate of <5 ml/min per 1.73 m^2 (Kausz et al., 2000). We also reviewed one study on the predictors of suboptimal pre-dialysis care that used hypoalbuminemia, hematrocrit of <28%, and erythropoietin usage as measures of suboptimal care (Obrador et al., 1999).

The studies reviewed were located in five countries, each with different national health care systems: three studies were conducted in Canada, eight in the United States (U.S.), three in the United Kingdom (U.K.), and one each in France and Australia. The studies also varied in size of patient sample or population studied (ranging from $n = 55$ to $N = 155,076$) and the number and type of potential determinants analyzed. The determinants most frequently studied were demographic (age, gender and race/ethnicity), followed by socioeconomic status, comorbidities and predisposing disease, and geographical and health service characteristics (proximity to care, and renal centre/network). We located only one prior study that considered the potential impact of patients' social support (i.e. marital status – Kinchen et al., 2002).

We begin our literature summary with findings related to the predictive effect of renal patients' health conditions (comorbidities and predisposing disease). These are followed by a discussion of findings related to demographic, socioeconomic and social support indicators and, finally, geographic/health services characteristics (proximity to treatment, and renal centre or network).

Prior Health Conditions
A diagnosis of diabetes has often been found to have a protective effect against late referral (Holland & Lam, 2000; Schmidt et al., 1998; Winkelmayer

et al., 2001), presumably due to the close physician monitoring that diabetics are likely to undergo. In contrast, a number of studies have not found diabetes to be protective against late referral (Arora et al., 1999; Curtis et al., 2002; Ratcliffe et al., 1984). Obrador et al. (1999) found diabetes to be associated with sub-optimal pre-dialysis care when testing the effect of diabetes on hypoalbuminemia, but found no such association when testing the effect of diabetes on suboptimal care defined by a hematocrit level of <28%. However, Obrador et al. (1999) did find diabetes to be protective against suboptimal pre-dialysis care when testing the effect of diabetes on erythropoietin usage.

There is similar conflicting information regarding the impact of patients' comorbid conditions – i.e. an equal number of late-referral studies found a relationship between comorbidity (type or severity of) and late referral (Holland & Lam, 2000; Kinchen et al., 2002) as did not (Arora et al., 1999; Roderick et al., 2002). In addition, an association between comorbidity and early referral has been reported by Winkelmayer et al. (2001) and Kausz et al. (2000) found an association between comorbidity and early dialysis initiation.

The findings related to cause of end-stage renal disease (ESRD) are equally contradictory: two studies found an association between cause of ESRD and late referral (Jungers et al., 1993; Ratcliffe et al., 1984) and four studies did not (Arora et al., 1999; Holland & Lam, 2000; Ifudu et al., 1999; Roderick et al., 2002). Schmidt et al. (1998) found an association between diabetic renal failure and early referral; however, Kausz et al. (2000) found an association between cause of ESRD (diabetes) and late dialysis initiation.

Demographics, SES and Social Support

Relevant studies on a variety of social determinants also reported inconsistent findings. The majority of these studies found increasing age to be associated with greater risk of late referral (Curtis et al., 2002; Holland & Lam, 2000; Letourneau et al., 2003; Ratcliffe et al., 1984; Roderick et al., 2002; Winkelmayer et al., 2001); however, Steel and Ellis (2002) found persons of younger age to be more likely to be late referred. A number of studies did not find an association between age and late referral (Arora et al., 1999; Jungers et al., 1993; Kinchen et al., 2002; Schmidt et al., 1998), and Ifudu and colleagues (1999) found conflicting results depending on how late referral was defined (i.e. they found increased age to be associated with a poor serum creatinine level, but not with <12 months of referral). On the other hand, Kausz et al. (2000) reported younger age to be associated with late dialysis initiation, but Iofel et al. (1998) did not find age to be related to late dialysis initiation, and Obrador et al. (1999) did not find an association between increased age and suboptimal pre-dialysis care.

The overwhelming majority of late referral studies that included gender as part of the analysis did not find an association between patient gender and late referral (Arora et al., 1999; Curtis et al., 2002; Ifudu et al., 1999; Jungers et al., 1993; Kinchen et al., 2002; Roderick et al., 2002; Schmidt et al., 1998; Steel & Ellis, 2002). However, a few studies found female gender to be associated with late referral (Holland & Lam, 2000), delayed dialysis initiation (Kausz et al., 2000) and suboptimal pre-dialysis care (Obrador et al., 1999). Only one study (Winkelmayer et al., 2001) found male gender to be a factor in late referral (i.e. for males <65 years of age).

Nearly all of the studies that included race/ethnicity as a predictor found non-whites and/or blacks to have a greater probability of late referral, delayed dialysis initiation or sub-optimal pre-dialysis care (Ifudu et al., 1999; Iofel et al., 1998; Kausz et al., 2000; Kinchen et al., 2002; Obrador et al., 1999; Winkelmayer et al., 2001). Two studies did not find an association between race/ethnicity and late referral (Arora et al., 1999; Schmidt et al., 1998), and Ifudu et al. (1999) found conflicting results depending on how late referral was defined (non-whites were found to have a greater probability of late referral measured by serum creatinine concentration; however, race/ethnicity was not a factor in <12 months referral).

Socioeconomic status was variously defined as level of health insurance (U.S. studies) education, urban areas of disadvantage/advantage, and a measure of high/middle/low income. Two studies found a relationship between lower SES and late referral (Cass et al., 2003; Kinchen et al., 2002); however, two other studies did not (Jungers et al., 1993; Winkelmayer et al., 2001), and Arora et al. (1999) found that HMO U.S. patients had a greater chance of late referral than Medicare patients. Low SES was, however, found to be linked to late dialysis initiation (Kausz et al., 2000) and sub-optimal pre-dialysis care (Obrador et al., 1999).

Marital status as a measure of social support was included in only one study (Kinchen et al., 2002) and was not found to be related to late referral. No additional measures of social support were located within the literature reviewed.

Geographic and Health System Characteristics
A number of late referral studies included measures of proximity to, or availability of, renal care services; however, none were found to be associated with late referral (Cass et al., 2003; Holland & Lam, 2000; Schmidt et al., 1998). Two studies did, however, find a patient's renal network (i.e. renal services provider) to be associated with late dialysis initiation (Kausz et al., 2000) and suboptimal pre-dialysis care (Obrador et al., 1999).

In summary, the research findings on impact of prior health conditions are mixed. The majority of studies found increasing age, non-white or Black race/ethnicity, and lower SES to be associated with late referral, late dialysis initiation or suboptimal pre-dialysis care; however, the same was not true of gender. Although social support (as measured by marital status) was not found to be associated with late referral, this finding is based on the strength of one study only. Proximity to care was not found to be predictive of late referral; however, other studies on the likelihood of whether a patient would ever be referred to nephrology care have reported a relationship between proximity to care and nephrology referral (Boyle et al., 1996; Mendelssohn et al., 1995). Patients' renal care network/service, while not studied in relation to late referral, was predictive of late dialysis initiation or suboptimal pre-dialysis care.

In short, the majority of existing studies on late nephrology referral lack complexity by overlooking important variables that should be included from a determinants-of-health perspective. This lack of complexity and inconsistency in reported findings necessitates further research that is robust in its inclusion of potential variables and involves analysis of statistically generalizable data. The study reported on below is a step in this direction.

Study Hypotheses

Hypotheses derived from our review of the relevant literature and related to those determinants available for study based on our utilization of existing data on BC renal patients are presented in Table 1. Hypotheses regarding the predictive effect of patients' age, race/ethnicity, and SES were straightforward, given the prior research findings discussed above. Although the findings on prior health conditions

Table 1. Research Hypotheses.

Determinant	Research Hypotheses
Prior health condition	1. ESRD cause is directly related to LR and/or LR/AS.
	2. Diabetes is protective against LR and/or LR/AS.
Age	3. Increasing age is directly related to LR and/or LR/AS.
Gender	4. Female gender is directly related to LR and/or LR/AS.
Race/Ethnicity	5. Ethnic minority status is directly related to LR and/or LR/AS.
SES	6. Low SES is directly related to LR and/or LR/AS.
Social support	7. Presence of a spouse/partner or next-of-kin is directly related to ER.
Proximity to care	8. >1 hour drive to regional renal centre is directly related to LR and/or LR/AS.
Renal centre	9. Regional renal centre is directly related to LR and/or LR/AS.

Note: ER = early referral; LR = late or no referral with no acute start; LR/AS = late/no referral with acute start.

were contradictory, we hypothesized that cause of ESRD would impact the timing of patient referral, and that a diagnosis of diabetes would be found to have a protective effect against suboptimal referral. Similarly, although previous findings regarding gender were contradictory, where a significant association was found it was consistently associated with female gender; therefore, we constructed a hypothesis to this effect. Because social support has been generally ignored in prior studies, we decided to include it in our model. We hypothesized a relationship between reduced social support and late referral. Given prior research findings regarding the impact of a patient's renal network or dialysis centre, we surmised there may be differences in the type of referral experienced by patients accessing different renal care centres in BC. Finally, despite contradictory prior findings about proximity to care, given the size and geography of BC,[3] we hypothesized that reduced proximity to care is associated with late referral, and defined reduced proximity as >1 hour's drive, which coincides with the definition used by Schmidt et al. (1998). The relationship between the independent variables and dependent variable, including potential interaction effects between independent variables, is represented in Fig. 1.

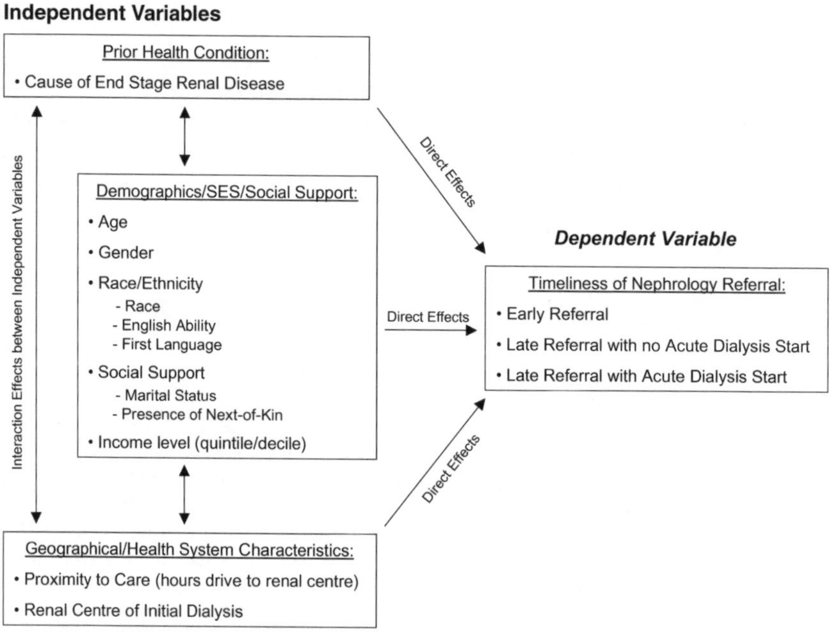

Fig. 1.   Relationship Between Independent and Dependent Variables.

METHODS

Data and Sample

The research hypotheses have been tested with existing data provided by the British Columbia Provincial Renal Agency (BCPRA) on the total number of new renal patients who initiated dialysis during the period April 1, 2000 to March 31, 2003 ($N = 2,001$). Only known CKD patients at time of nephrology referral or acute start onto dialysis were included in the dataset; those classified as ARF were not included. Data on CKD patients' socioeconomic status (income quintile and decile data from Statistics Canada) were obtained through the British Columbia Linked Health Database (BCLHD) maintained by the Centre for Health Services and Policy Research at the University of British Columbia. Income data for the year 2001 were used for the majority of patients; however, in instances where patient postal codes had been retired, 1996 income data were substituted where possible ($n = 44$ cases).

Measures

The determinants of health included in our study, based on the availability of existing provincial data (i.e. prior health conditions, demographics, socioeconomic status, social support, and geographic/health system characteristics), are presented in Table 2. These datasets restricted the research design to data elements currently recorded (e.g. the approximate measure of patient socio-economic status is based on aggregate-level income quintile/decile[4] data derived from the Canada Census). Despite such shortcomings, we believe the research findings provide a crucial first step in identifying the potential impact of multiple health determinants on renal patients' initial access to nephrology care.

Analytical Technique

Our research employs a retrospective cross-sectional design. Multinomial logistic regression analysis was performed using the program SAS (Statistical Analysis for the Social Sciences) to study the impact of the independent on dependent variables of interest – i.e. the direct and interaction effects of renal patients' health determinants (e.g. availability of social support, adequacy of income, age, ethnicity, etc.) on their nephrology referral experience. The use of multinomial logistic regression was appropriate for our three-category dependent variable (early

Table 2.   Measures Operationalized.

Determinant	Operationalized Measure	Type of Variable	
		IV	DV
Type of referral	Early referral; late or no referral without an acute start; late/no referral with acute start		X
Prior health condition	Cause of ESRD (primary diagnosis)	X	
Age	Age at dialysis initiation	X	
Gender	Male, female	X	
Race/Ethnicity	Race/ethnicity	X	
	English ability	X	
	First language	X	
SES	Income quintiles/deciles (Census data)	X	
Social support	Marital status	X	
	Presence of next-of-kin	X	
Proximity to care	Hours drive to regional renal centre	X	
Renal centre	Regional renal centre where patient referred and initially dialyzed)	X	

Note: IV = independent variable; DV = dependent variable.

referral, late referral with no acute start onto dialysis, or late referral with an acute start), and included all variables identified in Table 3.

Data recodes were performed to deal with small cell issues and missing values within patient records. Missing values were recoded to an "unknown" category for each variable and maintained in the analysis; no attempt was made to attribute values for missing ones. Although there were more complex statistical methods for dealing with missing values, coding them to a separate category was preferable to deleting these cases altogether. We employed a late referral definition of <3 months for our analysis, since it was one of the most often used definitions and has been used in two prior Canadian late referral studies (Curtis et al., 2002; Letourneau et al., 2003). In contrast to prior late referral studies, we separated the acute starters from other late referred patients and put them into a distinct category. In addition, we re-ran our analysis using alternate late referral cut-offs (i.e. <1, <4, <6 and <12 months referral) to report on potential differences in the significance of health determinant effects on patients' referral type. When testing the impact of patient age, we tested for a possible curvilinear effect, and retained the original one-year age increments for greater statistical sensitivity. Geographic proximity to care was measured using MapQuest (www.mapquest.com), which enabled us to calculate the driving distance between a patient's city of residence and postal code to the street address of their regional renal centre. Finally, two and three-way interactions between the independent variables (e.g. gender by marital status) were included in our model to test for potential interaction effects.

Table 3. Descriptive Statistics: Determinants of Patient Referral.

Variable	Type of Patient Referral – Frequency Distribution							
	ER		LR		LR/AS		Total Patients	
	N	%	*N*	%	*N*	%	*N*	%
Type of referral	969	48.4	803	40.1	229	11.4	2001	100
Cause of ESRD								
Diabetes	279	65.3	130	30.4	18	4.2	427	100
Glom/AID	162	58.5	90	32.5	25	9.0	277	100
Nephropath.	12	54.6	6	27.3	4	18.2	22	100
Renal Vasc.	98	53.3	70	38.0	16	8.7	184	100
Congenital or polycystic	83	73.5	29	25.7	1	0.9	113	100
Other	53	34.0	74	47.4	29	18.6	156	100
Unknown	282	34.3	404	49.2	136	16.6	822	100
Gender								
Male	580	49.4	452	38.5	143	12.2	1175	100
Female	389	47.1	351	42.5	86	10.4	826	100
Race/Ethnicity								
Caucasian	426	56.8	270	36.0	54	7.2	750	100
Other than Caucasian	263	52.9	184	37.0	50	10.1	497	100
Unknown	280	37.1	349	46.3	125	16.6	754	100
English ability								
Proficient	619	54.7	401	35.4	112	9.9	1132	100
Less than proficient	138	49.8	112	40.4	27	9.8	277	100
Unknown	212	35.8	290	49.0	90	15.2	592	100
First language								
English	304	56.3	179	33.2	57	10.6	540	100
Other than English	125	50.4	96	38.7	27	10.9	248	100
Unknown	540	44.5	528	43.5	145	12.0	1213	100
SES								
Income Quintile								
1 (lowest)	243	50.0	198	40.7	45	9.3	486	100
2	228	51.7	165	37.4	48	10.9	441	100
3	176	45.1	168	43.1	46	11.8	390	100
4	148	48.1	118	38.3	42	13.6	308	100
5 (highest)	134	48.6	111	40.2	31	11.2	276	100
Unknown	40	40.0	43	43.0	17	17.0	100	100
Income Decile								
1 (lowest)	125	46.1	129	47.6	17	6.3	271	100
2	118	54.9	69	32.1	28	13.0	215	100
3	127	52.3	94	38.7	22	9.1	243	100
4	101	51.0	71	35.9	26	13.1	198	100
5	86	41.4	95	45.7	27	13.0	208	100

Table 3.   (*Continued*)

Variable	Type of Patient Referral – Frequency Distribution							
	ER		LR		LR/AS		Total Patients	
	N	%	N	%	N	%	N	%
6	90	49.5	73	40.1	19	10.4	182	100
7	79	50.0	58	36.7	21	13.3	158	100
8	69	46.0	60	40.0	21	14.0	150	100
9	71	46.1	67	43.5	16	10.4	154	100
10 (highest)	63	51.6	44	36.1	15	12.3	122	100
Unknown	40	40.0	43	43.0	17	17.0	100	100
Social support								
Marital status								
Married/Common law	338	57.8	213	36.4	34	5.8	585	100
Divorced/Separated	22	48.9	19	42.2	4	8.9	45	100
Single	73	62.9	39	33.6	4	3.5	116	100
Widowed	46	52.9	33	37.9	8	9.2	87	100
Unknown	490	42.0	499	42.7	179	15.3	1168	100
Presence of next of kin								
No	15	44.1	17	50.0	2	5.9	34	100
Yes	380	54.9	254	36.7	58	8.4	692	100
Unknown	574	45.0	532	41.7	169	13.3	1275	100
Proximity to care								
≤1 hour drive	787	49.9	608	38.6	181	11.5	1576	100
>1 hour drive	176	44.0	180	45.0	44	11.0	400	100
Unknown	6	24.0	15	60.0	4	16.0	25	100
Dialysis centre								
Dialysis centre A	161	54.6	92	31.2	42	14.2	295	100
Dialysis centre B	213	50.5	134	31.8	75	17.8	422	100
Dialysis centre C	11	57.9	8	42.1	0	0.0	19	100
Dialysis centre D	185	48.6	180	47.2	16	4.2	381	100
Dialysis centre E	50	30.9	58	35.8	54	33.3	162	100
Dialysis centre F	154	50.8	145	47.9	4	1.3	303	100
Dialysis centre G	49	46.7	48	45.7	8	7.6	105	100
Dialysis centre H	29	43.9	35	53.0	2	3.0	66	100
Dialysis centre I	34	44.2	34	44.2	9	11.7	77	100
Dialysis centre J	58	47.2	48	39.0	17	13.8	123	100
Dialysis centre K	25	52.1	21	43.8	2	4.2	48	100

Note: ER = early referral; LR = late or no referral with no acute start; LR/AS = late/no referral with an acute start.

Data sources: BCPRA Patient Records, Outcome and Management Information System (PROMIS); Statistics Canada for income quintile/decile data, provided by the BC Centre for Health Services and Policy Research.

FINDINGS

Descriptive Statistics

Descriptive statistics regarding the relationship between patient characteristics and type of nephrology referral are presented in Table 3. Of the 2001 persons with CKD who began dialysis in British Columbia during the period April 1, 2000, to March 31, 2003, 229 or 11.4% experienced late referral with an acute start onto dialysis (i.e. zero referral time and an emergent dialysis start). A further 473 patients (23.6%) also experienced zero referral time but did not acute start onto dialysis, making for a total of 702 patients (35.1%) who had no prior exposure to a nephrologist before their dialysis initiation. This is in line with Canadian referral estimates provided by Levin (2000) who reported that 20–50% of new renal patients enter onto dialysis without a period of previous exposure to a nephrologist.

In addition to the 11.4% of new patients who experienced late (no) referral with an acute dialysis start, an additional 40.1% were late referred to nephrology assessment based on a late referral definition of <3 months. This means that fully 51.5% of new renal patients in BC were referred to a nephrologist less than 3 months before they required dialysis (percentage includes acute starters), which is higher than the 35% reported in a previous Canadian study that involved 15 renal centres across seven provinces and also defined late-referral as <3 months (Curtis et al., 2002). When we re-ran the analysis using alternate definitions of late referral (i.e. from <1 month to <12 months) we found that, in addition to the 11.4% who acute started, between 31% and 62% experienced late referral to nephrology assessment prior to initiating dialysis. The above descriptive data hint at a major problem in regard to timely access to care for persons with CKD, seriously affecting their chronic illness pathways and reducing their overall quality of health.

Logistic Regression Statistics

Our multinomial logistic regression results indicated that a number of the health determinants studied had a statistically significant effect on renal patients' referral experience (see Table 4). The overall likelihood ratio test of significance for the model was: $\chi^2 = 557.8601$, df $= 88$, $p > \chi^2 = < 0.0001$, allowing us to reject the null hypothesis that none of the independent variables exerted significant effect on the dependent variable "type of referral." A statistical significance level of $p \leq 0.05$ indicated the importance of the following determinants found to have independent effect on patients' referral experience: cause of ESRD ($p = < 0.0001$), age (linear effect, $p = < 0.0001$), race/ethnicity ($p = 0.0019$),

Table 4.   SAS Type III Analysis of Effects on Patient Referral (Late Referral
Defined as <3 Months).

Independent Variable	Significance of Effect on Referral		
	df	Wald Chi-Square	Pr > Chi-Square
Cause of ESRD	12	120.7098	<0.0001
Age	2	21.6973	<0.0001
Gender	2	4.2543	0.1192
Race/Ethnicity	4	17.0228	0.0019
English ability	4	12.2179	0.0158
First language	4	5.0636	0.2808
Income decile	20	25.1923	0.1942
Marital status	8	18.1413	0.0202
Next of kin	4	4.1430	0.3870
Hours drive to care	4	12.9013	0.0118
Regional renal centre	20	147.3184	<0.0001
Age by first language[a]	4	11.2008	0.0244

Note: A "Pr > Chi-Square" of ≤ 0.05 is considered significant.
[a] Interaction effect.

English ability ($p = 0.0158$), social support (marital status, $p = 0.0202$), proximity to care ($p = 0.0118$), patient's regional renal centre ($p = < 0.0001$), and age by first language (interaction effect, $p = 0.0244$). In contrast, the following variables were found to have no significant effect: gender, first language, income quintile or decile, and availability of next-of-kin. When we re-ran the analysis using the alternate late referral definitions, we found the following differences in statistical significance of determinants: (1) for a definition of <1 month referral, in addition to the variables that were significant at <3 months, availability of next of kin became significant ($p = 0.0308$); (2) for <4 months referral, the identical determinants were found to be significant as were found for a <3 months definition; (3) for <6 months referral, the determinants English ability and proximity to care were no longer found to have a significant effect on timing of referral; and (4) for <12 months referral, English ability, proximity to care, as well as age and the age by language interaction were no longer found to have significant effect; however, income decile attained statistical significance as a predictor of timing of referral ($p = 0.0353$).

Parameter estimates from the multinomial regression analysis (for a late referral definition of <3 months) were converted to expected probabilities (e.g. the expected probability of experiencing an acute start onto dialysis if one is married or in a common-law relationship) and are presented in Table 5. These findings are

Table 5. Expected Probabilities for the Impact of Determinants on Patient Referral.

Determinant (Independent Variable)	Referral Experience		
	ER	LR	LR/AS
Cause of ESRD			
Diabetes	0.521	0.470	0.008
Glom/AID	0.489	0.491	0.019
Nephropath.	0.518	0.446	0.035
Renal Vasc.	0.401	0.576	0.023
Congenital or polycystic	0.593	0.405	0.002
Other	0.269	0.691	0.040
Unknown	0.267	0.706	0.027
Age			
10	0.208	0.776	0.016
20	0.244	0.740	0.016
30	0.284	0.700	0.016
40	0.328	0.656	0.016
50	0.374	0.609	0.016
60	0.424	0.560	0.016
70	0.474	0.510	0.016
80	0.526	0.459	0.015
90	0.576	0.409	0.015
Race/Ethnicity			
Caucasian	0.455	0.530	0.015
Other than Caucasian	0.480	0.507	0.013
Unknown	0.370	0.609	0.022
English ability			
Proficient	0.488	0.493	0.018
Less than proficient	0.435	0.555	0.010
Unknown	0.379	0.597	0.023
Interaction: Age by first language			
English			
Age			
10	0.221	0.766	0.012
20	0.262	0.724	0.013
30	0.308	0.678	0.014
40	0.358	0.628	0.014
50	0.411	0.574	0.015
60	0.466	0.519	0.015
70	0.522	0.463	0.015
80	0.577	0.408	0.015
90	0.630	0.355	0.014
Other than English			
10	0.112	0.879	0.009

Table 5.   (*Continued*)

Determinant (Independent Variable)	Referral Experience		
	ER	LR	LR/AS
20	0.146	0.843	0.011
30	0.188	0.798	0.014
40	0.238	0.745	0.017
50	0.297	0.683	0.020
60	0.363	0.614	0.023
70	0.434	0.540	0.026
80	0.507	0.464	0.029
90	0.579	0.390	0.031
Unknown			
10	0.334	0.636	0.030
20	0.355	0.620	0.025
30	0.377	0.602	0.021
40	0.399	0.583	0.018
50	0.421	0.564	0.015
60	0.443	0.544	0.012
70	0.466	0.524	0.010
80	0.489	0.503	0.009
90	0.511	0.481	0.007
Marital status			
Married/Common law	0.447	0.539	0.014
Divorced/Separated	0.427	0.558	0.015
Single	0.493	0.498	0.009
Widowed	0.419	0.560	0.021
Unknown	0.385	0.586	0.029
Proximity to care			
≤1 hour drive	0.556	0.432	0.013
>1 hour drive	0.455	0.528	0.017
Unknown	0.302	0.679	0.019
Dialysis centre			
Dialysis centre A	0.601	0.345	0.054
Dialysis centre B	0.437	0.449	0.114
Dialysis centre C	0.486	0.514	0.000
Dialysis centre D	0.416	0.561	0.023
Dialysis centre E	0.335	0.474	0.191
Dialysis centre F	0.541	0.455	0.004
Dialysis centre G	0.393	0.559	0.048
Dialysis centre H	0.306	0.678	0.016
Dialysis centre I	0.361	0.557	0.082
Dialysis centre J	0.353	0.551	0.096
Dialysis centre K	0.352	0.622	0.027

Note: ER = early referral; LR = late or no referral with no acute start; LR/AS = Late/no referral with acute start.

subsequently discussed using the following abbreviations for the "type of referral" categories: ER = early referral; LR = late (or no) referral without an acute start onto dialysis; LR/AS = late (no) referral with an acute start.

Determinants of Health Results

Prior Health Conditions

Individuals' genetic endowment and biological make-up are primary determinants of health (CIHI, 2004). Our data were limited to the extent that we had no information on genetic and most biological determinants of the study population, although we did have information on certain physical health characteristics that gave some indication of the association between other disease occurrences, chronic kidney disease and referral to specialized care.

The expected probability of a patient experiencing LR/AS varied from between 0.2% for patients with congenital or polycystic disease as their cause of ESRD, to 4.0% for those identified as having an "other" unnamed cause. Persons with "other" or "unknown" cause also had the highest expected probabilities for LR (69.1 and 70.6% respectively), and the lowest expected probabilities for ER (26.9 and 26.7%). For persons whose cause of ESRD was known, those with "congenital or polycystic" disease had the lowest expected probability of LR (40.5%), and the highest expected probability of ER (59.3%). Next to the "other" category, persons with nephropathy had the highest expected probability of LR/AS (3.5%), and, next to the "other" and unknown categories, persons with renal vascular disease had the highest expected probability of LR (57.6%). As expected, being diabetic was found to have a somewhat protective effect against LR/AS (0.8% expected probability) and LR (47% expected probability).

Demographics

(a) Age

Our expected probability calculations indicated the opposite relationship to what we predicted with our age hypothesis – i.e. a person's expected probability of LR substantially decreased with increasing age, and LR/AS minimally decreased for those aged 80 and 90. As can be seen in Table 5, persons aged ≤30 had a 70% or greater expected probability of LR, in comparison to those aged 60+ who had a 56% or lesser probability of LR. The relationship was not as evident for the referral category LR/AS; however, those aged 80+ had a slightly reduced probability of LR/AS. The expected probability of ER increased with age.

(b) Race/Ethnicity

Similar to our findings on age, the expected probability calculations for race/ethnicity indicated the opposite relationship to what we predicted – i.e. Caucasians were found to have a slightly higher expected probability of both LR and LR/AS compared to persons of other known racial background. However, since there were a substantial number of missing values for this variable (754 out of 2001 patients), it was not known whether these cases would shift the balance of our results – i.e. patients in the "unknown" category had the highest expected probability of LR (60.9% compared to 53% for Caucasians and 50.7% for "others") and LR/AS (2.2% compared to 1.5% for Caucasians and 1.3% for "others").

The expected probability findings for English ability somewhat mirrored those for race/ethnicity – i.e. those who were English proficient had a higher expected probability of LR/AS than those who were less proficient in English (1.8% compared to 1.0% respectively); however, the relationship was reversed for LR, where those who were less than proficient in English had a 55.5% expected probability compared to 49.3% for those who were English proficient. Persons with unknown English ability ($n = 592$) had the highest probability of LR/AS and LR (2.3 and 59.7%), and those who were English proficient had the highest probability of ER (48.8% compared to 43.5 and 37.9% for the less than English proficient and unknowns).

(c) Interaction Effect: Age by First Language

When we included potential two and three-way interactions in our multinomial logistic regression model, patients' first language attained significance when paired with patient age ($p = 0.0244$). The resulting expected probabilities for the "age by first language" interaction provided more in-depth information than what was found by looking solely at the results for the individual variables "age," "race" or "English ability" above. Unlike the age results, the expected probabilities for "age by first language" indicated that the probability of LR/AS increased with age for those whose first language was English or other than English, and decreased with age for those whose first language was unknown. For those whose first language was English, there was a slightly reduced expected probability of LR/AS for those aged 90 compared to those aged 50–80. Similar to the age results reported above, for each of the three categories of first language, the probability of LR decreased with age; however, the probability of LR at almost every age was higher for those whose first language was other than English compared to those whose language was English or unknown (i.e. expected probabilities were lower only at ages 80 and 90 compared to those for whom language was unknown) – this agreed with the above finding for English ability, where those who were less than proficient at English were found to have a higher expected probability of LR than those who were English proficient. Again, similar to the age results, for each of the three categories of first language the expected probability of ER increased with age; however, the expected probability of ER was higher at every age for those whose first language was English compared to those whose first language was other than English (this was also similar to the English ability results above, where those who were English proficient were found to have a higher expected probability of ER than those who were less than English proficient).

Social Support

The availability and extent of a person's social support network are primary determinants of health (CIHI, 2004). Although we had access to data on patients' marital status and the presence of next-of-kin (Y/N), additional data were not available to quantify the extent and quality of other supportive networks likely experienced by some/most patients (e.g. the supportive networks of adult children, other relatives, neighbors and/or community support groups). However, our measures provided some indication of the association between social support and renal patients' referral experience.

As expected, the presence of a spouse or common-law partner was found to have a protective effect against LR or LR/AS; however, somewhat surprisingly, single persons were found to have the lowest expected probabilities of LR and LR/AS (49.8 and 0.9% respectively, compared to 53.9 and 1.4% for married/common law, 55.8 and 1.5% for divorced/separated, 56 and 2.1% for widowed, and 58.6 and 2.9% for persons of unknown marital status). The results suggest that a person's loss of prior social support in the form of a marital/common-law partner may increase their probability of LR or LR/AS; however, the high proportion of unknown values for this variable (1168 out of 2001 cases) makes such a generalization somewhat problematic. When we ran a cross tabulation of marital status by gender, the distribution of male and female cases for patients of unknown marital status most closely approximated the divorced/separated category; however, it was not possible to infer with certainty which category(s) the unknown cases match to.

Geographical and Health Service Characteristics

The physical environment and geographical location of populations is a key social determinant of health. Poor environments include exposure to polluted air, water and/or soil. Physical environments can also be inadequate because of over-crowding, poor indoor air quality, inordinate noise and lack of basic amenities, including access to primary and specialized health care services (CIHI, 2004). Our data included measures of geographic proximity and a limited measure of health care service – the regional renal centre to which a patient was referred for nephrology care and initial dialysis treatment (i.e. ongoing dialysis could possibly be accessed at a community dialysis centre, depending on a patient's health condition and location of residence).

(a) Geographic Proximity

As expected, persons with a greater than one hour drive to their regional renal centre were found to have a greater expected probability of LR and LR/AS than persons located one hour or less from renal care. Again, those in the unknown category experienced the greatest expected probability of LR or LR/AS; however, there were only 25 out of 2001 patients for whom geographic proximity was unknown.

(b) Regional Renal Centre

Our expected probability findings indicated significant variation in patients' type of referral across BC's regional renal centres. Persons who initially access renal centre E (Greater Fraser Valley region) had the highest expected probability of LR/AS (19.1%), compared to those centres where patients had the lowest expected probability of LR/AS: renal centre C (0% – however, a very small number of patients access this centre in the Vancouver Mainland region), and renal centre F (0.4% – Vancouver Island Region). Persons who access renal centre A (Lower Mainland region) had the lowest expected probability of LR (34.5%) and the highest expected probability of ER (60.1%), and persons who initially access renal centre H (Southern Okanagan region) had the highest expected probability of LR (67.8%) and the lowest expected probability of ER (30.6%).

DISCUSSION

This study set out to determine why a substantial proportion of new renal patients in the province of BC, Canada, were referred late in the progression of their chronic illness to a nephrologist for assessment, and why a portion of these late-referred patients experienced an acute start onto dialysis. As noted in the introduction, prior research indicated that late referral to nephrology care was associated with delayed dialysis initiation, reduced opportunities for more ambulatory modes of renal replacement therapy and for delaying or halting disease progression, increased patient morbidity and hospitalization, and premature death (Iofel, 1998; Jungers, 2002; Levin, 2000). Given the lack of research into potential non-medical explanations for observed disparities in patients' initial access to the renal care system (as well as the lack of robust data on a variety of these key health determinant variables), we used available province-wide data on patients who initiated dialysis in BC between April 2000 and March 2003 to research the impact of patients' health conditions, demographics, socioeconomic status, social support, and geographical and health system characteristics on their differential referral experience. We believe our study and analysis to be unique in considering the acute-starters separately from other late-referred renal patients.

The results of our study add to the determinants of health literature in which a range of factors (demographic characteristics, socioeconomic status, social support, equity of access to health care services, environmental exposures and personal health practices) have been shown to interact in complex ways with genetic predispositions to influence population health (see, e.g. Evans et al., 1994; Williams, 2003). Our results also augment the growing body of research that has been conducted into the predictors of late referral to nephrology care. Late-referral studies have defined late referral in a number of ways and have to varying degrees incorporated the following potential predictors of late referral into their analyses: comorbidity and/or cause of ESRD, age, gender, race/ethnicity, socioeconomic status, marital status (1 study only), geographic proximity to care, and renal service/network. In one of these studies, Holland and Lam (2000) point out that the variables in their model predicted only 16% of the variability in referral of patients to nephrology care in one facility in Ontario, Canada, and state that other yet-to-be-determined factors may account for a significant amount of the variation. The scope of our study therefore included available indicators on patients' social support, socioeconomic status, geographic and health service characteristics, effectively linking the existing late-referral research to the "determinants of health" literature, and bringing a sociological focus to the study of predictors of observed disparities in renal patient access to this chronic life support service.

Our descriptive and logistic regression results presented above demonstrate the utility of using a determinants-of-health framework to understand differential access to renal care in a region of Canada where such specialized health services are free at the point of delivery. The descriptive statistics indicated that 11.4% of new renal patients acute started onto dialysis during the period April 2000 to March 2003, and a further 31–62% were late referred to nephrology assessment depending on the definition of late referral used (from <1 to <12 months referral). Fully 35% of new renal patients had no prior exposure to a nephrologist prior to requiring dialysis, a figure that is in keeping with Canadian estimates (Levin, 2000). A recent Canadian study by Curtis et al. (2002) indicated that up to 10% of persons with chronic kidney disease may have no advance symptoms of their disease prior to requiring nephrology care. It was therefore possible that the 11.4% who acute started in BC were asymptomatic (unfortunately, patient symptom data were not available for our study); however, Jungers et al. (1993) found that only 18% of their late referred patients were asymptomatic, or approximately 5% of their total patients. By translation, this could mean that only half of the acute starters in our study were asymptomatic. In addition, our study findings indicated that a number of health determinants (social and otherwise) also had an impact on the probability of whether a patient would experience late referral or late referral accompanied by an acute start onto dialysis.

The logistic regression results and presentation of expected probabilities calculations indicated that the following health determinants had a statistically significant effect on the timing of referral experienced by renal patients: prior health condition (cause of ESRD), age, race/ethnicity (racial category and English ability), age by first language (interaction effect), social support (marital status), geographic proximity to care (hours drive), and health system characteristics (regional renal centre where patient is referred and receives initial dialysis).

Our analysis indicated that a patient's expected probability of ER, LR or LR/AS varied according to their diagnosed cause of ESRD, which concurred with our hypothesis that cause of ESRD had a direct effect on LR or LR/AS. For example, persons with a diagnosis of nephropathy or "other" disease were found to have the highest expected probabilities of LR/AS (3.5 and 4.0% respectively) compared to different causes of ESRD. Prior late referral studies were mixed in their results regarding the relationship between ESRD cause and type of referral; our finding regarding the significance of cause of ESRD confirmed findings reported by Jungers et al. (1993) and Ratcliffe et al. (1984). Our hypothesis that being diabetic would be protective against LR or LR/AS was largely born out in our analysis, which concurs with half of the studies we located that examined the effect of diabetes on late referral (Holland & Lam, 2000; Schmidt et al., 1998; Winkelmayer et al., 2001). The protective effect of diabetes was likely due to the more rigorous physician monitoring that a diabetic was likely to undergo. In other words, those patients in frequent contact with the public health care system were more likely to be diagnosed with other chronic care conditions such as renal insufficiency.

Our analytical results regarding patient age indicated the opposite relationship to what we expected; i.e. rather than increasing age having a direct effect on LR or LR/AS, younger patients were found to have a greater expected probability of LR or LR/AS. In contrast, the majority of prior studies we reviewed (including three conducted in Canada) found increasing age to be a significant predictor of late referral (Curtis et al., 2002; Holland & Lam, 2000; Letourneau et al., 2003; Ratcliffe et al., 1984; Roderick et al., 2002; Winkelmayer et al., 2001). However, our age results confirmed those reported by Steel and Ellis (2002), who found younger age to be associated with late referral, and with Kausz and colleagues (2000), who found younger age to be associated with late dialysis initiation. It is possible that younger persons with CKD may delay nephrology referral and dialysis initiation due to competing employment/other commitments, or may be more likely to be generally healthy and had no prior health care crises. Further research is required to confirm these and other possible explanations regarding the effect of younger age on LR and LR/AS in BC renal patients.

Our prediction that females experience greater LR and LR/AS was not born out in our analysis, a finding that agrees with the majority of prior studies that assessed the effect of gender on late referral (Arora et al., 1999; Curtis et al., 2002; Ifudu et al., 1999; Jungers et al., 1993; Kinchen et al., 2002; Roderick et al., 2002; Schmidt et al., 1998; Steel & Ellis, 2002). Although we tested for potential interactions between gender and other variables (e.g. income), none were found to be statistically significant.

Our findings regarding patients' race/ethnicity indicated that Caucasians had a higher expected probability of LR and LR/AS compared to persons of other known race/ethnicity. These results were the opposite of what we expected, given the overwhelming prior findings in the literature that non-whites or Blacks had a greater risk of late referral, late dialysis initiation or sub-optimal pre-dialysis care (Iofel et al., 1998; Ifudu et al., 1999; Kausz et al., 2000; Kinchen et al., 2002; Obrador et al., 1999; Winkelmayer et al., 2001). In addition, the excessive burden of renal disease reported in Aboriginal compared to non-Aboriginal populations in Canada (Dyck, 2001; Young et al., 1989), and in Black compared to White populations in the United States (Kutner & Brogan, 2000; Livingston, 1993; Nzerue et al., 2002), as well as prior findings that indicated that race/ethnicity had played a role in Blacks' ability to obtain equitable access to organ transplantation (Gordon, 2002), together led us to expect that those who were "other than Caucasian" would have a greater expected probability of LR and LR/AS. It is possible that the large proportion of missing values for our race/ethnicity indicator (754 out of 2001 patients) would either alter or corroborate our finding that Caucasians are more likely to experience LR or LR/AS than non-Caucasians. However, it is also possible that the Canadian health care system is doing a fairly good job of providing comparable access to this specialized health service for otherwise disadvantaged groups, such as women, persons of lower SES, and non-white minorities (despite the greater burden of renal disease found in many minority populations). Potential interactions that we tested between race and other variables (e.g. income) were not found to be statistically significant. Teasing out the differential effect of race/ethnicity on renal patient access is an intriguing problem that warrants further research, including the effect of different cultural ideas about illness and health seeking behavior.

Our findings regarding patient race/ethnicity were somewhat mirrored by the expected probability calculations for patients' English ability, whereby English-proficient patients were found to have a higher expected probability of LR/AS than those who are less than English proficient; however our findings were reversed for LR. Our "age by first language" interaction results generally agreed with and provided additional clarification regarding the expected probabilities calculated individually for the "age" and "English ability" variables. Again, although the number of missing values for "English ability" and "age by first language" may have hampered the generalizability of our findings, as noted above, other reasons may exist for the differences found between patient groups that warrant more extended research.

Contrary to our expectation, patient income level (measured by income quintile or decile data) was not found to be directly related to LR or LR/AS. Our result confirmed a prior finding by Jungers et al. (1993) who also used an income-specific indicator of SES (high, medium or low income) and found that low SES was not related to late referral. The majority of prior studies reviewed did not use an income-specific indicator for SES but reported a relationship between lower SES (measured variously as level of health insurance, education, or area of urban disadvantage) and late referral, late dialysis initiation or sub-optimal pre-dialysis care (Cass et al., 2003; Kausz et al., 2000; Kinchen et al., 2002; Obrador et al., 1999). These prior studies were conducted in either the United States or Australia, where different national health care systems may be responsible for the predictive effect of low SES. Therefore, although we cannot be sure in the absence of further research, it is possible that the Canadian health care system is working comparably well at providing equitable access to renal care across income groups. Further research is warranted on this variable as well.

As hypothesized, the presence of a spouse or common-law partner was found to exert a protective effect against LR or LR/AS; however, patients who are single were found to have the lowest expected probability of LR or LR/AS. This finding suggests that the loss of a patient's prior marital/common-law partner may contribute to their probability of experiencing LR or LR/AS; however, these results were hampered by the large proportion of missing data in patient cases. The only other prior study we found on the effect of marital status on late referral (Kinchen et al., 2002) did not find a significant effect; however, that study population was relatively small for a U.S. national study (828 cases), in comparison to the substantially larger size of our provincial study (2001 cases). In addition, Kinchen and colleagues (2002) categorized marital status as "unmarried" and "married" only. Our increased number of marital status categories (including common-law partnership) may be responsible for greater sensitivity in pulling out a marital status connection with patient referral. Additional support for our marital status findings was found in prior literature on the relationship between social support and the health status of chronic disease patients, which indicates that received or perceived support influences patients' health or course of disease (Kriegsman et al., 1995; Kutner, 1987). Additional non-renal research similarly points to the importance of other measures of social support networks (including adult children, friends, neighbors and community organizations) to decreased morbidity (see, for example, Arber & Evandrou, 1993; Dean & Tausig, 1986; Procidano & Heller, 1983). Such measures were not possible to include in our present study and are thus worthy of further investigation in research related to the health determinants of late nephrology referral.

Our hypothesis regarding the predictive effect of availability of next-of-kin on LR and LR/AS was not born out in our analysis. It is probable that the large proportion of missing values for this indicator (1,275 out of 2,001 cases) hampered the ability to tease out potential significance regarding its predictive effect.

Patients' proximity to their regional renal centre was found to be directly related to a LR or LR/AS experience, verifying our hypothesis. This finding differs from prior late referral studies that found no association between the proximity or availability of health services and late referral (Cass et al., 2003; Holland & Lam, 2000; Schmidt et al., 1998). However, our finding confirmed other studies that reported a relationship between proximity to care and whether a patient would ever be referred for nephrology care (Boyle et al., 1996; Mendelssohn et al., 1995). Geographical proximity to care is one of the most vexing problems facing the research site as well as most other provinces in Canada. It is a problem that BC and other provinces have struggled to address in recent years through restructuring health care services under regional "health authorities," and through creating incentives to encourage the system's gatekeepers, physicians, to relocate to more sparsely populated areas and inner cities. This problem remains very real at the point of writing (see, e.g. Benoit et al., 2002; Evans et al., 1994). Additional studies, such as a representative panel of renal patients by geographical region followed over time, would shed light on the generalizability of this preliminary finding.

Similar to our results on proximity to care, our expected probability calculations verified our hypothesis of regional renal centre differences in LR and LR/AS. This confirmed a prior finding by Ganz et al. (1997) who reported differences in patients' clinical outcomes between BC's regional dialysis centres. Our finding similarly reinforced earlier findings on the predictive impact of a patient's renal care network on late dialysis initiation (Kausz et al., 2000) and suboptimal pre-dialysis care (Obrador et al., 1999). In fact, in our study, a patient's regional renal centre offered the *greatest* predictive effect of all indicators included in our conceptual model in determining a patient's acuity of referral experience. It is possible that some of the impact can be explained by service capacity issues that have been faced by various regions in the past few years; however, theoretically, the absence of an available dialysis machine should not impact on whether a patient can be assessed by a nephrologist in advance of requiring treatment. It is also possible that regional renal centre differences in referral type may reflect differing referral practices by general practitioners. It is noteworthy in this regard that the BC renal community has stepped up efforts to educate physicians regarding the signs of chronic renal disease and when to refer potential patients for nephrology assessment. Again, this preliminary finding requires further examination before any definitive conclusions can be drawn.

CONCLUSION

This study began with the question as to why some people with chronic kidney illness residing in one area of Canada fare better than others, by studying the case example of timing of patient referral to nephrology care. The results of our research begin to fill a void in the literature regarding the impact of health determinants on renal patients' initial access to renal care services, in a health care system where such services are free at the point of delivery. Sociologists of health in recent years have argued that researchers would do well to focus attention not only on what physicians and hospital authorities recommend as important for patient care but also on the complex web of background characteristics that affect people's health and access to crucial primary care as well as specialized services for chronic health problems. The results of our research indicate that such an inquiry is definitely fruitful and yet much more needs to be done before we can clearly separate out genetic/biological factors and the broad array of social and other determinants that shape health and health care access for persons facing a chronic illness.

Our findings at the same time provide some practical information to BC renal patients, their health care providers and, perhaps more immediately, to the regional and provincial authorities responsible for effective planning of renal services. The research provided a test of the strength of BC's provincial renal database to support population health research of this nature. In addition, the findings have a practical benefit in helping the BC Provincial Renal Agency to develop strategies to reach more renal patients early on in their illness careers, and at the same time to initiate dialogue with key stakeholders to help explain variation in physician referral patterns that may be affecting access to renal care, as well as differences among the regional renal centres themselves. Finally, further prospective study with renal patients, their social support networks and renal care providers is required to confirm and build on our study's findings, and to thereby enhance our current limited understanding of how the determinants of health impact renal patient access to initial and ongoing renal care.

NOTES

1. "Acute start" refers to persons who have chronic kidney disease (CKD), and should not be confused with non-CKD patients who may experience a sudden acute temporary requirement for dialysis that is often able to be reversed when an underlying disease/condition has been treated.

2. This study forms the first phase of an ongoing research project that will also assess the impact of patients' health determinants and initial referral experience on their risk of excess morbidity. The results of these further phases of analysis will be available in later 2004.

3. British Columbia is the westernmost province of Canada. Large areas of the central and northern parts of the province are sparsely settled. In fact, nearly three fourths of the population resides in the southwest coastal tip which includes the largest city and chief port of Vancouver and the provincial capital, Victoria, located on Vancouver Island.

4. Income quintiles/deciles are relative measures based on census summary data at the Enumeration Area (1996) or Dissemination Area (2001) level. BC quintiles/deciles are calculated to be area-specific (i.e. by Census Metropolitan Area, Census Agglomeration, or provincial residual area not in any CMA or CA), "to minimize the effect on household welfare of large differences in housing costs" (Statistics Canada, 2001). The 2001 quintile/decile data may be affected by a problem identified with the postal code conversion to DA; therefore, data may not always reconcile with data produced in future releases/reports (CHSPR, personal communication, April 7, 2004).

ACKNOWLEDGMENTS

This research has been co-sponsored by a 2003/2004 research trainee award from the Michael Smith Foundation for Health Research and the British Columbia Medical Services Foundation. Access to renal patient data from the Patient Records, Outcome and Management Information System (PROMIS), as well as support in analytical interpretation, was provided by Adeera Levin, Director, British Columbia Provincial Renal Agency (BCPRA), and Ognjenka Djurdjev, Head, Data Management Centre, BCPRA. Access to income quintile and decile data was provided by the British Columbia Ministry of Health Services and the Centre for Health Services and Policy Research (CHSPR). Special thanks as well to Doug Baer and Mikael Jansson for their insightful comments on our analysis.

REFERENCES

Arber, S., & Evandrou, M. (1993). *Aging, independence and the life course*. London: Taylor & Francis.

Arora, P., Obrador, G. T., Ruthazer, R., Kausz, A. T., Meyer, K. B., Jenuleson, C. S., & Pereira, B. J. G. (1999). Prevalence, predictors, and consequences of late nephrology referral at a tertiary care center. *Journal of the American Society of Nephrology, 10*, 1281–1286.

Benoit, C. (2003). The politics of health-care policy: The United States in comparative perspective. *Perspectives in Biology and Medicine, 46*(4), 592–599.

Benoit, C., Carroll, D., & Millar, A. (2002). But is it good for non-urban women's health? Regionalizing maternity care services in British Columbia, Canadian Review of Sociology. *Canadian Review of Sociology & Anthropology, 39*(4), 373–395.

Blomqvist, A., & Brown, D. (Eds) (1994). *Limit to care: Reforming Canada's health care system in an age of restraint.* Toronto: C. D. Howe.

Boyle, P. J., Kudlac, H., & Williams, A. J. (1996). Geographical variation in the referral of patients with chronic end stage renal failure for renal replacement therapy. *Quarterly Journal of Medicine, 89*, 151–157.

Broyles et al. (1983). The use of physician services under a national insurance scheme. *Medical Care, 21*, 1037–1054.

Canadian Institute for Health Information (CIHI) (2004). *Improving the health of Canadians.* Ottawa: Canadian Institute for Health Information.

Canadian Population Health Initiative (CPHI) (2002). Webpage: About population health. Canadian Institute for Health Information (CIHI) website, accessed 29/10/2002. http://secure.cihi.ca/cihiweb/dispPage.jsp?cw_page=cphi_aboutph_e.

Cass, A., Cunningham, J., Snelling, P., Wang, Z., & Hoy, W. (2003). Urban disadvantage and delayed nephrology referral in Australia. *Health and Place, 9*, 175–182.

Cass, A., Cunningham, J., Wang, Z., & Hoy, W. (2001, August). Social disadvantage and variation in the incidence of end-stage renal disease in Australian capital cities. *Australian and New Zealand Journal of Public Health, 25*(4), 322–326.

CHSPR (Centre for Health Services and Policy Research), located at the University of British Columbia, 429–2194 Health Sciences Mall, Vancouver, BC, Canada, V6T 1Z3, Tel: (604) 822–1949, Fax: (604) 822–5690, Website: http://www.chspr.ubc.ca.

Curtis, B. M., Barrett, B. J., Jindal, K., Djurdjev, O., Levin, A., Barre, P., Bernstein, K., Blake, P., Carlisle, E., Cartier, P., Clase, C., Culleton, B., Deziel, C., Donnelly, S., Ethier, J., Fine, A., Ganz, G., Goldstein, M., Kappel, J., Karr, G., Langlois, S., Mendelsohn, D., Muirhead, N., Murphy, B., Pylpchuk, G., & Toffelmire, E. (2002). Canadian survey of clinical status at dialysis initiation 1998–1999: A multicenter prospective survey. *Clinical Nephrology, 58*(4), 282–288.

Dean, A., & Tausig, M. (1986). Measuring intimate support: The family and confidant relationship. In: N. Lin, A. Dean & W. Ensel (Eds), *Social Support, Life Events, and Depression* (pp. 117–128). Orlando, FL: Academic Press.

Dyck, R. F. (2001). Mechanisms of renal disease in indigenous populations: Influences at work in Canadian indigenous peoples. *Nephrology, 6*, 3–7.

Evans, R. G., Barer, M. L., & Marmor, T. R. (Eds) (1994). *Why are some people healthy and others not?* New York: Aldine de Gruyter.

Fored, C. M., Ejerblad, E., Fryzek, J. P., Lambe, M., Lindblad, P., Nyren, O., & Elinder, C.-G. (2003). Socio-economic status and chronic renal failure: A population-based case-control study in Sweden. *Nephrology Dialysis Transplantation, 18*, 82–88.

Ganz, G., Singh, S., Djurdjev, O., & Levin, A. (1997, September). Current dialysis practices in British Columbia a cross-sectional study. *Journal of the American Society of Nephrology, 8* (Supplement: AO898).

Garg, P. P., Diener-West, M., & Powe, N. R. (2001, July). Income-based disparities in outcomes for patients with chronic kidney disease. *Seminars in Nephrology, 21*(4), 377–385.

Gordon, E. J. (2001). Patients' decisions for treatment of end-stage renal disease and their implications for access to transplantation. *Social Science & Medicine, 53*, 971–987.

Gordon, E. J. (2002). What "race" cannot tell us about access to kidney transplantation. *Cambridge Quarterly of Healthcare Ethics, 11*, 134–141.

Hirsch, D. J., West, M. L., Cohen, A. D., & Jindal, K. K. (1994, March). Experience with not offering dialysis to patients with a poor prognosis. *American Journal of Kidney Diseases, 23*(3), 463–466.

Holland, D. C., & Lam, M. (2000). Predictors of early vs. late referral among a retrospective cohort of pre-dialysis patients. *Dialysis and Transplantation, 29*(9), 526–534.

Ifudu, O., Dawood, M., Iofel, Y., Valcourt, J. S., & Friedman, E. A. (1999). Delayed referral of Black, Hispanic, and older patients with chronic renal failure. *American Journal of Kidney Diseases, 33*(4), 728–733.

Iofel, Y., Dawood, M., Valcourt, J. S., & Ifudu, O. (1998, September–October). Initiation of dialysis is not delayed in Whites with progressive renal failure. *ASAIO Journal, 44*(5), M598-M600.

Jungers, P. (2002). Late referral: Loss of chance for the patient, loss of money for society. *Nephrology Dialysis Transplantation, 17*, 371–375.

Jungers, P., Zingraff, J., Albouze, G., Chauveau, P., Page, B., Hannedouche, T., & Man, N. K. (1993). Late referral to maintenance dialysis: Detrimental consequences. *Nephrology Dialysis Transplantation, 8*, 1089–1093.

Kasiske, B. L., Snyder, J. J., Matas, A. J., Ellison, M. D., Gill, J. S., & Kausz, A. T. (2002). Preemptive kidney transplantation: The advantage and the advantaged. *Journal of the American Society of Nephrology, 13*, 1358–1364.

Kausz, A. T., Obrador, G. T., Arora, P., Ruthazer, R., Levey, A. S., & Pereira, B. J. G. (2000). Late initiation of dialysis among women and ethnic minorities in the United States. *Journal of the American Society of Nephrology, 11*, 2351–2357.

Kinchen, K. S., Sadler, J., Fink, N., Brookmeyer, R., Klag, M. J., Levey, A. S., & Powe, N. R. (2002, September 17). The timing of specialist evaluation in chronic kidney disease and mortality. *Annals of Internal Medicine, 137*(6), 479–486.

Kjellstrand, C. M., & Moody, H. (1994). Hemodialysis in Canada: A first-class medical crisis. *Canadian Medical Association Journal, 150*(7), 1067–1071.

Kriegsman, D. M. W., Penninx, B., W. J. H., & van Eijk, J. Th. M. (1995). A criterion-based literature survey of the relationship between family support and incidence and course of chronic disease in the elderly. *Family Systems Medicine, 13*(1), 39–68.

Kutner, N. G. (1987). Social ties, social support, and perceived health status among chronically disabled people. *Social Science and Medicine, 25*(1), 22–34.

Kutner, N. G., & Brogan, D. (2000). Race, socioeconomic status, and risk of a catastrophic health condition in later life. *Health, Illness and Use of Care: The Impact of Social Factors, 18*, 151–165.

Kutner, N. G., & Gray, H. L. (1981, July). Women and chronic renal failure: Some neglected issues. *Journal of Sociology and Social Welfare, 8*(2), 320–333.

Letourneau, I., Ouimet, D., Dumont, M., Pichette, V., & Leblanc, M. (2003, March–April). Renal replacement in end-stage renal disease patients over 75 years old. *American Journal of Nephrology, 23*(2), 71–77.

Levin, A. (2000). Consequences of late referral on patient outcomes. *Nephrology Dialysis Transplantation, 15*(Suppl. 3), 8–13.

Livingston, I. L. (1993). Renal disease and Black Americans: Selected issues. *Social Science & Medicine, 37*(5), 613–621.

Marmot, M. (2003). Understanding social inequalities in health. *Perspectives in Biology and Medicine, 46*(3, Suppl.), S9–S23.

Marmot, M. G., & Wilkinson, R. G. (Eds) (1999). *Social determinants of health.* Oxford: Oxford University Press.

McCauley, J., Irish, W., Thompson, L., Stevenson, J., Lockett, R., Bussard, R., & Washington, M. (1997, December). Factors determining the rate of referral, transplantation, and survival on dialysis in women with ESRD. *American Journal of Kidney Diseases, 30*(6), 739–748.

McKenzie, J. K., Moss, A. H., Feest, T. G., Stocking, C. B., & Siegler, M. (1998). Dialysis decision making in Canada, the United Kingdom, and the United States. *American Journal of Kidney Diseases, 31*(1), 12–18.

Mendelssohn, D. C., Kua, B. T., & Singer, P. A. (1995, December 11–25). Referral for dialysis in Ontario. *Archives of Internal Medicine, 155*(22), 2473–2478.

Nzerue, C. M., Demissachew, H., & Tucker, J. K. (2002). Race and kidney disease: Role of social and environmental factors. *Journal of the National Medical Association, 94*(8, Suppl.), 28S–38S.

Obrador, G. T., Ruthazer, R., Arora, P., Kausz, A. T., & Pereira, B. J. G. (1999). Prevalence of and factors associated with suboptimal care before initiation of dialysis in the United States. *Journal of the American Society of Nephrology, 10*, 1793–1800.

Perneger, T. V., Whelton, P. K., & Klag, M. J. (1995, June 12). Race and end-stage renal disease. Socioeconomic status and access to health care as mediating factors. *Archives of Internal Medicine, 155*, 1201–1208.

Procidano, M., & Heller, K. (1983). Measures of perceived social support from friends and from family: Three validation studies. *American Journal of Community Psychology, 11*(1), 1–24.

Ratcliffe, P. J., Phillips, R. E., & Oliver, D. O. (1984, February 11). Late referral for maintenance dialysis. *British Medical Journal, 288*, 441–443.

Roderick, P., Jones, C., Drey, N., Blakeley, S., Webster, P., Goddard, J., Garland, S., Bourton, L., Mason, J., & Tomson, C. (2002). Late referral for end-stage renal disease: A region-wide survey in the south west of England. *Nephrology Dialysis Transplantation, 17*(7), 1252–1259.

Salvalaggio, G., Kelly, L., & Minore, B. (2003, Winter). Perspectives on health: Experiences of First Nations dialysis patients relocated from remote communities for treatment. *Canadian Journal of Rural Medicine.* Contents available at http://www.cma.ca.

Schmidt, R. J., Domico, J. R., Sorkin, M. I., & Hobbs, G. (1998, August). Early referral and its impact on emergent first dialyses, health care costs, and outcome. *American Journal of Kidney Diseases, 32*(2), 278–283.

Segall, A., & Chappell, N. (2000). *Health and health care in Canada.* Toronto: Pearson Canada.

Sekkarie, M., Cosma, M., & Mendelssohn, D. (2001, July). Nonreferral and nonacceptance to dialysis by primary care physicians and nephrologists in Canada and the United States. *American Journal of Kidney Diseases, 38*(1), 36–41.

Shortt, S., & Shaw, R. (2003, February 18). Equity in Canadian health care: Does socioeconomic status affect waiting times for elective surgery? *Canadian Medical Association Journal (CMAJ), 168*(4), 413.

Statistics Canada (2001, August). *PCCF + Version 3G user's guide (Geocodes/PCCF): Automated geographic coding based on the statistics Canada poster code conversion files including postal codes to June 2001.* Ottawa: Statistics Canada. Catalogue No. 82F0086-XDB.

Steel, J., & Ellis, P. (2002, October–December). Do demographic variables affect the timing of referral to the nephrologist? *EDTNA/ERCA Journal, 28*(4), 185–187.

Turner-Musa, J., Leidner, D., Simmens, S., Reiss, D., Kimmel, P. L., & Holder, B. (1999). Family structure and patient survival in an African-American end-stage renal disease population: A preliminary investigation. *Social Science & Medicine, 48*, 1333–1340.

Wenger, N. S., Lynn, J., Oye, R. K., Liu, H., Teno, J. M., Phillips, R. S., Desbiens, N. A., Sehgal, A., Kussin, P., Taub, H., Harrell, F., & Knaus, W. (2000). Withholding vs. withdrawing life-sustaining treatment: Patient factors and documentation associated with dialysis decisions. *Journal of the American Geriatrics Society, 48*(5, Suppl.), S75–S83.

Williams, G. H. (2003). The determinants of health: Structure, context and agency. *Sociology of Health & Illness, 25*, 131–154.

Wilson, R., Godwin, M., Seguin, R., Burrows, P., Caulfield, P., Toffelmire, E., Morton, R., White, P., Rogerson, M., Eisele, G., & Bont, G. (2001, July). End-stage renal disease: Factors affecting referral decisions by family physicians in Canada, the United States, and Britain. *American Journal of Kidney Diseases, 38*(1), 42–48.

Winkelmayer, W. C., Glynn, R. J., Levin, R., Owen, W. F., & Avorn, J. (2001, December). Determinants of delayed nephrologist referral in patients with chronic kidney disease. *American Journal of Kidney Diseases, 38*(6), 1178–1184.

Young, E. W., Mauger, E. A., Jiang, K.-H., Port, F. K., & Wolfe, R. A. (1994). Socioeconomic status and end-stage renal disease in the United States. *Kidney International, 45*, 907–911.

Young, T. K., Kaufert, J. M., & McKenzie, J. K. (1989, June). Excessive burden of end-state renal disease among Canadian Indians: A national survey. *American Journal of Public Health, 79*, 756–758.

WHO ADVOCATES FOR PATIENTS WHEN HEALTH CARE SYSTEMS FAIL? ENSURING ACCESS TO ESSENTIAL MEDICINES IN SOUTH AFRICA (AND THE U.S.)

Melanie E. Campbell and Peri J. Ballantyne

ABSTRACT

Public health policy often excludes access to essential medicines. Drawing on an in-depth case study examining access to essential medicines in the context of the HIV/AIDS pandemic in South Africa, and more briefly, making reference to the U.S. diabetes epidemic, we highlight the relationship between the need for essential medicines in world populations, and the role of groups external to government in promoting access to essential medicines in public health policy. We consider how, in the context of health stratification, the activities of patient advocacy groups, and "third way" social policies of the pharmaceutical industry generate "social capital," creating enhanced access to essential medicines for a few, and promoting the ideal of the right to access for all. The implications for the development of public health policy inclusive of essential medicines are discussed.

Chronic Care, Health Care Systems and Services Integration
Research in the Sociology of Health Care, Volume 22, 239–260
Copyright © 2004 by Elsevier Ltd.
All rights of reproduction in any form reserved
ISSN: 0275-4959/doi:10.1016/S0275-4959(04)22012-9

INTRODUCTION

Use of medicines is of increasing importance for the management of certain diseases. Effective use of some medicines can dramatically change both the quality of life and life expectancy of patients afflicted with certain diseases. There are a number of diseases where this is the case. Two that have reached epidemic proportions – namely HIV/AIDS in South Africa and diabetes in the U.S. – are discussed in this paper. Access to essential medicines – those that prolong life and prevent further disease progression or deterioration (Tamblyn et al., 2001) – has become a highly politicized issue, as disease risks are polarized between, and within, the developed and developing world.

The impact of the medicinal treatment of HIV/AIDS is illustrated by changes in HIV/AIDS mortality statistics in the developed world. For example, in the U.S., deaths reported in adults with HIV infection decreased 67%, coincident with the implementation of highly active antiretroviral therapy (HAART) (McNaghten et al., 1999; Palella et al., 1998; Selik et al., 2002) the number of children who died with HIV infection annually decreased 81% from 1994 to 1999, attributable to both HAART and the prevention of perinatal HIV transmission using antiretroviral therapy (Lindegren et al., 1999; Selik & Lindegren, 2003). A European study of changes in mortality rates among HIV-1 infected patients reported a decline in death rates amounting to a mortality risk in 1998 that was one-fifth the relative risk of death in 1995; these changes were also attributed to the effectiveness of combination therapy for HIV/AIDS (Mocroft et al., 1998). The authors of a Swiss study reporting a 49% drop in HIV-related hospital admissions between 1994 and 1999 noted the association of the decline in admissions to the advent of HAART (Nuesch et al., 2002).

However, for many, HIV/AIDS remains a terminal illness. In a recent BBC interview, experts reported that in Britain, "of all the people who will die this year with AIDS-related illnesses, a third will do so just three months after diagnosis – because they tested too late for treatments to be effective" (British Broadcasting Corporation, 2003). In the developing world, where access to testing or any form of treatment is extremely limited, HIV remains a death sentence. For example, 35–59% of HIV+ African children die by their second birthday(Dabis & Ekpini, 2002). Thus, while there have been significant advances in the science of using medicines to treat very serious diseases such as HIV/AIDS, socio-political forces determine who benefits from them; who lives and dies.

This is not just the case of treatment of diseases in the developing world. The polarization of risk of disease associated with access to essential medicines also occurs in developed world settings. This can be attributed to market failures in the pharmaceutical and health (and drug) insurance industries, such as, in the former, a lack of price competition and patent protection, and in the latter, fragmented drug insurance coverage, and prohibitive prices for those most in need (Frank, 2002; Henry & Lexchin, 2002). Thus, capacity to pay (out-of-pocket, or by rules of access of typically limited private and public drug benefit insurers) ultimately determines access to essential medicines for the majority of people in the developing world, and for all but the most vulnerable (who are public insurance beneficiaries) in the developed world. With growing need and encumbered access to essential medicines in specific populations and nations, extra-governmental involvement in enhancing access to essential medicines has been growing.

In two case studies that follow, we describe the activities of several groups, in two world contexts (SA & the U.S.), directed toward the urgent need for medicines in specific patient populations. In the context of governments' failure to act on behalf of citizens in need of essential medicines, we discuss the actions (and activism) of these groups in reference to the sociological concept *social capital*. There are many definitions of social capital, but for our purposes, we use it to refer to "an asset through which people are able to widen their access to resources and other actors" (Bebbington, 1999, p. 2021), which has "relational, material and political aspects" (Hawe & Shield, 2000, p. 873). Also relevant to the present analysis, we note that social capital refers both to the *availability of resources* (presence or absence for individuals, households, communities and societies), and to *the capacity* (of individuals, households, communities and societies) *for social capital*, which can be built and generated through intervention (Bebbington, 1999; Hawe & Shield, 2000). In the present analysis then, we refer to the ways extra-governmental groups generate social capital in ways that: (1) directly affect individuals' and groups' (patient populations) access to medicines; and that (2) has (or demonstrates) the potential to become a movement to promote the ideal of a *citizen's right to essential medicines*, in response to institutional deficits regarding this aspect of health equity (Gilbert & Walker, 2002; Nathan et al., 2002).

Finally, drawing on Hawe and Shield's insight that (having relational, material and political aspects) social capital may have positive *or* negative effects (Hawe & Shield, 2000), we consider how, in the context of health stratification, the activities of the pharmaceutical industry related to pharmaceutical donation programs, might be construed as "third way" social policy – shown to enable (or to create it, as in the U.S. case) access to essential medicines, at the same time as (potentially) *constraining or deflecting* discussion and action around the pursuit of the principle of the right to access (to essential medicines) that democratically elected governments ought to pursue on behalf of their citizens.

We draw primarily on a recently completed case study conducted in South Africa during the fall, 2002 (Campbell, 2003), to describe the perspective of three groups that influenced government decision-making and policy re-development around the issue of a specific drug marketed to reduce mother-to-child transmission of HIV/AIDs. These groups included an international pharmaceutical company that manufactured the drug in question; a sophisticated HIV/AIDS treatment advocacy group within SA, and (some of) the medical-research community in that country. We examine how these groups influenced the South African national government's plans to implement a broad access program for both the prevention of mother-to-child transmission of HIV/AIDS, and for antiretrovirals needed in the larger HIV-infected population.

Following the presentation of the SA case study, we briefly consider another setting and epidemic involving limited access to essential medicines. With rising numbers of U.S. citizens living with diabetes, and with the absence of a national (or state-based) drug benefit program, two groups have acted to influence the problem of limited treatment access for this population. We note that, as with the SA case, a national diabetes advocacy group, and the pharmaceutical industry have both participated in enhancing drug treatment access for U.S. diabetes patients. The activities of these extra-governmental groups may help to reinforce an ideal of patients' right to essential medicines, and (may) have the potential to drive (or suppress) national initiatives that guarantee such a right to all citizens.

ADVOCACY AND ACTIVITIES IN REPONSE TO A NATIONAL GOVERNMENT'S FAILURE TO ACT: SOUTH AFRICA'S HIV/AIDS EPIDEMIC

In 2003, South Africa was home to more than 4.5 million persons with HIV/AIDS, the largest number of HIV-positive people living in any one country (Doctors Without Borders, 2003). In 2002, the prevalence rate in the adult population was 20.1%, with the disease burden greater for women than for men (Gilbert & Walker, 2002). Prevalence is greater in poorer, mainly black areas. Prevalence rates at antenatal clinics in SA range from 8.7 to 36.2% depending on where the clinic is located (Adler & Obed, 1999; UNAIDS, 2002). Next only to transmission via heterosexual intercourse, mother-to-child transmission (MTCT) is the second leading mode of transmission of the HIV virus (UNAIDS, 1998), accounting for 70,000 HIV+ babies, or 6% of total births in South Africa each year (Treatment Action Campaign, 2001b; UNICEF, 2002).

The efficacy of the antiretroviral drug Nevirapine, requiring one dose given to mothers while in labor, and a second dose given to babies within 72 hours of delivery, is approximately 50%. That is, it reduces the natural rate of MTCT from approximately 30 to 15% (Guay et al., 1999; McIntyre & Gray, 2002). In 2000, Boehringer Ingelheim, the manufacturers of Nevirapine, offered to provide it for free for five-years in many developing countries for use in PMTCT programs. While PMTCT *prevents* the transmission of HIV/AIDS, in this paper, we emphasize the link between the PMTCT struggle in SA and the fight for long-term antiretroviral treatment (HAART) undertaken by the same activists. It is the availability of HAART that allows HIV-infected persons to live with it as a chronic, manageable condition, rather than face imminent death from the disease.

Governments were slow to take up the Boehringer Ingelheim offer (Anonymous, 2001), and in SA, the reasons for this are complex (Campbell, 2003). Because of a still-inequitable health care system, there are serious obstacles preventing the implementation of a comprehensive Nevirapine program. In post-Apartheid South Africa, governments have been struggling to build a public health care system that can meet the needs of all of its citizens (Benatar, 1997). In 1994, after the first democratic elections in South Africa, the new national government, the African National Congress (ANC), tabled a national health plan for South Africa. The plan was founded on the basis of equity and the right to health; it emphasized primary health care services; and a comprehensive, equitable, and integrated national health system (African National Congress; UNICEF; and World Health Organization, 1994). The ANC was applauded for recognizing that a broad primary care system would better meet the needs of the majority of South Africans who are relatively poor and live in rural areas with little health care infrastructure (Benatar, 1997). However, a comprehensive, primary care system has not been achieved. Rural South Africans continue to have poor access to health care, while wealthy urban dwellers have access to private health care that ranks among the best in the world (Benatar, 1997). With respect to the opportunity provided by free access to Nevirapine for PMTCT, and in spite of its constitutional responsibility for public health and mounting public pressure, the South African national government balked at implementing a broad-access Nevirapine program. Instead, in January 2001, the SA national government initiated a limited, 18-site PMTCT pilot program (kaisernetwork.org, 2001; Smith, 2001).

Boehringer Ingelheim

In 2000, the German pharmaceutical company, Boehringer Ingelheim, issued an imperative for South Africa's governments to act, when it offered to provide Nevirapine at no cost. A Boehringer Ingelheim representative indicated that the motivation for his company's offer to SA and other African nations was based on the moral imperative to get the drug to populations in need, and he suggested that the need in Africa was unique (for the most part) to the developed world, as explained in the following excerpt:

The motivation came from the fact that Viramune (Nevirapine) . . . appeared to be ideally suited to mother-to-child transmission in the developing world environment. It's obviously not the drug of choice in the [normal] environment (because . . . HIV+ pregnant woman would be identified and would get triple-therapy, but in South Africa . . . pregnant women come to the clinics very late, they come also in labour, and if you can give a tablet to the mother in labour and if you can give a small dose to the baby within 72 hours then that is a proven regimen, if you like, to reduce the transmission . . . So based on the fact that the drug was sort of ideal . . . that was the motivation (Campbell, 2003, Case ID 012).

The Boehringer Ingelheim representative indicated that the company was ill-prepared for the (lack of) response to the donation program they offered. The company representative surmised that this was due to the fact that acceptance of the medicine would imply an intent to deliver it, yet in SA there was insufficient capacity for a comprehensive delivery program:

. . . one has to admit that we went into the donation program . . . a little bit inexperienced because . . . of the infrastructure required to accept a donation . . . we met with the Lesotho Government, for example, in February 2001, and it was only just recently that their request was submitted and approved because they didn't have that infrastructure that was required to perform a good program that respects the rights of the mother, makes sure that the patients are tested for HIV and (if) they turn out positive that they are counselled as well, you know, that type of thing (Campbell, 2003, Case ID 012).

While critics argue that pharmaceutical donation or price reduction programs are both laudable and morally unsustainable (Schüklenk & Ashcroft, 2002), in making the donation offer, Boehringer-Ingelheim effectively shifted responsibility to the recipient governments to either accept the offer, or to find a rationale for its rejection. As described in Campbell (2003), until only recently, the SA national government resisted acknowledging there was any need to accept the offer, and instead expressed a suspicion that AIDS itself was part of a "conspiracy against Africans, either from the country's white conservatives or from the pharmaceutical industry" (Fassin & Schneider, 2003) and challenged the claims of efficacy and safety of Nevirapine and other antiretrovirals (kaisernetwork.org, 2002a).

While having made its offer to provide the drug in 2000, by December 2002, Boehringer Ingelheim had made no donation to the SA national government. Indeed, for the purposes of the SA pilot project involving Nevirapine, the government was *purchasing* the drug, not receiving it through donation (Campbell, 2003).

The TAC

In response to the AIDS pandemic in South Africa, the Treatment Action Campaign (TAC) was established on December 10, 1998, to raise public awareness and understanding of issues related to the availability, affordability and use of HIV treatments, to advocate for greater access to HIV treatment for all South Africans, and to campaign against the view that AIDS is a "death sentence" (Treatment Action Campaign, 2002). The TAC's founding campaign was for access to antiretroviral drugs for PMTCT (Treatment Action Campaign, 2001a). At that time, the TAC's call was for AZT; Nevirapine was not yet indicated for PMTCT. When Nevirapine was recognized as uniquely valuable for PMTCT in the developing world setting, the Boehringer Ingelheim offer helped to publicly strengthen the TAC's case for a comprehensive PMTCT intervention strategy. Since its inception, TAC has continued to push relentlessly for PMTCT interventions as well as to access to long-term antiretrovirals (Schneider, 2002; Treatment Action Campaign, 2001a).

Health activists, led by the TAC, took issue with the national government's limited-access pilot program, and the inequity in access for citizens with private and public health insurance. The TAC charged that [the pilot program] was irrational and arbitrary, creating "an untenable inequality which discriminates against the poor ... and ... inevitably amounts to discrimination on grounds of race as well" (Treatment Action Campaign, 2001c). Further, the TAC claimed that the government's PMTCT pilot-program policy constituted "a profound threat to the fundamental rights of South Africans, such as access to health care services, including reproductive health care; basic health care services for children; life; human dignity; equality; and psychological integrity, including the right to make decisions regarding reproduction" (Treatment Action Campaign, 2001c).

In August 2001, the Treatment Action Campaign took its case for a comprehensive PMTCT program to the Pretoria High Court, and later, through appeal, to the South African Constitutional Court. In documents submitted for this case, and on the basis of constitutionally defined responsibilities for health, the national government and all nine South African provincial governments are named (Later, following the roll out of separate province-wide Neviripine programs, charges against three provinces – Western Cape, KwaZulu-Natal and Gauteng – were dropped) (Treatment Action Campaign, 2001b). After a series of decisions and appeals, in July 2002 the Constitutional Court of South Africa ruled in favor of the TAC, and charged the South African National Government with the responsibility of rolling out a comprehensive PMTCT (kaisernetwork.org, 2002b; Sidley, 2002). Recently, the South African government has also announced that they will begin to provide access to antiretrovirals for long-term use within the year (kaisernetwork.org, 2003), illustrating that the struggle for PMTCT contributed to the broader strategy of pushing for access to long-term treatment.

TAC's activities and eventual success can be examined in terms of two types of activism: "elite activism" and grassroots mobilization. In terms of elite activism, it is instructive to consider both the era as well as the membership of the newly formed

TAC. TAC was shaped through the anti-Apartheid struggle, and its operations and strategies were informed by the legal and human rights framework that permeated the work of the SA AIDS Law Project (ALP), a group that existed prior to the TAC, and continues it advocacy work on behalf of individual cases. Further, the TAC had formed coalitions with most of the various organizations dealing with AIDS in South Africa and elsewhere. This included close links with the ALP, the National Association of People Living with HIV/AIDS (NAPWA), and the international humanitarian group Médecins Sans Frontières (MSF). Globally TAC had alliances with many of the major players involved in AIDS activism and treatment advocacy, such as ACT-UP (AIDS Coalition to Unleash Power), Health GAP (Health Global Access Project), Consumer Project on Technology (CPTech), and MSF. The TAC was also a founding member of the Pan-African HIV/AIDS Treatment Access Movement. It was within this context involving a broad pro-treatment network of associations that the TAC case against the SA government(s) was undertaken, in reference to the national government's own constitution and human rights aspirations.

At a grassroots level, TAC's strategies included building a massive TAC membership by developing networks and alliances with unions, employers, religious bodies, women and youth organizations, lesbian and gay organizations and other interested sections of the community. TAC established and maintained visibility in communities, through posters, pamphlets, meetings, street activism and letter writing. TAC worked in schools, at rallies and public events, and maintained offices in communities such as Khayelitsha township, a poor area near Capetown, interacting with Médecins Sans Frontières (MSF) to bring treatment to that community (Campbell, 2003).

Although the activities of TAC have helped get drugs to individual patients, these small-scale programs were never intended to replace the government's responsibility for the treatment needs of its population. The TAC never abandoned its strategy of activism to force government action around broad access to PMTCT interventions and long-term antiretrovirals.

Physician/Researchers

Physician/researchers also played an important role in challenging the South African government on PMTCT issues, and in acting on behalf of HIV patients. In addition to supporting the TAC through the writing of affidavits for the court case, and increasing pressure on government through letter writing and op-ed pieces, physicians/researchers covertly bypassed the government's limited access Nevirapine policy by attempting to get life-saving drugs to small numbers of patients. Some of the perspectives and activities of a subset of physicians/researchers directly involved in PMTCT are described below.

First, many physicians who were interviewed for this case study had quite interesting philosophical ideas about AIDS care in South Africa, and these ideas motivated their desire to do more than official policy permitted. One physician explained the parallels in outcomes of restrictive treatment policy for AIDS and the differential rights of citizens under Apartheid:

> Why does someone with chronic liver disease get everything (in terms of needed care and treatment), but someone with chronic immune deficiency disease gets nothing? Is it because the person is a child? Is it because you stick a label of HIV on that patient? Is it because most of them are black? Is this patient being given less because there are many others that have the same problem? What is it that makes us regard this patient (differently)? Under Apartheid it was quite clear it was color. Now I think that it's maybe more complicated but it's there, some people are being treated as less than human despite our Constitution's bill of rights. Who would of thought that a new disease would emerge that's as stigmatizing and as dehumanizing as Apartheid (Campbell, 2003, Case ID A).

This physician emphasized the ethical responsibilities of the profession of medicine in the face of this new "Apartheid":

> On the issue of government making policy, the profession failed to address the injustices under Apartheid. Now during the AIDS era, the profession is failing again to limit the injustices of the present system, and I see really serious annuities there; we have a duty to critique government policy ... (Campbell, 2003, Case ID A).

Another physician felt the appropriate role of the physician and scientist should be less critical and activist-oriented, and more that of a neutral technical expert:

> I've spent my professional life in the country and have been involved in many initiatives against Apartheid, so I have considerable belief in what activism can achieve. But I think that we physicians and scientists have a very special role that goes beyond activism, I think what we have best to offer is dispassionate and high level analysis – the science and scientific argument. That doesn't discount the importance of activism like that of people in the Treatment Action Campaign, but, they depend on good scientists ... (Campbell, 2003, Case ID B).

On the basis of the ideal that patients should be treated equally, and out of the helplessness experienced by some clinicians because they weren't able to offer treatment to patients with AIDS, some physicians found ways around policy, sometimes undertaken covertly, for fear of being stopped or reprimanded. For example, physician-participants in this study had set up or initiated programs that contravened government policy, and did so because they felt it was their only option:

> The one thing we have realized, beyond a shadow of a doubt is that both PMTCT and antiretrovirals are absolutely essential. It has revolutionized our care, before, as I said, it was a demoralizing, totally nihilistic kind of thing. But, suddenly, (with) being able to do something positive, it turns that all around and that has strengthened us to say, "well, blow you, if we don't

get support from you, we'll just finance it ourselves and we'll keep our heads down, and we'll go for it" ... (but) we're very careful to not play the party politics game, to not be seen to be manipulating, we inform, we keep it fairly low profile, we don't make a big rah rah of it and that's been our strategy, to try and just get it done (Campbell, 2003, Case ID C).

Conveying a similar story, another physician had found funding and set up an antiretroviral program. This individual described how national policy (that prevented the formal distribution of antiretrovirals in this community) was circumvented:

To give you an idea of how it works, I was up at a meeting with (other physician colleagues) ... and we were discussing (this) project (we were involved in) and X was sitting behind me and I told him ... "there's this (foreign) charity that's going to give me three quarters of a million Rand a year, and I can buy treatment but I can't use it in the hospital service (because of national policy), how must I solve the problem?", and X got on his cell phone basically and two minutes later, literally, he said "what you must do is ... write (a) research proposal" (Campbell, 2003, Case ID D).

This physician was able to provide antiretrovirals to patients outside an "official" pilot site, since providing antiretrovirals under the guise of research was not in contravention of official government policy at that time.

The physicians had varied ideas about whether they considered themselves activists or subversives, and they described a range of views about the appropriate role of a physician, both in this case and other similar situations. One physician supported the idea of *more* action and advocacy by the medical community in dealing with AIDS, and in legitimizing demands for nation-wide access to treatment for PMTCT:

I think physicians in this country, as everywhere in the world, have been, in the majority, much too conservative, not very concerned about the issue – except the few hundreds that have been very actively involved in advocacy (Campbell, 2003, Case ID G).

However, another took a different view, asserting that most physicians ought to work within the status quo; that acceptance of the fact that interventions were not available was necessary in order for (some) practitioners to cope with the contradiction they faced in their role as a health care provide during the era of HIV/AIDS:

There are people who are perfectly content to see patients everyday in the office and they just work within the status quo. And it's great, you know, when I get sick I want to go to a doctor's office and find that the person is interested primarily in my health (Campbell, 2003, Case ID H)

Finally, with respect to future needs around AIDS and health-care related rights, one physician had very clear ideas about what physicians should be doing:

I think HIV has taught us that there needs to be quite a lot of advocacy and that it is not sufficient to say, "The leaders won't do it, well, we'll just sit by". One of our roles (as physicians) is advocacy, and I think that advocacy has to happen in two ways. On the one hand, we have to be out there standing on our soap boxes saying this is the right thing to do, but on the other hand, I think we need to be encouraging our patients, our clients or the people we interact with, to do the same ... so I see part of my role as informing my patients, my clients what their rights are and almost inciting them, to also be demanding their rights, to join TAC, to back up organizations that are pushing for these things. But then I also have a responsibility to write editorials, and, (to speak) in any meeting where I have the opportunity ... in this field, we have no choice ... just sitting back waiting for the government to do something is not acceptable (Case ID C).

In summary, while describing a range of responses the profession has had to the HIV/AIDS epidemic, these physicians were nearly unanimous in their agreement that, by virtue of their relatively powerful status in society, the profession has an added responsibility to challenge the status quo. As with the TAC's small-scale treatment programs, the significance of the work of these physicians is not limited to the provision of drug treatment to a small number of patients *per se*, but is demonstrated in the wider effect such efforts have in raising awareness among patients and other citizens. Furthermore, in assisting the TAC, and in advocating to government directly, these physicians (whose views may not be representative of all physicians/researchers in South Africa) upheld an ideal that governments are responsible for assuring access to essential medicines for all.

The South African case-study illustrates the complexity of, and the (potentially) diverse sources of pressure on health policy making. In the SA case, we described the activities of groups that, while external to formal decision-making bodies, acted to promote HIV/AIDS treatment in general, and PMTCT in particular, and influenced the specific series of (re)actions by the SA national government, resulting most recently in the national government's stated commitment to roll out a broad ARV program in that country.

The analysis of the external pressures on formal health-care policy development can be applied in other contexts, and may add further to an understanding of how national epidemics compel action among non-government actors and interest groups. As an illustration, we briefly consider another national health crisis where medicinal treatment is essential – that is, the diabetes epidemic in North America.

ADVOCACY AND ACTIVITIES OF NON-GOVERNMENTAL ACTORS IN RESPONSE TO THE U.S. DIABETES EPIDEMIC

Reporting that an estimated 135 million people worldwide had diagnosed diabetes in 1995, and projecting 300 million cases by the year 2025, a recent paper describes diabetes as a major public health problem and an emerging pandemic (Venkat Narayan et al., 2000). Health Canada reported that in 1999, approximately 1.2–1.4 million Canadians aged 12 and over have diabetes (4.9–5.8% of this population) (Health Canada, 1999). In the U.S., the American Diabetes Association reports that approximately 17 million people have diabetes, representing 6.2% of the population; of these, approximately 90–95% have Type 2 and 5–10% have Type 1 diabetes, and approximately one-third of cases are undiagnosed (American Diabetes Association, 2003a).

The issue of undiagnosed diabetes is material to the current discussion of the imperatives to deliver essential medicines to diabetes patients, as is the issue of sub-optimal treatment. Diabetes is reported to be the leading cause of new cases of blindness, end-stage renal disease, and lower-extremity amputation (Bjork, 2001) and it is a major contributor to cardiovascular death in the U.S. (Egede & Zheng, 2002). Early diagnosis and aggressive treatment is essential to the management of the disease and its progression, including pharmacological management of both Type 1 and Type 2 diabetes. However, Chan and Abrahamson (2003) note that, with respect to Type 2 Diabetes, the most prevalent form of the disease:

> Despite better understanding of the . . . disease mechanisms, the expanded armamentarium of targeted oral antidiabetic drugs and the conclusive evidence of the benefits of stringent glycemic control, actual treatment outcomes in clinical practice remain suboptimal relative to established treatment goals (Chan & Abrahamson, 2003, p. 459).

Further, Skyler and Oddo (2002) pronounce that there is urgent need for improved diabetes care in the U.S. Citing several studies examining diabetes treatment and outcomes, these authors charge that diabetes management in the U.S. is in need of improvement:

> It is the view of the authors that if one were to rank the overall effectiveness of diabetes care systems on an arbitrary gradient scale of one to four (with one being primitive and four being comprehensive), the U.S. would deserve a rank of two. In contrast, the diabetes care in Nordic countries would deserve a rank of four. Clearly, the U.S. needs to provide more comprehensive care (Skyler & Oddo, 2002, S25).

The U.S. has a mixed health insurance system with most of the population under the age of 65 covered by either individual insurers or group policies purchased by small and large businesses and their employees. A public system provides basic health care services to the elderly and disabled (Medicare) and the indigent (Medicaid) (Iglehart, 1999). In 2002, 43.6 million people, or 15.2% of the U.S. population were without health insurance coverage during the entire year (U.S. Census Bureau, 2003). Up to the present time, Medicare has only provided coverage for the costs of prescription medications provided in hospital (The Henry J. Kaiser Family Foundation, 2003), while Medicaid programs – operated at the state level – provide beneficiaries only limited access to prescription medicines (The Henry J. Kaiser Family Foundation, 2003).

The American Diabetes Association (2003b) reports that the level of coverage for diabetes benefits in the different U.S. health insurance plans varies. It reports that 46 states have laws requiring comprehensive coverage of diabetes supplies, services and medications by the individual and small-group health insurance market, and that Medicare is required by law to cover blood glucose monitoring supplies, insulin pumps and diabetes education services, but not oral medications, insulin or syringes. It reports that the Medicaid program covers most diabetes medications, but does not always cover diabetes education services or insulin pumps, and that in large-group and special health insurance markets (where some states have created purchasing pools to enable small business and individuals to group together in buying insurance), employers have the option to cover specific needs, such as diabetes services and medications (American Diabetes Association, 2003b). The Association's emphasis on advocacy for improvements in prescription drug insurance coverage indicates that, at the present time in the U.S., such coverage for diabetic patients is inadequate.

The availability of medication insurance, and the out-of-pocket costs of treatment (direct payment, insurance co-payments and deductibles) influence the population's use of medications for the treatment of diabetes. For example, in a recent study examining the effect of out-of-pocket expenditures on the utilization of recommended diabetes preventive services, Karter et al. (2003) concluded that a co-payment requirement and full cost services were associated with lower use of recommended preventive care services including dilated eye exams, attendance at health education classes and performance of daily self-monitoring of blood glucose (SMBG). In a related study, Karter et al. (2000) found that SMBG practices were reduced with increasing out-of-pocket costs. Brown et al. (2003) reported that among Medicare managed care beneficiaries (65+) with diabetes mellitus, all of whom had the same pharmacy benefit, there were low rates of use of evidence-based therapies overall and substantially lower use of statins (cholesterol lowering medication) by poorer persons. In general, cost-sharing in drug benefit programs is demonstrated to reduce the use of at least some discretionary and essential medicines (see Harten & Ballantyne, 2004, for a Canadian perspective) and general health care (Fortess et al., 2001; Soumerai et al., 1987; Soumerai et al., 1994; Stuart & Zacker, 1999). Thus, the direct costs of diabetes medications borne by patients in the U.S. may account, in part, for the sub-optimal medication regimes reported in many studies. For example, in one study discussing mortality trends in Type 1 diabetes, the authors report that "*the reasons for a higher mortality in the U.S. may relate to the costly health care system for diabetics*" (Nishimura et al., 2001, p. 825).

Our preliminary investigation of medication access for diabetes patients in the U.S. suggests that when it comes to treatment "activism" on behalf of U.S. diabetes patients, the American Diabetes Association, a national advocacy group, and pharmaceutical manufacturers represent two key players – the former through advocacy to national and state governments for enhanced or comprehensive coverage of diabetes education and treatment services; the latter through patient-assistance (to medicines) programs.

Advocacy by the American Diabetes Association is primarily related to the quest for improved prescription drug insurance for diabetic patients, as indicated in the following except from its website:

> The Association is advocating before Congress for a comprehensive Medicare prescription drug benefit for senior Americans living with diabetes. Additionally, it is working in Washington, DC and in state capitals across the country to ensure that all health plans provide comprehensive diabetes benefits as part of a basic benefits package. Third, the Association continues to advocate for health insurance reforms like "community rating" that will make health insurance affordable for Americans living with diabetes. Fourth, the Association is working with several members of Congress to dramatically improve the public health system in the United States (American Diabetes Association, 2003b, p. 3).

The American Diabetes Association takes (partial) credit for national- and state-government level incursions into the massive health insurance machine in the U.S., for example, those that resulted in coverage for selected diabetes health care in the national Medicare program, and legal protections for diabetic patients covered by small and individual market health insurance, in 46 states.

U.S. diabetic patients without insurance coverage can seek access to diabetes medications through one or more of a growing number of medication assistance programs. These programs, sponsored by individual pharmaceutical companies, provide (eligible) indigent and uninsured Americans access to prescription medications. The Pharmaceutical Research and Manufacturers Association (PhRMA) reported that, in 2002, assistance was provided to 5.5 million U.S. patients, who received 14 million free prescriptions through these programs (PhRMA, 2003). The PhRMA describes the industry's medication assistance to the poor as a philanthropic program, and reports a growing number of assistance programs in a Directory of Prescription Drug Patient Assistance Programs. We highlight the availability of such programs as a means to demonstrate that the activities of one group – in this case, the pharmaceutical industry – help to address a significant limitation of health care in the U.S., related to gaps in insurance coverage.

While the assistance programs appear to help fill an important gap – for example, Chisholm and DiPiro (2002) reported that approximately 53% of the top 200 prescribed medications in 1999 were offered through medication assistance programs to the indigent – there are many U.S. citizens who fall through the cracks of the health insurance system. Consider, for example, the 15% without health insurance in 2002 (U.S. Census Bureau, 2003). Further, much of the current political rhetoric addressing the problems of access to drug-benefit insurance is focused on enhanced access for the elderly and disabled, and not on the population as a whole. The recently passed Medicare Prescription Drug Improvement and Modernization Act, in December 2003, serves as an example of this point. This focus on Medicare beneficiaries (which sets the elderly and disabled apart from the remainder of the population as "deserving" of public benefits), is also found on the Eli Lilly internet documentation of its donation program *LillyAnswers*. One of the questions it poses on this program's web page is "Does Lilly support Medicare reform as it applies to prescription drugs?" Its response is reproduced below:

> Lilly believes drug coverage for all Medicare beneficiaries is long past due and that its design is critical. We believe that market-based prescription drug coverage for all Medicare beneficiaries is the best long-term solution to provide all seniors access to the medicines they need. We are moving forward with LillyAnswers because even legislation enacted tomorrow will take significant time – perhaps years – to implement. Between now and then, we are committed to two things: to help seniors in greatest need and to do whatever we can to support the speedy enactment of Medicare reform that benefits all seniors (Eli Lilly & Company, 1994–2003).

It is not our intent here to debate the adequacy of its scope, or the motivation or politics of the industry's programs, but only to note that an important gap left by the limitations of government health care policy is being partially filled by the industry's contributions to *eligible* low-income applicants without prescription drug insurance.

DISCUSSION

The analysis of two national settings illustrates the complexity of, and the (potentially) diverse sources of pressure on public health policy-making. In the SA case, we described the activities of three extra-governmental groups – Boehringer Ingelheim, the TAC and (some of) the SA medical community – that acted to promote HIV/AIDS treatment in general, and PMTCT in particular. In our analysis of access to drug treatment for diabetes in the U.S., we note that the American Diabetes Association advocates directly on behalf of the diabetes population, seeking comprehensive coverage for essential diabetes education, services and medicinal treatment, while the pharmaceutical industry hosts a large, and growing number of medication assistance programs to which low income persons living with diabetes may be eligible. In both national settings, we note that the effect of these groups' activities has been to acknowledge a population's *need* for essential medicines (as in the U.S. case study), if not explicitly to address the *right of access* to them (as in the SA case study).

In the context of governments' failure to act on behalf of citizens in need of essential medicines, we distinguish among the types and effects of activities undertaken by extra-governmental groups, in reference to the sociological concept *social capital*. Referring to "an asset through which people are able to widen their access to resources and other actors" (Bebbington, 1999, p. 2021), which has "relational, material and political aspects" (Hawe & Shield, 2000, p. 873), we focus on the enhanced material capital generated through the *direct provision of medicines* to people in need (as provided through the grass roots efforts of the TAC, and the medical/research community in SA, and through pharmaceutical donation programs in the U.S.), and the enhanced relational and political capital generated through the *representation of patient interests* by SA physician-activists, the TAC, and the American Diabetes Association.

We distinguish the *activism or advocacy* of the TAC, the Diabetes Association and SA physicians (effecting a change the status quo) from the *activity* of the pharmaceutical industry (effecting the maintenance of it). For example, the Treatment Action Campaign used the donation offer from Boehringer-Ingelheim and drew on the national government's own constitutional aspirations for (health-) equity for all citizens to make a case for universal access to essential medicines for the prevention or treatment of HIV/AIDS. The TAC meets most of the "domains of capacity" described by Nathan et al. (2002), in their assessment of the capacity of NGOs to advocate for health equity, including credibility and a track record (globally and within SA), having grass roots connections, having a strong membership base, bi-partisanship, being fair and representative, supporting claims and having expertise (with assistance from the medical research committee, as noted in the case study), and the absence of conflicts of interest or vested interests (Nathan et al., 2002).

In the U.S., the responsibility of the national (or state) government to provide health care is not constitutionally or legally mandated. There is, therefore, a need to consider the (inclination and) capacity of those governments to impede the economic "freedoms" of the market-based insurance and pharmaceutical products industries, as may be necessary to create a public health program that provides access to essential (health care and) medicines. Drawing on the insights of those who view social capital from an institutions or network approach, we consider the potential costs as well as the benefits of particular social network configurations or institutional relations (Hawe & Shield, 2000; Muntaner et al., 2001; Woolcock, 1998). The network analysis approach to social capital derives from the Weberian tradition in sociology that acknowledges the existence of stratification (power structures) within and among network members or groups, as well as the potential negative effects of strong networks for communities, such as, in the current discussion, the relationship of the pharmaceutical industry to the state, reflected in favourable arrangements related to patent laws and pricing regulation.

Given its (assumed) interest in maintaining this favoured position, the question of whether the pharmaceutical industry's actions are philanthropic is highly contested (Schüklenk & Ashcroft, 2002). One concern is that donation programs help to legitimize an industry that reaps significant profits while large populations (in developed as well as developing nations) face health adversity related to low income or poverty status, and lack of access to necessary medicines (Henry & Lexchin, 2002). In the U.S. context, the PhRMA's donation programs might be viewed as a type of "third way" social policy, an example of social capital functioning as a health policy alternative to large-scale government re-distrubution (Muntaner, 2001). In the U.S. and Europe, third way policies are seen to represent a retreat from social democracy and a reduced role for the state (Navarro, 1994), as reflected in increased reliance on assistance and means tested programs, privatization of social services, labor market flexibility, and modern philanthropy (Muntanner et al., 2001). In the context of health stratification, the activities of the pharmaceutical industry related to pharmaceutical donation programs, shown to enable (in the SA case) or to directly enhance a population's access to medicines (as in the U.S. case) may at the same time *constrain or deflect* any discussion and action around a democratically elected government's responsibility to pursue its citizens' right to access (to essential medicines).

Further, philanthropy provided by an industry with vested interests in (profits from) its products presents a problem of sustainability. That is, while the pharmaceutical industry's medication assistance programs are meeting the immediate needs of millions of U.S. citizens requiring medicines, the nation's reliance on corporate-based social-assistance means that increasing numbers of people are vulnerable to a decision by the industry that its medication assistance programs are not sustainable, or to changes in eligibility rules, undertaken as the result of increased demand. In the U.S. setting (and in SA, and other developing countries where HIV/AIDs rates continue to rise), growing demand is a real concern. For example, according to the PhRMA (2003), in 2002, assistance was provided to 5.5 million U.S. patients, who received 14 million free prescriptions through these programs (PhRMA, 2003). This contribution is significantly greater than in 1999, where assistance was provided to approximately 1.5 million persons, who filled some 2.7 million prescriptions (cited in Chisholm et al., 2000, p. 1131). Thus, the pharmaceutical industry faces credibility or legitimacy challenges as "advocates" for the public's health (Nathan et al., 2002), because of its commercial interest in the product it is promoting and lack of long-term (patient) advocacy goals.

The presentation in this paper is preliminary only. We are not able to comment on what might be an optimal relationship between community advocacy and action and government response. As the Campbell (2003) case study demonstrates, there are many approaches that members of a community can take to demonstrate the need for and feasibility of drug treatment programs. However, the success of such approaches will depend on the strength of other groups' interests in maintaining the status quo, and their relative influence over government policy making. Perhaps the next question will be to focus our attention on the effects of a comprehensive, advocacy-driven HIV/AIDS treatment program in SA, and of the continuation of a corporate-controlled drug-benefit system in the U.S.

ACKNOWLEDGMENTS

We thank Dr. Solomon Benatar and Professor Jennie Jacobs Kronenfeld for their reviews of the manuscript, and for helpful insights and comments. Ms. Mayce Al-Sukhni provided excellent research assistance. Professors Richard Lee, Terry Sullivan, Beverly Chalmers, and Solomon Benatar, who made up the Masters thesis committee for, and who assisted Melanie Campbell in the completion of the SA case study described in this paper, need also be acknowledged and thanked!

REFERENCES

Adler, G., & Obed, Q. (1999). *HIV/AIDS and STDs in the South African health review*. Health Systems Trust Archives. Retrieved June 7, 2002 (http://www.hst.org.za/sahr/99/chap22.htm).

African National Congress, UNICEF, and World Health Organization (1994). *A National Health plan for South Africa*. Johannesburg, South Africa: African National Congress.

American Diabetes Association (2003a). *Basic diabetes information*. Retrieved January 6, 2004 (www.diabetes.org/info/diabetesinfo.jsp).

American Diabetes Association (2003b). *Health insurance for people with diabetes*. Retrieved January 6, 2004 (www.diabetes.org/info/diabetesinfo.jsp).

Anonymous (2001). Giving away HIV drugs is not as easy as it seems. *AIDS Alert, 16*(11), 137, 143–144.

Bebbington, A. (1999). Capitals and capabilities. A framework for analyzing peasant viability, rural livelihoods and poverty. *World Development, 27*, 2021–2044.

Benatar, S. R. (1997). Health care reform in the new South Africa. *New England Journal of Medicine, 336*, 891–895.

Bjork, S. (2001). The cost of diabetes and diabetes care. *Diabetes Research and Clinical Practice, 54*(suppl. 1), S13–S18.

British Broadcasting Corporation (2003). *HIV drugs boost 10-year survival*. Retrieved October 17, 2003 (http://news.bbc.co.uk/1/hi/health/3198326.stm).

Brown, A. F., Gross, A. G., Gutierrez, P. R., Jiang, L., Shapiro, M. F., & Mangione, C. M. (2003). Income-related differences in the use of evidence-based therapies in older persons with diabetes mellitus in for-profit managed care. *Journal of the American Geriatrics Society, 51*, 665–670.

Campbell, M.E. (2003). *Women's access to Nevirapine to prevent mother-to-child transmission of HIV: A case study of policy development in South Africa.* Unpublished Masters thesis, University of Toronto.

Chan, J. L., & Abrahamson, M. J. (2003). Pharmacological management of type 2 diabetes mellitus: Rationale for rational use of Insulin. *Mayo Clinic Proceedings, 78*, 459–467.

Chisholm, M. A., & DiPiro, J. T. (2002). Pharmaceutical manufacturer assistance programs. *Archives of Internal Medicine, 162*, 780–784.

Chisholm, M. A., Reinhardt, B. O., Vollenweider, L. J., Kendrick, B. D., & DiPiro, J. T. (2000). Medication assistance programs for uninsured and indigent patients. *American Society of Health System Pharmacists, 57*(12), 1131–1136.

Dabis, F., & Ekpini, E. R. (2002). HIV-1/AIDS and maternal and child Health in Africa. *The Lancet, 359*, 2097–2104.

Doctors Without Borders (2003). *Bringing antiretroviral therapy to South Africa.* Retrieved November 2003(http://www.doctorswithoutborders.org/publications/voices/khayelitsha_2003.shtml).

Egede, L. E., & Zheng, D. (2002). Modifiable cardiovascular risk factors in adults with diabetes: Prevalence and missed opportunities for physician counseling. *Archives of Internal Medicine, 162*, 427–433.

Eli Lilly and Company (1994–2003). *LillyAnwers. Questions and answers.* Retrieved January 6, 2004 (www.lillyanswers.com/questions_answers.html).

Fassin, D., & Schneider, H. (2003). The politics of AIDS in South Africa: Beyond the controversies. *British Medical Journal, 326*, 495–497.

Fortess, E., Soumerai, S., McLaughlin, T., & Ross-Degnan, D. (2001). Utilization of essential medications by vulnerable older people after a drug benefit cap: Importance of mental disorders, chronic pain, and practice setting. *Journal of the American Geriatric Society, 49*(6), 793–797.

Frank, R.G. (2002). Prescription drug prices. Why do some people pay more than others? *Health Affairs* (March/April), 115–128.

Gilbert, L., & Walker, L. (2002). Treading the path of least resistance: HIV/AIDS and social inequalities – A South African case study. *Social Science and Medicine, 54*, 1093–1110.

Guay, L. A., Musoke, P., Fleming, T., Bagenda, D., Allen, M., Nakabiito, C., Sherman, J., Bakaki, P., Ducar, C., Deseyve, M., Emel, L., Mirochnick, M., Fowler, M. G., Mofenson, L., Miotti, P., Dransfield, K., Bray, D., Mmiro, F., & Jackson, J. B. (1999). Intrapartum and neonatal single-dose Nevirapine compared with Zidovudine for prevention of mother-to-child transmission of HIV-1 in Kampala, Uganda: HIVNET 012 randomised trial. *The Lancet, 354*, 795–802.

Harten, C., & Ballantyne, P. (2004). Impact of cost-sharing within provincial drug benefit programs: A review. *Journal of Pharmaceutical Finance, Economics and Policy, 13*(1), 35–53.

Hawe, P., & Shield, A. (2000). Social capital and health promotion. A review. *Social Science and Medicine, 51*, 871–885.

Health Canada (1999). *Diabetes in Canada. National statistics and opportunities for improved surveillance, prevention and control.* Ottawa, Canada. Minister of Public Works and Government Services (Catalogue No. H49-121/1999).

Henry, D., & Lexchin, J. (2002). The pharmaceutical industry as medicines provider. *The Lancet, 260*, 1590–1595.

Iglehart, J. K. (1999). The American health care system – Expenditures. *New England Journal of Medicine, 340*(1), 70–76.

Kaisernetwork.org (2001). *South Africa to provide Nevirapine to HIV-positive pregnant women in 'Pilot Project'*. Kaisernetwork.org archives. Retrieved June 20, 2003 (http://www.kaisernetwork.org/daily_reports/rep_index.cfm?hint=1&DR_ID=2506).

Kaisernetwork.org (2002a). *South African health minister calls Nevirapine 'Poison'; Observers worry Government will continue to fight court order mandating distribution of the drug*. Kaisernetwork.org archives. Retrieved July 9, 2002 (http://www.kaisernetwork.org/daily_reports/rep_index.cfm?hint=1&DR_ID=12205).

Kaisernetwork.org (2002b). *In the courts: Constitutional court denies South African Government's right to appeal high court ruling on Nevirapine distribution*. Kaisernetwork.org archives. Retrieved July 05, 2002 (http://www.kaisernetwork.org/daily_reports/rep_index.cfm?hint=1&DR_ID=12057).

Kaisernetwork.org (2003). *Drug access: South African cabinet approves national antiretroviral distribution plan*. Retrieved November 20, 2003 (http://www.kaisernetwork.org/daily_reports/rep_index.cfm?DR-ID=20950).

Karter, A. J., Ferrara, A., Darbinian, J., Ackerson, L. M., & Selby, J. V. (2000). Self-monitoring of blood glucose: Language and financial barriers in a managed care population with diabetes. *Diabetes Care, 23*, 477–483.

Karter, A. J., Stevens, M. R., Herman, W. H., Ettner, S., Marrero, D. G., Safford, M. M., Engelgau, M. M., Curb, J. D., & Brown, A. F. (2003). Out-of-pocket costs and diabetes preventive services. *Diabetes Care, 26*(8), 2294–2299.

Lindegren, M. L., Byers, R. H., Jr., Thomas, P., Davis, S. F., Caldwell, B., Rogers, M., Gwinn, M., Ward, J. W., & Fleming, P. L. (1999). Trends in perinatal transmission of HIV/AIDS in the United States. *Journal of the American Medical Association, 282*, 531–538.

McIntyre, J., & Gray, G. (2002). What can we *do* to reduce mother-to-child transmission of HIV? *British Medical Journal, 324*, 218–221.

McNaghten, A. D., Hanson, D. L., Jones, J. L., Dworkin, M. S., & Ward, J. W. (1999). Effects of antiretroviral therapy and opportunistic illness primary chemoprophylaxis on survival after AIDS diagnosis. *AIDS, 13*, 1687–1695.

Mocroft, A., Vella S., Benfield, T. L., Chiesi, A., Miller V., Gargalianos, P., d'Arminio Monforte, A., Yust, I., Bruun, J. N., Phillips, A. N., & Lundgren, J. D. for the EuroSIDA study Group (1998). Changing patterns of mortality across Europe in patients infected with HIV-1. *The Lancet, 352*, 1725–1730.

Muntaner, C., Lynch, J., & Davey Smith, G. (2001). Social capital, disorganized communities, and the third way: Understanding the retreat from structural inequalities in epidemiology and public health. *International Journal of Health Services, 31*(2), 213–237.

Nathan, S., Rotem, A., & Ritchie, J. (2002). Closing the gap: Building the capacity of non-governmental organizations as advocates for health equity. *Health Promotion International, 17*(1), 69–78.

Navarro, V. (1994). *The politics of health policy. The U.S. reforms, 1980–1994*. Oxford, UK: Blackwell.

Nishimura, R., LaPorte, R. E., Dorman, J. S., Tajima, N., Becker, D., & Orchard, T. J. (2001). Mortality trends in type 1 diabetes. The Allegheny county (Pennsylvania) registry 1965–1999. *Diabetes Care, 24*(5), 823–827.

Nuesch, R., Geigy, N., Schaedler, E., & Battegay, M. (2002). Effect of highly active antiretroviral therapy on hospitalization characteristics of HIV-Infected Patients. *European Journal of Clinical Microbiology & Infectious Diseases, 21*, 684–687.

Palella, F. J., Jr., Delaney, K. M., Moorman, A. C., Loveless, M. O., Fuhrer, J., Satten, G. A., Aschman, D. J., & Holmberg, S. D. (1998). Declining morbidity and mortality among patients with advanced Human Immunodeficiency Virus Infection. *New England Journal of Medicine, 338,* 853–860.

Pharmaceutical Research and Manufacturers of America (2003). *Quick facts.* Retrieved January 6, 2003 (www.phrma.org/).

Schneider, H. (2002). On the fault-line: The politics of AIDS policy in contemporary South Africa. *African Studies, 61,* 145–167.

Schüklenk, U., & Ashcroft, R. E. (2002). Affordable access to essential medication in developing countries: Conflicts between ethical and economic imperatives. *Journal of Medicine and Philosophy, 27*(2), 179–195.

Selik, R. M., & Lindegren, M. L. (2003). Changes in deaths reported with Human Immunodeficiency Virus Infection among United States children less than thirteen years old, 1987 through 1999. *Pediatric Infectious Disease Journal, 22*(7), 635–641.

Selik, R. M., Byers, R. H., Jr., & Dworking, M. S. (2002). Trends in diseases reported on U.S. death certificates that mentioned HIV infection, 1987–1999. *Journal of Acquired Immune Deficiency Syndromes, 29,* 378–387.

Sidley, P. (2002). South African government forced to give mothers antiretroviral drug. *British Medical Journal, 325,* 121.

Skyler, J. S., & Oddo, C. (2002). Diabetes trends in the USA. *Diabetes Metabolism Research and Reviews, 18,* S21–S26.

Smith, C. (2001). Antiretroviral medication will soon be available for HIV-positive pregnant women and mothers at state hospitals. *Mail and Guardian* (January 26) Retrieved March 12, 2002 (http://www.sn.apc.org/wmail/issues/010126/OTHER38.html).

Soumerai, S., Avorn, J., Ross-Degnan, D., & Gortmaker, S. (1987). Payment restrictions for prescription drugs under medicaid. *New England Journal of Medicine, 317*(9), 550–556.

Soumerai, S., McLaughlin, T., Ross-Degnan, D., Casis, C., & Bollini, P. (1994). Effects of limiting medicaid drug-reimbursement benefits on the use of psychotropic agents and acute mental health services by patients with schizophrenia. *New England Journal of Medicine, 331,* 650–655.

Stuart, B., & Zacker, C. (1999). Who bears the burden of medicaid drug co-payment policies? *Health Affairs, 18*(2), 201–212.

Tamblyn, R., Laprise, R., Hanley, J. A., Abrahamowicz, M., Scott, S., Mayo, N., Hurley, J., Grad, R., Latimer, E., Perreault, R., McLeod, P., Huang, A., Larochelle, P., & Mallet, L. (2001). Adverse events associated with prescription drug cost-sharing among poor and elderly persons. *Journal of the American Medical Association, 285*(4), 421–429.

The Henry J. Kaiser Family Foundation (2003). *Medicare and prescription drugs.* Medicare Fact Sheet #1583–06. April 2003 (www.kff.org).

Treatment Action Campaign (2001a). *Mother-to-child transmission: A history of TAC activities until August 2000.* TAC Archives. Retrieved June 9, 2003 (http://www.tac.org.za/Documents/ MTCTPrevention/mtcthist.rtf).

Treatment Action Campaign (2001b). *TAC founding affidavit filed on 21 August 2001 at Pretoria High Court.* TAC Archives. Retrieved April 20, 2002 (http://www.tac.org.za/Documents/ MTCTCourtCase/ccmfound.rtf).

Treatment Action Campaign (2001c). *TAC's reply to the department of health's response: Heads of argument.* TAC Archives. Retrieved February 4, 2002 (http://www.tac.org.za/ Documents/MTCTCourtCase/Tachead1.txt).

Treatment Action Campaign (2002). *About TAC.* TAC Archives. Retrieved February 4, 2002 (http://www.tac.org.za/about.htm).

UNAIDS (1998). *Report on the global HIV/AIDS epidemic*. Retrieved February 10, 2002 (http://hivinsite.ucsf.edu/InSite.jsp?page=pr-02-01&doc=2098.3ce0).

UNAIDS (2002). *Report on the global HIV/AIDS epidemic*. Geneva: UNAIDS.

UNICEF (2002). *Statistical data: South Africa*. UNICEF. Retrieved June 4, 2003 (http://www.unicef.org/statis/Country_1Page146.html).

U.S. Census Bureau (2003). *Health insurance coverage in the United States: 2002. Current population reports*. U.S. Department of Commerce Economics and Statistics Administration, U.S. Census Bureau, Issued September 2003.

Venkat Narayan, K. M., Gregg, E. W., Fagot-Campagna, A., Engelgau, M. M., & Vinicor, F. (2000). Diabetes – A common, growing, serious, costly, and potentially preventable public health problem. *Diabetes Research and Clinical Practice, 50*(Suppl. 2), S77–S84.

Woolcock, M. (1998). Social capital and economic development: Toward a theoretical synthesis and policy framework. *Theory and Society, 27*, 151–208.

AT FIRST YOU WILL NOT SUCCEED: NEGOTIATING FOR CARE IN THE CONTEXT OF HEALTH REFORM

I. L. Bourgeault, S. Lindsay, E. Mykhalovskiy,
P. Armstrong, H. Armstrong, J. Choiniere,
J. Lexchin, S. Peters and J. White

ABSTRACT

In the majority of the literature on the social organization of care work, care is often defined in more traditional terms to refer to work on or directly related to the body. In this paper, we would like to venture beyond the body to elaborate upon a particular type of care work – negotiating care – that involves negotiations and sometimes petitions for the purpose of securing care. It is a concept that was salient in a comparative study of the experiences of health care providers with the increasing management of health care in Canada and the United States. For physicians and nurses in both settings we find a sense of the increasing burden of negotiating for care for patients – particularly textually mediated negotiations – as the access to and amount of care is increasingly limited through managed care policies. Moreover, the contexts for these negotiations are continually in flux exacerbating the time devoted to negotiate care. It is in the U.S. context, however, that textual negotiation of care is most extensive and differs in terms of audience – insurers as opposed to providers – and purpose – securing payment and not just care.

Chronic Care, Health Care Systems and Services Integration
Research in the Sociology of Health Care, Volume 22, 261–276
© 2004 Published by Elsevier Ltd.
ISSN: 0275-4959/doi:10.1016/S0275-4959(04)22013-0

INTRODUCTION

The conceptualization of care and the social organization of care work have garnered a resurgence of interest amongst academic scholars from a variety of disciplines (Aronson & Neysmith, 1996, 1997; Christopherson, 2001; McKie & Bowlby, 2001; Meyer, 2000; Reverby, 1987). Although a great deal of this literature focuses on informal care within the private sector, largely provided by families and women in families in particular, in what constitutes women's "third shift" (Gerstel, 2000), a growing body of literature also examines formal care within the public sector of paid employment. In both cases, however, care is often defined in more traditional terms to refer to work on or directly related to the body (cf. Isaksen, 2002).

In this paper, we would like to venture beyond the body and traditional care work to elaborate upon a particular type or aspect of care – *negotiating care*. The increasing importance of negotiating care was salient in a comparative study we conducted of the experiences of health care providers with the management of health care in Canada and the United States. It refers primarily to the negotiations and in some cases petitions that health care providers undertake with the expressed purpose of securing care for their patients. It involves negotiations not only between providers but also increasingly between providers and health care decision-makers (be they insurance companies or health care managers). Similar to other forms of care work, this kind of work is relatively invisible, is not acknowledged as a formal skill to be taught in medical or nursing school and is generally devalued despite its increasing pervasiveness. Elaborating on this concept enables better linkages to be made between the literatures on carework and inter-professional negotiations, particularly within the context of managed care.

CARE, MANAGED CARE AND NEGOTIATING CARE

Feminist scholarship has had a notable impact in expanding upon the concept of "care" both in the literature and on the public policy agenda. Although much of this has focused on unpaid care work done in the home, some attention has begun to focus on the caring that women do as a feature of paid work (Davies, 1994). One of the first theorists to begin to conceptualize the public provision of care is Susan Reverby's (1987) portrayal of nurses "caring dilemma." She describes this dilemma as the imposition of a duty to care in a society that devalues caring. At the heart of this dilemma is a tension between altruism and professional autonomy. Specifically, female care providers (and nurses in particular) feel obliged to provide care without having the decision-making power to determine how that care is to be provided.

What is implicit in Reverby's depiction of the caring dilemma and what has been made explicit by many other authors is that care work is an inherently gendered act that, for the most part, women do (Abel & Nelson, 1990; Christopherson, 2001; Gerstel, 2000; Thomas, 1993). Indeed, some go so far as to define care as women's work. Thomas (1993) for example states, "care involves work activities and feeling states and is provided on either a paid or unpaid basis *by women* to both able-bodied adults and children in either the public or domestic spheres, and in a variety of institutional settings" (p. 654; emphasis added). Because caring is gendered in this manner, the tendency is for it to be bound up with the subservient position of women in society; thus, carework tends to be devalued.

While there has been an emphasis on the gendered aspects of care work, there has been less attention paid in this literature to the restructuring of care within the public sphere. Davies (1994), for example argues, "the carework discussion has barely been noted in the debate about the new managerialism in the public sector" (p. 1). When delved into further, one finds that the restructuring of care is rooted in a contradiction between greater public expectation for higher quality care and a drive by funders to reduce the costs of that care (Christopherson, 2001) which can be considered a new variation on Reverby's caring dilemma. Indeed, the changing organization of caring work is making it more difficult to actually provide care and to compose a career around caring work (Christopherson, 2001). This is particularly the case when we look at the restructuring of health care work under systems of managed care.

Negotiating Care Under Managed Care

Managed care has become the dominant mode of health care delivery in the United States and to a lesser extent in other countries like Canada that have adopted some of its policies. Broadly defined, it is a system of health care decision-making that controls costs through closely monitoring and controlling the decisions of health care providers. As a result, it has transformed the roles of various health care providers, often leaving them with little control over the way in which care is delivered (Deuben, 1998; McKay, 1999). Physicians in particular have been a target of constraints and incentives to reduce the costs of their clinical care and administrative decisions (Grembowski et al., 2002; Hunter, 1996).

One of the key complaints that physicians (American physicians in particular) have with the system of managed care is its increasing administrative burden. Warren et al. (1999), for example, found that physicians working in States with high managed care participation reported greater problems with paperwork and with patients moving in and out of their practices because of changes in their insurance coverage or plan. Similarly, Spicer (1998) argues that juggling the administrative hassles of managed care means staying on top of credentialing paperwork, reimbursement arrangements, co-payment collection and ever-changing patient eligibility lists. But in addition to this, physicians increasingly find themselves being expected not just to work within wide-ranging systems but to teach patients how to do it too. Indeed, having to explain and re-explain to patients what their insurance will cover (and the constant changes to their coverage) illustrates what some physicians see as the biggest hassle of managed care (Spicer, 1998). Kassirer (1998) succinctly summarizes, "physicians' time is increasingly consumed by paperwork that they view as intrusive and valueless, by meetings devoted to expanding clinical-reporting requirements, by the need to seek permission to use resources, by telephone calls to patients as formularies change and by the complex business activities forced on them by the fragmented health care system" (p. 1543).

In addition to being a personal bother, many U.S. physicians cite administrative complexity as a major problem that adversely affects patient care with ever increasing frequency (Bailey et al., 1998). Derlet and Hamilton (1996), for example, not only analysed the total time required to complete a call to get approval for patient care – which varied from 20 minutes to 2.6 hours – they noted that authorization calls caused several kinds of problems including delays in care, denials and increased patient recidivism. This in turn, results in increasing frustration among physicians in their attempts to deliver ideal care (Kassirer, 1998).

Nurses also feel the impact of managed care policies both directly and through their impact on physicians. Brandi (2000), for example, argues that "the impact of managed care on physicians was making life harder for nurses" (p. 375). One of the primary reasons for this is that physicians increasingly attempt to delegate these mounting administrative tasks to nurses. Indeed, many nurses describe burdensome demands of paperwork. Corey-Lisle et al. (1999) described how

[a]s an example of the perceived prioritization of paperwork over quality patient care, a nurse wrote that she spent 'four hours one day trying to get prior approval from Medicaid for a package of adult diapers.' Another said, 'We are currently sinking under bureaucratic paperwork and regulations . . . If I ever leave nursing, it will be because I spent so much time writing [that] I couldn't properly care for my patients!' One nurse described '. . . the stress of getting everything on paper-lawyer perfect – rather than taking care of a sick patient who is depending on you and healthcare for answers' (p. 33–34).

These authors argue further that the increasing demand to negotiate care made it difficult for nurses to provide the kind of patient care they were educated to give. Similarly, Harrison (1999) describes that one of the greatest threats to their work perceived by nurses were the hassles involved in seeking authorization for care. In fact, "telephone nursing practice" (Huber & Blanchfield, 1999) has become a major nursing activity in ambulatory care settings. In all, nurses feel particularly frustrated by recent managed care reforms because they influence their ability to provide quality "care" (Gilliland, 1997).

In the data we gathered from nurses and physicians in California and British Columbia, we find similar themes that have arisen in this recent, largely U.S.-based literature on caring in the context of managed care. Specifically, we find that although inter-professional negotiation has been a longstanding feature of the daily lives of these health care providers in both settings, a greater proportion of time spent and new forms of negotiations have emerged as a direct result of "managed care" policies. These new features involve increasing textually mediated negotiations with non-health care providers to determine the limits of the accessibility to and amount of care that can be provided and how those limits can be appealed, if at all. In both settings, providers lament how negotiative care increasingly infiltrates the amount of time that providers can give direct care to ailing bodies (i.e. what is usually identified in the literature as carework); however, it is within the U.S. where there has been a greater penetration of managed care policies that this is most salient. What we add to this literature is not only a comparative lens but also a link between the literature on care work and the literature of working under managed care through our depiction of negotiating for care.

METHODS

Our focus on the issue of negotiating care emerged as a key theme from a larger study our research team undertook of the experiences of health care providers with the increasing management of care in Canada and the United States. One of our primary objectives of that larger study was to "test" the claims made by managed care organizations – specifically that it would result in greater integration and continuity; greater accountability for appropriate, quality care; and an enhanced focus on health promotion and disease prevention – against the everyday experiences of those who provided care.

Data for this study were gathered via individual interviews with physicians and facilitated focus groups with nurses following a similar semi-structured, qualitative interview guide. Participants were selected through a combination of purposive and snowball sampling. Our interview guide generally took the form of having health care providers detail how a patient would move through their particular segment of the health care system from gaining access through to discharge. A total of 52 individual interviews were conducted with physicians and focus groups with 81 nurses from a variety of health care settings and specialties from two U.S. states (New York & California) and two Canadian provinces (Ontario & British

Columbia). All interviews were tape-recorded, transcribed verbatim and entered into QSR-NUDIST 5.0 to manage the data for thematic analysis.

In this paper we focus on data from 35 nurses and 17 physicians from California and from 39 nurses and 14 physicians from British Columbia. These participants were specifically probed about the issue of negotiating care for their patients during the course of their interview following its emergence as an issue in previous interviews. These probes were inserted into our line of questioning that followed a patient through their various care organizations. For example, when discussing how a patient would seek care from the provider, participants were then probed for the types of negotiations this involved and with whom.

From a sub-sample of eight interviews (two from each group – nurses from California and British Columbia, and physicians from California and British Columbia) a draft coding scheme was developed jointly by the first and second author and then applied and further refined by the second author in coding the remaining interviews. Random reliability checks of the application of the coding scheme to the data were conducted by the first author. When necessary, recoding was conducted to ensure accuracy and consistency of the analysis of the data.

The data we present in the following section address the main conceptual categories of the coding scheme. We begin first with the impact of the increasing management of care on the ways in which care is negotiated both inter-professionally and textually and how this has evolved into a new variant of carework.

RESULTS

Our respondents in general and nurses in particular commented that negotiating care was not a particularly new element of their work. Indeed, a good deal of inter-professional negotiation has always been necessary to effectively orchestrate care for patients. What has changed, however, in response to the ever-persistent presence of the management of dwindling care resources is the proportion of health care providers' *time* devoted to negotiating care; the extent to which this has begun to infiltrate *medical* practice; and particularly in the U.S., the *audience* for and *form* of these negotiations.

Negotiating Care – Similarities Across Providers and Settings

There were many similarities that arose in the responses of our participants across provider groups and settings insofar as the negotiation of care was concerned. For example, health care providers in both California and British Columbia discussed at length the level of bureaucracy in care and the administrative "hoops" they had to jump through:

> We're *drowning in paper* and over directives from government and everything's in triplicate and quadruplicate and you know you get memo after memo and we certainly have a lot more forms to fill out now – Doctor from British Columbia.

> It takes a *lot more paperwork*. If you've got to sort through the [insurance] companies it takes a lot more time – Nurse from California.

Sometimes this requires negotiation between providers as to who will actually get the approval. This could be between physicians or between physicians and nurses:

> I think it applies to a lot of the referrals. So I won't order a whole battery of neurological tests. I'll ask a neurologist to see it and let him decide. So I think that's how a lot of our stuff is managed – Doctor from British Columbia.

> And you see the problem begins is that some of the specialists don't even bother doing that. They send that responsibility back to the primary care physician and say 'hey you get the approval for the surgery. I've already done my job'. I already evaluated surgery. And vice versa it happens with primary care physicians because there's no reimbursement that goes on there – Doctor from California.

What is implicit in these quotes is that these approvals in the Canadian context are primarily for *securing care* whereas in the U.S. context it is for *securing payment* for services. This may be partly due to the way the health care systems are differently organized – being a public, single-payer insurance system in British Columbia and a predominantly private, multiple-payer system in California. It is also important to note that with the increasing discontinuity of doctor-patient relationships in California, which is a direct result of continual shifts in insurance plans, companies, etc., it becomes much more difficult for physicians there to take a special interest or time to go this "extra mile":

> *Many physicians just won't put the time in to go through that.* So when they deny, their initial response is we're going to deny that procedure or deny that consult, often that's what happens and the patient doesn't get the procedure. It takes that extra effort on my part you know – Doctor from California.

> If you do not have the money, the resources to buy insurance you can at least provide your own primary care physician, then you have a relationship established. At least you have a doctor that knows you, knows your history; *he's more likely to take a personal and a professional interest in getting the care you really need* and advocating for you – Nurse from California.

Moreover, what once used to require a simple phone call now requires a fax or other form of text-mediated negotiations. Physicians often delegate such negotiative tasks (e.g. phoning, faxing) to others, particularly nurses:

It was forms to fill out and call backs to make to insurance companies, some of which I didn't do but *I would have to initiate and instruct someone else to do* – Doctor from California.

You still have to jump through all the hoops and spend all that time doing this administrative work when eventually they'll say okay. But there's this sort of effort that goes in, that I put in, *my nurse practitioner, she bears the brunt of all of this* – Doctor from California.

This ability to delegate, however, seems to be more readily available to those physicians working in large groups; that is, those who could collectively afford a staff to delegate these tasks to. For example, one former family physician in private practice in California noted:

I thought, I've got to get out of this situation. I am the staff. I'm the secretary. I'm the receptionist. You know. I do the faxes. I do my own typing. I am it. And so I was doing that and in the beginning, I think that's why I saw it so clearly because other physicians in other specialties were somewhat protected from it. They didn't get it. They had a buffer. They had a staff that was dealing with all this stuff. But it was right in my face – Doctor from California.

Moreover, as we shall see below, the ability to delegate many of the administrative tasks associated with the negotiation of care is increasingly being curbed by specific managed care policies.

Negotiating Care – Differences Across Providers and Settings

Although there are many similarities in the form and content of negotiative care that nurses and physicians do in both settings, there are some interesting differences that emerge in our comparative analysis as well. As noted above, negotiating access to and organizing care with other health care providers has always been an important element of health care work. With the increasing scarcity of resources, which has paralleled the increasing management of care in both settings, these inter-professional negotiations have taken on new meaning.

Purpose
In Canada, the increase in the level of negotiative care tends to be a consequence of *shortages* in the health care system. This is usually manifest in negotiations over access to beds:

There's such pressure in the system now that there's . . . this huge amount of time involved in sorting out who gets in and who doesn't – Doctor from British Columbia.

What is actually happening here on an informal basis is that care is being controlled or limited by bed numbers and by the restrictions placed on one by managers as to how you can, where you can direct your patients? – Nurse from British Columbia.

Accessing beds can sometimes be manipulated by "who knows who" or also through other means drawing upon social relationships:

> We have good relationships with all the pediatricians there, or other sub-specialists. And that means the pediatricians get a sense of what we want and what we like and they find a referral for us, conversation to us is easy cause they know who we are – Doctor from British Columbia.

> In theory you can phone up the admitting department and say, 'I have Mrs. X who has this and I would like her admitted. And they say we'll put her on a wait list . . . Then, there's the negotiation on a day-to-day basis of how to get the patients in. So we have a . . . fantastic lab [tech] here . . . whose job is to suck up to the ambulance drivers so they can have coffee and donuts when they get here and they'll hang around and get these people back and forth . . . There's negotiations all the time with those folk cause that makes the place run – Doctor from British Columbia.

As a result of health care restructuring, which has come to involve the closure of units to mergers of entire hospitals, many of these social networks have become severed. This has made the context for negotiating care that much more difficult. The flattening of professional hierarchies and the loss of head nurses, which is another consequence of health care restructuring in British Columbia, was a particularly salient issue for some of the nurses there:

> They've changed the rules, they've reduced the supervisory role in our facility for the second time in $3\frac{1}{2}$ years – Nurse from British Columbia.

> I have to talk to 15 different people on three different shifts to get the message across . . . But if I'd had head nurses I could have talked to six people all at once – Nurse from British Columbia.

In contrast to British Columbia, negotiations that California health care providers partake in tend to be over *coverage*; that is, the resources are usually there in terms of availability of hospital beds. However, what California providers tend to have to negotiate is who has the coverage to access services, for how long and how, when, and whether reimbursement for providing care will be forthcoming. Indeed much time was noted by providers being spent dealing with responding to denials of coverage or payment for services:

> Individual denials were the worst thing. You know, you did a procedure and then they say they wouldn't pay for it. It was a random non-payment of services that I think was institutionalized as part of the way they did their business where they would automatically deny a certain percentage of all claims with the full knowledge most doctors' offices are very inefficient and would never be able to really appeal those –Doctor from California.

> People are ignorant of what they're denied . . . We don't really know what we're allowed to have and what we're not allowed to have until we come up against it and then, or in the insurance company itself we can choose our providers, they'll say oh that wasn't covered and not pay for it. And if you argue and say yes it was and you have to pay for this, eventually they will. It might take a year and most people have given up long before that . . . I mean I talk to nurses all the time. I say just keep harassing them – Nurse from California.

Some were particularly concerned with what they regarded as being a policy on the part of insurers of denying all claims submitted the first time around:

> Sometimes they flat out don't approve it . . . We found one [insurance] group in particular was denying, well what appeared to us to be literally every claim, every single thing. Even if we sent in copies of the authorization, it came back denied. We finally sent someone from our office to that building with a stack of denied claims in their hand saying 'what is going on'? And believe it or not, we found an honest employee at this managed care organization and this employee finally said to us 'look, they told us every claim that comes in, the first submission just deny it. Categorically deny it.' . . . Usually if I'm willing to spend the time to get approval for whatever, it is . . . but that takes time – Doctor from California.

The constant questioning of the clinical decision-making of professionals, which is one of the key elements of "managed care," exacerbated the amount of negotiating for care that health care providers had to do:

> There was a tremendous amount of having to negotiate and try to get them to cover this or that and try to get enough payment – Doctor from California.

> I feel I spend a lot of time in a day advocating for patients for level of care or quality of care. I spend an awful lot of time on the phone like with disability people or the MediCal people or the specialists or the whatever, you know, because if I just let the system take care of it, the patient will never get seen. They'll never get their procedure done or it'll never get approved – Doctor from California.

Indeed, in some cases, direct medical contact was deemed necessary for an approval to be forthcoming. This was all the more frustrating to physicians because they felt that the persons making the decision did not have the health care background necessary to assess the request for coverage of care. It was regarded as just another hoop to go through to help improve the company's bottom line:

> The calls I'd have to make to people to try to justify things, and they almost always gave you what you wanted anyway. It's just you had to go through all these hoops – Doctor from California.

Such a policy also prevented physicians from attempting to delegate this negotiative care to nurses and other auxiliary staff. Moreover, providers in California noted the impact of how the context of negotiations constantly shifted largely as a result of changes in coverage:

> Our formulary usually encompasses what major insurance companies keep on their formulary. The problem is that they change their formulary quicker than we have a chance to change ours. So you're playing this catch up battle all the time – Doctor from California.

In brief, whereas the context of negotiations in British Columbia tends to be a result of shortages, the context of negotiations in California was regarding coverage. Overlapping these contextual features of negotiative carework in the two settings was also a difference in the audiences for negotiations.

Audience

The audience for the negotiation of care in British Columbia tended to be of a more traditional nature; that is, with other health care providers. For example, one physician explained that:

> When the beds are tight I have to actually broker this through someone else and that is a physician admitting officer. So there is a set of individuals who maintain and monitor the utilization – Doctor from British Columbia.

In the quotes by health care providers in British Columbia highlighted above, the audience for negotiations largely entailed other health care providers – e.g. pediatric specialists for referral assistance, and ambulance drivers for quick assistance in the transportation of patients to ease the admissions process.

In contrast, the audience for negotiations in California not only entailed similar inter-professional negotiations, the more salient or perhaps the more problematic audience expressed by providers in our interviews were health care insurers. What was particularly frustrating for some of the health care providers was that the representatives of the insurance companies they were negotiating with often did not have the same kind of background that their colleagues did:

> They go to the doctor and the doctor makes a referral to the insurance company. And then the insurance company says no. And then you fight with this high school person on a computer that says this person with that diagnosis doesn't need this. And you're going, "But they're 83 years old and da da da." But they're looking into the computer and they don't have the capacity to understand – Nurse from California.

Thus the kind of negotiations that they were involved in differed in quality with the negotiations they had with fellow health care providers. Further, because there were multiple insurers for the various patients for which they were attempting to provide care, this exacerbated the amount of negotiations that they had to undertake:

> I have to fill out a form and the form differs for each insurance company and there are hundreds of insurance companies. I have to fill out a form asking permission to do that study and I have to fill out why I want the study . . . for some kinds of insurance I even have to fill out a form to see the patient again – Doctor from California.

> It takes a lot more paperwork. If you've got to sort through the companies it takes a lot more time – Nurse from California.

Although there were some clear similarities in complaints about administrative or negotiative care work by providers across both settings, there were also some salient differences in the context and audience of these negotiations. Before we discuss what these similarities and differences tell us about negotiating care conceptually, it is important to first highlight a few of the consequences of the increasing burden of negotiating for care.

A Brief Note About Consequences

Health care providers in both settings highlighted some of the consequences the ever increasing level of negotiations had on their ability to provide care on a daily basis. One of the most salient was how this took (or attempted to take) time away from providing direct care to patients:

> The administrative work takes time away from what could be spent learning, being with patients – Doctor from California.

> The system has made us believe that completing documentation has everything to do with our care. It doesn't. I'm going to give as much care as I can give. Whether or not the paper work is filled out is meaningless to me – Nurse from California.

One of the consequences for health care providers of attempting to bridge the gap between providing care and documenting and negotiating care was an increased risk of burnout:

> The reason I stopped clinical work wasn't only because I wanted to move on. I was basically burned out. I had huge numbers of charts. In order to go faster and faster, one of the things that would get left behind would be the charting – Doctor from California.

What is also salient in the quote above is that not only was the level of negotiating care increasing, there was a parallel increase in the expectations of amount of care that could be given by each provider. This in turn exacerbated the level of negotiations because there were now more patients to negotiate on behalf of as well as more insurers to negotiate with. This compounded already excessive workloads. Some health care providers began to question whether this has resulted in a system that is more managed than is providing care:

> It's extremely over managed. Obviously every little thing is listed in terms of what we'll pay for, what won't we, how much will we pay for it. And the hospitals and the managed care companies in turn you know they advertise we need more managed care, less paper work and stuff like that. Baloney. There's never been so much paper work – Doctor from California.

In sum, across physicians and nurses in both settings we find a sense among them of an increasing burden of negotiating care for patients as the access to (particularly in California) and amount of care resources is increasingly limited through managed care policies. Moreover, through restructuring and other cost-cutting measures, the contexts for these negotiations are continually in flux, exacerbating the time devoted to such negotiations. So in both settings there is generally more of the same kind of negotiations that has been going on prior to the onset of managed care along with an increase in textually mediated negotiations. It is in the California context, however, where there is a greater penetration of managed care – and perhaps as a result more flux in the system – that negotiating care through texts has evolved into a new variant in terms of audience and purpose.

DISCUSSION

The main purpose of our examination herein was not to determine whether there is an increase in health care providers' administrative burden as a result of managed care,[1] although our data do lend some support to this argument. Our primary motivation is to better understand how negotiations not just between providers, but also between providers and insurers, constitute a new dimension of care work and how this is salient for different provider groups across settings.

Our findings suggest that there is a qualitative difference between the kind of negotiative care that health care providers in British Columbia and California are doing. There may also be a quantitative difference as well in that we suspect that there is much less negotiation going on in Canada than in the U.S., despite an increase in both settings. This, however, is difficult to assess using our methodology. Some of the qualitative differences are more readily apparent. It was already noted that part of the context or purpose behind the negotiations in British Columbia was for care, whereas it was by and large for payment of services (and by extension care as well) in California. This is also related to the audience for these negotiative efforts – being primarily other health care providers in this Canadian Province and the tendency for it to be with insurers in this American State. So new dimensions of care work vary depending on the context. In British Columbia it tends to be more of the same personal/social methods of negotiating, but in California this has become more depersonalized, textually-based petitioning. In California, the context and audience leads us to conclude that this is new dimension of negotiating care that has evolved much more fully and rapidly.

Although this type of care work, may not be completely congruent with the traditional notion of care of bodies, it does entail some of the key characteristics of care work. For instance, it is work that is relatively invisible, not highly valued and it is delegated to others as much as possible, be it from physicians to nurses or to administrative staff. Consequently, it tends to be work accomplished mainly by women. Although we suspect that this occurs because of this delegation and the fact that nurses spend much more time with patients overall, they tend to be the ones negotiating much of the daily care for patients in comparison with physicians. This again is difficult to quantitatively assess with our methodology.

What is interesting, however, is how salient the increasing burden of negotiating care was to physicians, particularly those in California. This has also been echoed in some of the recent literature on physician's experiences with managed care, particularly their advocacy role (Mullan, 2001; Waitzin, 2000). Perhaps it is because their traditional methods of coping with this delegation was increasingly being curbed by the policies of some managed care organizations that now require direct physician involvement in the paperwork necessary to acquire care for their patients (see also Barker, 1996). This is particularly telling of the curbing of medical autonomy through managed care, which a great deal of the literature discusses. Thus, in contrast to some (e.g. Christopherson, 2001; Treiber, 2001) who argue that the privatization of care widens the gap between highly skilled professionals and lower-skilled workers who provide most of the basic hands-on care, our examination reveals that negotiative care work is starting to permeate higher skill levels. It will be interesting to see how this will be managed or problematized by physicians who heretofore have been able to avoid much of the burden of negotiating care.

The impact of the evolution of new variations of carework and its interconnection with gender may be subtle. Perhaps what we have uncovered here is how managerialism may be breaking down the gendered lines of caring work requiring medicine, a traditionally male-dominated profession, to increasingly partake in the act of negotiating care. It may also be that we have uncovered another dimension of the caring dilemma. No longer is it so much feeling obliged to provide care without having the decision-making power to determine how that care is to be provided. The dilemma may now result from having to spend more time negotiating the ability to provide care, which paradoxically takes away time from actually providing the care being negotiated.

NOTE

1. Indeed, some of the literature questions this widely held belief (Remler et al., 2000).

ACKNOWLEDGMENTS

The authors would like to acknowledge funding for this research project by the Social Sciences and Humanities Research Council of Canada through a Standard Research Grant. We would also like to acknowledge helpful comments made on an earlier draft of this paper by Deborah Stone and members of the Polinomics Research Support Group of the Centre for Health Economics and Policy Analysis at McMaster University.

REFERENCES

Abel, E., & Nelson, M. (1990). *Circles of care: Work and identity in women's lives.* New York: State University of New York Press.

Aronson, J., & Neysmith, S. (1996). The work of visiting homemakers in the context of cost cutting in long term care. *Canadian Journal of Public Health, 87*(6), 422–425.

Aronson, J., & Neysmith, S. (1997). The retreat of the state and long-term provision: Implementations for frail elderly people, unpaid family carers and paid home care workers. *Studies in Political Economy, 53*(Summer), 37–66.

Bailey, J. E., Bush, A. J., Bertran, P., & Somes, G. (1998). Physicians' experiences with Medicaid managed care: The Tennessee American College of physicians survey on TennCare. *Tennessee Medicine, 91*(8), 313–316.

Barker, C. (1996). Maximizing efficiency in the management of the physician practice: Survival under managed care. *Journal of Health Care Finance, 22*(4), 22–28.

Brandi, C. (2000). Relationships between nurse executives and physicians: The gender paradox in healthcare. *Journal of Advanced Nursing, 30*(7/8), 373–378.

Christopherson, S. (2001). Women in the restructuring of care-work: Cross national variations and trends in ten OECD countries. In: N. J. Hirschmann & U. Liebert (Eds), *Women And Welfare: Theory And Practice In The United States And Europe* (pp. 244–260). New Brunswick: Rutgers University Press.

Corey-Lisle, P., Tarzian, A., & Cohen, M. (1999). Healthcare reform: Its effects on nurses. *Journal of Nursing Administration, 29*(3), 30–37.

Davies, C. (1994). *Competence versus care? New managerialism meets nursing.* International Sociological Association.

Derlet, R., & Hamilton, B. (1996). The impact of health maintenance organization care authorization policy on an emergency department before California's new managed care law. *Academic Emergency Medicine, 3*(4), 338–344.

Deuben, C. J. (1998). The impact of managed care on labor substitution in the health care workforce. *Michigan Academician, 30*(1), 69–83.

Gerstel, N. (2000). The third shift: Gender and care work outside the home. *Qualitative Sociology, 23*(4), 467–483.

Gilliland, M. (1997). Workforce reductions: Low morale, reduced quality of care. *Nursing Economics, 15*(6), 320–322.

Grembowski, D., Cook, K., Patrick, D., & Roussel, A. (2002). Managed care and the U.S. health care system: A social exchange perspective. *Social Science and Medicine, 54*, 1167–1180.

Harrison, J. (1999). Influence of managed care on professional nursing practice. *Image – the Journal of Nursing Scholarship, 31*(2), 161–166.

Huber, D., & Blanchfield, K. (1999). Telephone nursing interventions in ambulatory care. *Journal of Nursing Administration, 29*(3), 38–44.

Hunter, D. (1996). The changing roles of health care personnel in health and health care management. *Social Science and Medicine, 43*, 799–808.

Isaksen, L. W. (2002). Toward a sociology of (gendered) disgust: Images of bodily decay and the social organization of care work. *Journal of Family Issues, 23*(7), 791–811.

Kassirer, J. (1998). Doctor discontent. *The New England Journal of Medicine, 339*(21), 1543–1545.

McKay, T. (1999). Managed care: A turning point for nursing. *Journal of Transcultural Nursing, 10*(4), 292.

McKie, L., & Bowlby, S. (2001). Caring and employment in Britain. *Journal of Social Policy, 30*(2), 233–258.

Meyer, M. (2000). *Care work: Gender labor and the welfare state*. New York: Routledge.

Mullan, F. (2001). Tin cup medicine. *Health Affairs, 20*(November/December, 6), 216–221.

Reverby, S. (1987). *Ordered to care*. Cambridge, MA: Cambridge University Press.

Spicer, J. (1998). Coping with managed care's administrative hassles. *Family Practice Management* (March), 1–11.

Thomas, C. (1993). Deconstructing concepts of care. *Sociology, 27*(3), 649–669.

Treiber, L. (2001). Health care organizations and devalued labor: Labor process control of caring work conference. *Southern Sociological Society*.

Waitzin, H. (2000). Changing patient-physician relationships in the changing health-policy environment. In: C. Bird, P. Conrad & A. Freemont (Eds), *Handbook of Medical Sociology* (5th ed.).

Warren, M., Weitz, R., & Kulis, S. (1999). The impact of managed care on physicians. *Health Care Management Review, 24*(2), 44–56.